The Human-Animal Bond and Grief

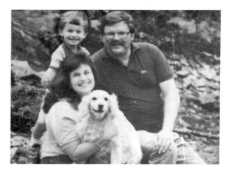

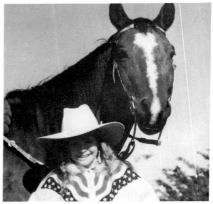

W.B. SAUNDERS COMPANY
A Division of Harcourt Brace & Company

Philadelphia   London   Toronto
Montreal   Sydney   Tokyo

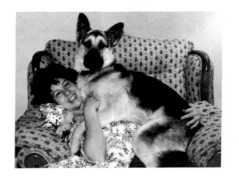

The Human-Animal Bond and Grief

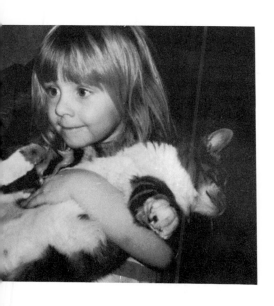

Laurel Lagoni, MS

Carolyn Butler, MS

Co-Directors, Changes: The Support for
  People and Pets Program
Colorado State University Veterinary
  Teaching Hospital
College of Veterinary Medicine and
  Biomedical Sciences
Fort Collins, Colorado

Suzanne Hetts, PhD

Animal Behavior Associates
Denver, Colorado

W.B. SAUNDERS COMPANY

A Division of Harcourt Brace & Company

The Curtis Center
Independence Square West
Philadelphia, PA 19106

Library of Congress Cataloging-in-Publication Data

Lagoni, Laurel S.
    The human-animal bond and grief / Laurel S. Lagoni, Suzanne Hetts,
Carolyn S. Butler.
        p.   cm.
    Includes bibliographical references and index.
    ISBN 0–7216–4577–1
    1. Pet owners—Psychology.   2. Pets—Death—Psychological aspects,
3. Veterinarian and client.   4. Bereavement—Psychological aspects.
5. Human-animal relationships.   I. Hetts, Suzanne.   II. Butler,
Carolyn S.   III. Title.
SF411.47.L34   1994
636.089′6029—dc20   93–39220

Cover art: Jennifer Robinson

THE HUMAN-ANIMAL BOND AND GRIEF   ISBN 0–7216–4577–1

Printed in the United States of America

Last digit is the print number: 9   8   7   6   5   4   3   2

Preface

In the last two decades, much has been learned about the human-animal bond and about the grief pet owners experience when beloved companion animals die. Less has been learned, however, about the roles veterinarians play in their clients' grief processes. This is due to two factors. First, the veterinarians' roles and levels of responsibility in matters concerning pet loss and client grief have not been well defined. Second, advances in medical technology and the race to stay abreast of them have nudged the human side of veterinary medicine out of many educational curriculums.

As a veterinarian, you probably possess a wealth of scientific knowledge regarding the potential *cure* of your animal patients. However, you probably possess very little knowledge regarding the *care* of your human clients. Survey after survey reinforces the fact that consumers of today's medical services want doctors to care about them more than they want doctors to cure them.[1] Without education and training in both client relations and effective communication techniques, you are at a distinct disadvantage when practicing contemporary veterinary medicine.

A survey conducted by Fogle and Abrahamson[2] uncovered this deficiency in veterinary training. Of the veterinarians they surveyed, 96 percent had received no training on how to explain terminal illness to clients, and 72 percent felt this training would be helpful. These statistics are even more significant when combined with survey results showing that 15 percent of former pet owners refrain from adopting other companion animals because their experiences with the deaths of their previous pets were too painful to repeat.[3]

Today, veterinary schools are beginning to recognize the importance of training students in human-animal bond studies, grief counseling, and effective communication techniques. To this end, they are striving to teach students about human emotions as well as veterinary diagnostics and treatment procedures. The University of Florida and the University of California at Davis, for instance, operate telephone hotlines through which student volunteers receive firsthand experience talking with grieving clients. The University of Minnesota, the University of Pennsylvania, Purdue, Texas A&M, Auburn, and Tufts, along with Kansas, Washington, and Louisiana State Universities, also address the issues of pet loss, grief, and client relations through various combinations of research, teaching, and direct support to clients. Some of these schools offer elective classes and experiential learning opportunities to veterinary students. Others offer formalized training in grief counseling and effective communication techniques within their professional veterinary curriculums.

Colorado State University (CSU) offers veterinary students all these learning opportunities. This is achieved primarily through classroom and clinical work conducted in conjunction with CSU's grief counseling service located at the Veterinary Teaching Hospital (VTH). This service is called Changes: The Support for People and Pets Program. We, the authors of this textbook, are the Changes Program's co-founders and current co-directors.

As counselors with the Changes Program, we assist in facilitating the emotional aspects of CSU's medical cases. This means we provide pet owners with grief education and support during emergencies, diagnoses, treatment procedures, decision-making processes, unexpected deaths, euthanasias, and bereavement follow-ups. Since the human side of veterinary medicine is consistently addressed at CSU, clinicians, technicians, and veterinary students have opportunities to experience various interdisciplinary approaches to case management. Due to CSU's commitment to and consistent involvement with subject matter related to the human-animal bond, the veterinary teaching hospital has evolved into what we call a "bond-centered" veterinary practice.

In simple terms, a bond-centered veterinary practice is one in which the relationships between people and their companion animals are recognized as significant and thus are always acknowledged and respected. Veterinarians who practice veterinary medicine with this attitude realize that certain human needs are created when the human-animal bond is changed or threatened, as it is during an animal's illness or death. In a bond-centered practice, caring for *both* clients and patients is viewed as a professional responsibility. Thus, when clients bring their pets to a bond-centered practice, they are simultaneously offered medical care for their animals and emotional care for themselves. During times of pet loss, this concurrent approach to the delivery of both medical-based and support-based veterinary services forms the philosophical base from which veterinarians reach out and attempt to build helping relationships with their grieving clients.

Veterinarians who see themselves as helpers must be skilled communicators. Through education and training, they have learned to anticipate and assess clients' needs and to use effective communication techniques to convey to pet owners that help and understanding are available to them.

As effective communicators, veterinarians have also come to realize the importance of providing clients with additional support services. Support-based services extend veterinary care beyond the medical treatment of companion animals. In terms of pet loss and client grief, for example, the provision of additional support services may mean collaborating with professional pet loss counselors or local pet loss support groups.

It is not the goal of this textbook to teach *you* to become a pet loss counselor or to lead a pet loss support group. Rather, the goal is to teach you to become a skilled communicator so you can use the basic communication techniques, known and used by paraprofessional helpers across the country, to build effective helping relationships with your clients. Effective communication is the cornerstone of any helping relationship. When you know how to build helping relationships with your clients, you can confidently and effectively intervene in situations that involve pet loss and provide comfort and support to grieving clients.

By adding the role of helper to your already multifaceted job description, you enhance the quality of the veterinary care you provide. You can most efficiently integrate this role into your professional identity within the context of a veterinary practice centered on acknowledging and promoting the human-animal bond. The core goal of this text is to teach you how to establish a bond-centered veterinary practice from which you can provide grief support to clients.

Since the beginning of the Changes Program in 1985, we have educated and counseled thousands of students and pet owners and, in the process, discovered dozens of ways to deal effectively with pet loss and client grief. In the classes we teach, we translate what we have learned from pet owners, students, and veterinary professionals into information that you, as a veterinarian, can apply to your own bond-centered veterinary practice. This text provides you with that information. It is divided into four sections and, generally, follows the organization of lecture material and clinical experiences as we present them within CSU's professional veterinary curriculum.

Section I orients you to the theories and rationales underlying the concept of helping within the context of a bond-centered veterinary practice. Section II discusses the effective use of a helping model and provides you with descriptions of a variety of communication techniques appropriate for use by veterinarians. Section III teaches you how to apply communication techniques during large- and small-animal euthanasia procedures and case follow-ups. The personal stress associated with caring for others is also addressed. Section IV examines practice management issues pertinent to contemporary veterinary medicine. It includes specific suggestions about helping in a variety of situations and with a variety of populations. The ethics of helping are also considered.

The book ends with a Resource Appendix. A roster of the classes we teach at CSU is included here. We hope the information and suggested curriculum become a valuable guide for those interested in teaching veterinary students about pet loss and client grief. We also hope this information acts as a catalyst for the evolution of many more classes and service programs focused on pet loss and client grief at veterinary schools across the nation. The time has come for enrollment and participation in human-animal bond-oriented classes and programs to move from elective to required status. As Dr. Alan Beck, Center for Applied Ethology and Human-Animal Interaction at the School of Veterinary Medicine at Purdue University, states,

> It is time to consider the appropriateness of including [Human-Animal Interaction] programs as being integral to veterinary medicine education, like epidemiology and pathology, and no veterinary school curriculum be considered complete without a core commitment to Human-Animal Interaction studies.[4]

Laurel Lagoni, M.S.
Carolyn Butler, M.S.
Suzanne Hetts, Ph.D.

REFERENCES

1. Peters, R.: Practical Intelligence. New York, Harper and Row, 1987, p. 96.
2. Fogle, B., and Abrahamson, D.: Pet loss: A survey of the attitudes and feelings of practicing veterinarians. *Anthrozoos*, 3(3):143–150, 1990.
3. Wilbur, R.H.: Pets, pet ownership, and animal control: Social and psychological attitudes. *In* Proceedings of the National Conference on Dog and Cat Control. Denver, Colo., National Association of Animal Control Officers, 1976.
4. Beck, A.M.: Teaching human-animal interactions in veterinary education. *In* Proceedings of the Delta Society Ninth Annual Conference. Houston, Tex., The Delta Society, 1990, p. 64.

Acknowledgments

We wish to thank the thousands of pet owners and companion animals who have made Changes: The Support for People and Pets Program a success. We sincerely hope that, with the education and support our clients have received, they have grown and benefited in some way from the experience of grieving. We also wish to extend our heartfelt thanks to Colorado State University's veterinarians, technicians, staff, and students. Without their continued support of the Changes Program, we would not be as well integrated as we are into the daily casework and classwork of both the hospital and the professional veterinary medicine curriculum.

Special thanks go to several key supporters of the Changes Program. They are CSU's Dean of the College of Veterinary Medicine and Biomedical Sciences, Dr. James Voss; the Head of the Clinical Sciences Department, Dr. Anthony Knight; the Director of the Veterinary Teaching Hospital (VTH), Dr. Wendell Nelson; the former Director of the VTH, Dr. Dennis McCurnin; and the Chief of the Comparative Oncology Service at the VTH, Dr. Steve Withrow. We also wish to thank the entire oncology faculty and staff, who have always been supportive of our efforts.

Our particular gratitude goes to Dr. Withrow. The Changes Program owes its life to him. Dr. Withrow was the first to recognize the need for a client support program, and from Day One of its inception, he has been its champion. Dr. Withrow has done everything possible to provide the Changes Program with stability and credibility. He has provided direction for its growth and development, mentored the directors of the program, and "gone to battle" to achieve adequate program funding. Much of the credit for the success of the Changes Program belongs to him.

Others have also contributed to the Changes Program over the years. They include many professionals and numerous corporate sponsors, each with a special interest in promoting the human-animal bond. We wish to acknowledge Drs. Alicia Cook and Keven Oltjenbruns, who first taught us about grief, encouraged us to take pet loss seriously, and provided us with professional and moral support along the way. We would also like to thank Dr. Bernie Rollin for inviting us to present our first guest lecture in his Ethics course in 1987, and Tamina Toray, Ph.D., Kristi Kleban, M.S., and Connee Pike, M.S., three of the Changes Program's original counselors.

The corporate sponsors we wish to acknowledge are Dr. Jack Mara and Hills Pet Products, Dr. John Albers and the American Animal Hospital Association, and the Ralston Purina Company. These sponsors helped us financially when the continuation of the Changes Program was in doubt. We remain grateful for their belief in us and in this aspect of veterinary medicine.

We also want to acknowledge our many human-animal bond and pet loss counseling colleagues, many of whom are active members of The Delta Society, an organization to which we also owe a great deal. Susan Cohen and Jamie Quackenbush pioneered the field of pet loss counseling and, in many ways, made providing grief education and support for pet loss credible. They willingly shared their ideas with us when we first began our program, and we are in their debt today. So many others, Lynette Hart, Ph.D.; Cecelia Soares, D.V.M, M.S.; Bonnie Mader, M.S.; Betty Carmack, Ph.D.; and Sandra Brackenridge, M.S., to name a few, continue to move the field forward and to keep the ideas about pet loss and client grief fresh today. It is our hope that we can all continue to work together to make even greater inroads into the field of veterinary medicine.

Several people who made direct contributions to this textbook deserve individual recognition. They include LaRue Johnson, D.V.M., Ph.D., for his expertise regarding llama medicine and the dozen or so equine practitioners, both at CSU and in private practice, who contributed to or reviewed the medical material in Chapter 9. We also want to thank CSU's pharmacists; staff photographers Charlie Kerlee and Jenger Smith; Susan Schneider, M.Ed., former staff counselor and contributor to the sections on helping models and codependency; Jean McBride, M.S., our friend and colleague who temporarily covered part of our caseload while we wrote this textbook; and the two student members of our Changes office staff, Janet O'Faolain and Dayna Edwards. Their help during the writing of this text was invaluable.

Our special gratitude goes to the many pet owners who supplied us with essays, photographs, and personal letters. We realize that, in some cases, these memorabilia were hard for our friends, clients, and colleagues to share as they restimulated losses all over again. Yet, because there is real emotion still attached to these pieces, they are all the more valuable to us as teaching tools. Therefore, we hope the personal accounts and revealing portraits included in this text will serve as lessons to our readers and as tributes to the human-animal bonds they describe.

Finally, it goes without saying that we are grateful to our editors at W.B. Saunders. Linda Mills took this book on as a personal project and cinched the contract for us with her considerable powers of persuasion. Ray Kersey took over and guided us to its successful completion. Both Linda and Ray were extremely patient with us as we struggled to work writing deadlines into our already crunched clinic schedules. Without the support of W.B. Saunders, our ideas and experiences would still be confined to the classrooms and hospital examination rooms of Colorado State University. We feel honored that, with this textbook, we have been given the opportunity to pass our ideas on.

PERSONAL ACKNOWLEDGMENTS

To my co-authors Carolyn Butler and Suzanne Hetts, I wish to extend my deepest feelings of affection and respect. During the course of developing the Changes Program and writing this textbook, I have been privileged to work with both of you. Together, we have worked extremely hard, but we have also had a lot of fun! I can't imagine what my life, this book, or the Changes Program would be like without you. Thank you for sharing your intelligence, enthusiasm, creativity, concern, and friendship with me. You are both very special.

I also wish to thank my wonderful husband, Pete, and my sweet daughter, Bryn, for their cooperation and encouragement during the writing of this book. I spent many hours away from my family, devoting myself to this project; and my family spent many hours away from me, wisely devoting themselves to "staying out of my way"! I have missed both of you.

Finally, I want to thank another member of my family, one whom I have yet to meet. I spent the end of this writing project several months pregnant. Baby Lagoni kept me company during the late nights and weekends in my office. I've been a bit preoccupied with finishing this book, Baby, but you have my full attention now. Grow healthy and strong. Your daddy, big sister, and I can't wait to see you!—L. L.

Thank you to my writing partners, Laurel and Suzanne. There is really no way I can adequately acknowledge the years of learning and collaboration with you. To Laurel, thanks for saying, "Let's write this book!" As senior author and friend, you made the writing process work. It has been productive, meaningful, and fun. To Suzanne, your expertise in all areas of the human-animal bond strengthened the book and made the writing easier.

Family and friends also have my deepest gratitude for their commitment to this book. My husband, Scott, supported me in words and in deeds and gave up many gorgeous Colorado weekends so I could write. His cooking and sense of humor carried me through the "rough spots." Special appreciation goes to my mom, and to my sisters and brothers, for their celebration of each completed step. Finally, thank you to my wonderful circle of friends who gave me support during times when I could not return it. To each and every one of you, thanks for helping us bring this project to completion.—C. B.

A special thank you to the animal owners I've talked with over the years who cared so much for their pets and who were willing to take the risk to share their feelings with me. I also owe a debt of gratitude to Laurel and Carolyn, whose friendship, knowledge, and perspectives on grief and life, in general, have enriched my life in uncountable ways. Love and thanks to my husband, Dan Estep, whose encouragement and support helps me accomplish things I never thought I could and who is always willing to "read this over and tell me what you think"!—S. H.

Introduction

The entire area of human-animal bond studies, with a particular focus on pet loss issues, is experiencing an explosion of interest within veterinary medicine. Until recently, veterinary medicine was "only" worried about animal health. We frequently overlooked the fact that there was an owner at the end of the leash who sometimes required more care than the pet. Veterinarians have traditionally been well equipped to deal with disease, but often woefully unprepared to deal with issues of human emotion. The recent introduction of pet loss counselors and related individuals to the practice of veterinary medicine has been an exciting advance in the profession. We can and must learn better techniques and strategies to be both humane and human.

Having graduated 20 years ago from a prestigious and progressive college of veterinary medicine, I felt I was trained for the medical challenges ahead. I never really thought about my ability to deal with distraught clients or with issues of pet loss. It seemed rather simple: Pets lived, pets died, and, in between, I tried to make things better for the animals. Although I was not free of interaction with owners, it was not considered part of my job description to dwell on their problems. Even if it was in my job duties, I had absolutely no exposure to the proper techniques and strategies I could use to deal with these issues. Times have changed, though, and now veterinary medicine must accept the challenge of meeting our clients' needs as well as caring for their pets.

Veterinarians *are* not and *should* not consider themselves qualified psychologists, psychiatrists, social workers, or grief counselors. We should, however, be informed and aware of the techniques of helping that can be used to assist our clients in times of need. In all honesty, I was initially skeptical of some of the data and science that emanated from the social sciences relative to pet owner issues. I was wrong. It has been my honor to help develop Changes: The Support for People and Pets Program at Colorado State University and to see its impact on students, residents, interns, nurses, and faculty—to say nothing of the impact it has had on our clients themselves. The Changes Program has rapidly become involved in teaching, service, and research and is now considered a crucial and vital part of the hospital, with staff members focusing their work on the alleviation of suffering, both physical and mental, of humans and animals.

This book brings together the true life experience of the authors who live and practice what they preach. I believe it encompasses both the theory and applied information specific to establishing bond-centered veterinary practices. As I said before, an awareness of our clients' needs and of the methods used to help them does not make us grief counselors or social workers. It does, however, help us deal with client emotion in a more scientific and compassionate manner. I encourage all animal health care providers and the members of their staffs to read, consider, and implement the ideas and concepts outlined in this book. You can only become a better person and professional for your efforts.

Stephen J. Withrow, D.V.M.
Chief, Comparative Oncology
Colorado State University
Co-Founder, Changes: The Support for People and Pets Program

Authors' Note

In the human-animal bond literature, when the veterinarian's role in issues of pet loss and pet owner grief is discussed, it is commonly referred to as "pet loss counseling." However, many veterinarians are reluctant to align themselves too closely with a counseling role. This is due, perhaps, to the fact that even the most sensitive and efficient veterinarians do not have the time, interest, or fee structure required to do counseling justice and to the concern that veterinarians will breach their legal and ethical boundaries if they are perceived to be providing their clients with some form of professional counseling.

Professional pet loss counseling for grieving pet owners is perhaps most effective in private veterinary practice when it is provided by an interdisciplinary team consisting of both veterinary and human service professionals. In terms of this textbook, the terms "pet loss counselor" and "pet loss counseling" are used in reference to the people and services aligned with the human service professions. The term "helper" is used to refer to veterinary professionals engaged in providing education, guidance, and support to clients.

Contents

xix

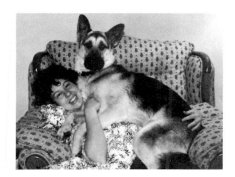

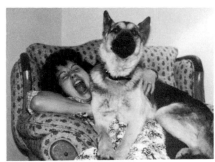

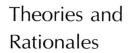

I

Theories and Rationales

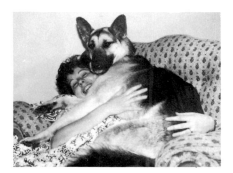

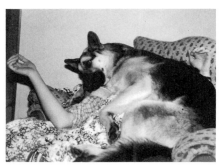

1

The Human-Animal Bond

Today, more people have pets (or, as they are more often called in the literature, companion animals) than they do children. According to a recent article in *Pet Business*, 229 million pets (cats, dogs, birds, fish, and small mammals) live in the United States alone.[1] One study has shown that 99 percent of cat and dog owners consider their pets to be full-fledged family members.[2] Another reports that 82 percent of cat owners, 73 percent of dog owners, and 63 percent of bird owners cite companionship as the major reason for owning their pets.[3]

There are other valid reasons for owning a pet. Research indicates that pets help maintain the health and well-being of their owners.[4] Studies have also indicated that pets act as social lubricants, making interpersonal conversations with the disabled, ill, or socially awkward person easier and more likely to occur.[5]

Pets are most often described by their owners as children, parents, best friends, partners, and confidantes. As companion animals, pets enhance and stabilize the lives of their owners with their constant presence and unconditional love. They also accept their owners regardless of appearances, feelings, or behaviors. During the numerous life transitions that people experience, it is not unusual for companion animals to be the constant factor in their changing lives. Therefore, because friendships with companion animals are always available to pet owners, the devotion that these animals show is often credited with pulling owners through the "rough spots" in their lives. Often the relationships pet owners enjoy with their dogs, cats, horses, birds, and other animals are among the strongest and most important in their lives.

People have had relationships with animals for thousands of years. Still, in the last three decades, the relationships between humans and certain species and breeds of animals have deepened and changed. Even the shift in the terminology used to describe the relationship between people and pets reflects this change in status. Animals who live with people have traditionally been called "pets." Although the term "pet" implies ownership of property, "companion animal" implies a mutual relationship, much more like friendship (Fig. 1-1).

With this change in the status of pets, relationships with animals are no longer relegated to the peripheries of people's lives. Today they often play key roles in people's daily routines. In fact, for many people, companion animals are the primary sources of emotional and social support. This results, in part, from the fact that the pressures of modern, mobile society have changed the nature of traditional support systems. In today's culture, divorced, widowed, never-married, and childless people make up larger segments of western society than ever before. Frequent moves and self-care situations for children of working parents are common. Later in life many men and women live alone and endure the hardship of loneliness. Without spouses, close friends, or sympathetic family members nearby, many people have begun to rely on animals for comfort and companion-

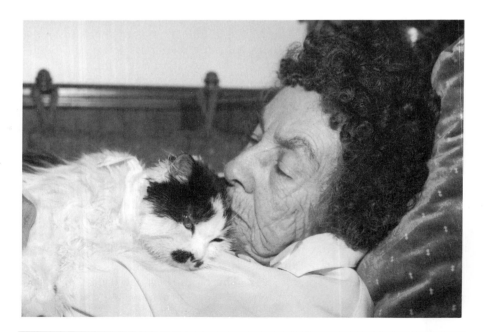

Figure 1-1   For many pet owners, the bonds with their companion animals grow stronger during difficult times.

ship. This deepened bond is depicted in the following letter, written about a special human-animal relationship.

> Socksy was more than "a pet." She was a best friend—a close buddy. She was always there to lick away our tears or to give us kisses when no one else was around. She loved to cuddle with us at night, with her head on a pillow and her body pressed close to one of ours. Socksy loved to sit in the bathroom when we would take showers and feel the mist on her face (though she never dared to go in)!
>
> Socksy's favorite activity was running. The sight of our running shoes and her leash made it impossible for Socks to control herself. She would sit by the door and wait for the words, "OK, Socksy, let's go for a run!" She would be out the door in a flash and begin prancing down the road like a queen, as if to say, "Look dogs, look at me! Hah!!!"
>
> Socksy is—and always will be—a part of the "Brumage Clan." She loved us all unconditionally, even up to the very end of her life. Socksy did not want to leave us. She fought hard for every last breath, until the pain on her face was too much for us to bear, and we had to make the decision to let her go.
>
> We will never forget our Baby Socks, our Socksy Anne, our Socker Ball. She is our forever friend—a part of our souls. We love you Socksy!!
>
> —From a tribute composed jointly by Jim, Joan,
> Laura, Lynne, and Karen Brumage

The thoughts and feelings expressed by the Brumage family in this letter reflect many of the traits and characteristics that endear pets to their human families. As the Brumages so eloquently described it, pets who enjoy full family-member status often share intimate times, take part in daily routines, and show behaviors commonly associated with close friendships. Like the Brumages, many families bestow their pets with special nicknames and anthropomorphic thoughts (Fig. 1-2). This practice tends to humanize pets and to strengthen the bonds between them and their owners.

In the last 10 to 15 years, the term "human-animal bond" has become a popular way of referring to the types of attachments and relationships that exist between people and their pets. The human-animal bond has also become an accepted area of scholarly research within the field of veterinary medicine. Most of us working in this area of study have readily used the term, yet a clear definition and a full understanding of the expression continue to elude us, perhaps because of the many dimensions and ramifications of the human-animal bond that are yet to be explored.

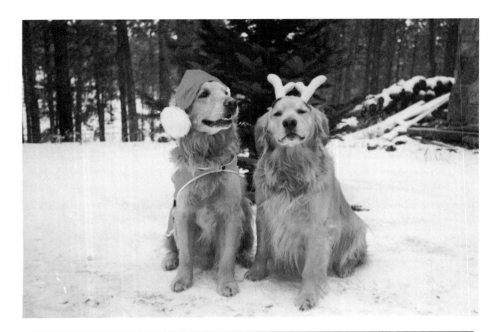

Figure 1-2 Some pet owners playfully dress their pets in costumes and enter them in parades, shows, or contests.

In attempts to better define the human-animal bond, experts are beginning to ask pertinent questions, including: "What is a bond?" "How are bonds between people and pets formed?" "What are the consequences of the bond for animals, for pet owners, and for veterinarians?" "Are human-animal bonds always beneficial or can they be damaging to either humans or animals?" and "What role does the human-animal bond play in the practice of veterinary medicine?" This chapter further examines these questions.

DEFINING A BOND

The concept of bonding or of forming attachments is not exclusive to people and their pets. In fact, a large body of literature exists on attachment theory as it applies to both humans and animals. Attachment was first investigated by studying the relationships between mothers and infants in humans,[6] nonhuman primates,[7] and other species of animals.[8] Further studies have shown, however, that social attachments also form between individuals other than mothers and infants. For instance, attachments form between members of the same species (conspecifics) as well as between individuals of different species (heterospecifics).

There are several ways to conceptualize how attachments form as they relate to the human-animal bond. For example, one theory has suggested that attachment is influenced by people's time and activities with pets, affect toward pets, knowledge about pets and their care, and behavioral responsiveness toward pets.[9] Miller and Lago[10] hypothesized that attachment is based on affectionate companionship, equal family-member status, mutual physical activities, and dominance and submissiveness factors. Ainsworth[11] defined attachment as an affectional tie that endures over time, and the Templer[12] pet attitude inventory focused on love and interaction, pets in the home, and joy of pet ownership as factors indicative of attachment. Estep and Hetts[13] postulated that an attachment forms when an individual acts to maintain proximity to the attachment object and shows signs of separation distress at involuntary separation.

Factors Influencing the Formation of the Human-Animal Bond

People can become attached to any animal, whether domestic or wild. The most common companion animals include dogs, cats, horses, llamas, pigs, goats, birds, fish, snakes and other reptiles, and small mammals such as guinea pigs, rabbits, mice, and hamsters. The strong attachments that people form with these animals are due to several factors including anthropomorphized behaviors, companion rather than utilitarian roles, easily misinterpreted communication signals, and living conditions (usually freedom from enclosures such as cages or pens) (Fig. 1-3), which allow animals

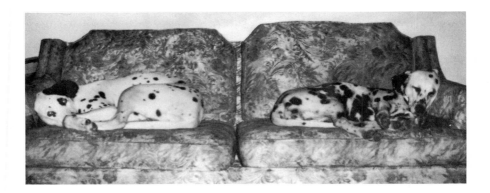

Figure 1-3 Strong attachments between pet owners and their pets are due, in part, to the fact that pets are free from cages or enclosures and can easily participate in their owners' lives.

to share daily routines and leisure-time activities with humans. Thus, no one factor accounts for attachment strengths. For example, although most birds are kept in cages, some can mimic human speech, a factor which gives, at least, the perception of shared communication. Also, although horses are historically thought of as utilitarian animals, they have the longest life-span of any companion animal, thus creating the potential to increase the development of strong attachments.

Veterinarians can gain a better understanding of the reasons for human-animal attachment by understanding the major factors that contribute to it. This book discusses domestication histories, anthropomorphism, neoteny, and allelomimetic behavior. First, let us examine the domestication history of the two most popular companion animals: the dog and the cat.

Domestication Histories

Dogs. Many species of animals have lived in association with humans for literally thousands of years. The dog (Fig. 1-4) is the oldest domesticated animal, having been domesticated at least 12,000 years ago[14] (Fig. 1-5). Although it has been postulated that our domestic dogs' wild canid

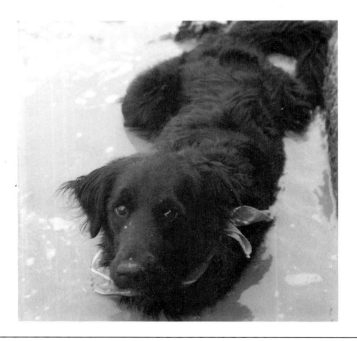

Figure 1-4 The dog, the oldest domesticated animal, may be hunter, protector, co-competitor, playmate, and friend.

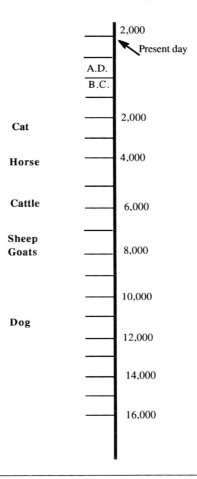

Figure 1-5 A domestication time-line. The dog is the oldest domesticated animal, having been domesticated as long as 15,000 years ago. The cat was domesticated relatively recently, approximately 4000 years ago. Differences in domestication histories partially explain the different types of bonds we develop with dogs and cats.

ancestors were encouraged to accompany early humans on hunting and scavenging expeditions, it is unlikely that dogs were domesticated solely for this purpose. Taming an unwilling animal to engage in an activity as intricate as mutual hunting would have required a huge time investment. The effort alone would probably have precluded its undertaking. It is more likely that the presence of wild canids was encouraged for the purpose of companionship. In the thousands of years since their domestication, dogs

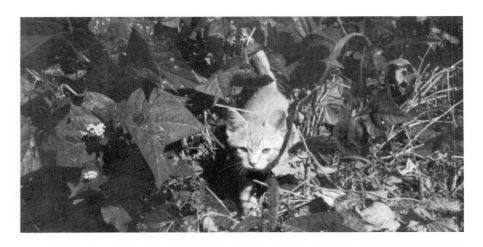

Figure 1-6 Because cats are the most recently domesticated mammal, they often resemble their wild ancestors both physically and behaviorally. Feline domestication began around 2000 B.C., whereas canine domestication began around 10,000 B.C.

have come to be bred and valued for both companionship and for various utilitarian functions.[15]

Cats.   Although cats have recently overtaken dogs as the most common and, hence, the most popular companion animal,[1] the domestication history of the cat is briefer than that of the dog. Cats (Fig. 1-6) are the most recently domesticated mammal, having been domesticated about 4000 years ago,[14] relatively late considering that they had lived in association with humans for at least 1000 years before that time. The selective breeding of cats for characteristics that facilitate their role as companion animals has occurred only during the last 100 years. Cats resemble their wild ancestors both physically and behaviorally, much more so than do their canine counterparts.

Before and after domestication, cats served the utilitarian function of rodent control. Later, they were worshipped and considered sacred. During the Middle Ages, however, cats became associated with witchcraft and were considered to be the symbol of Satan. Due to the dark side of cat ownership, they did not become extremely popular as pets until the nineteenth century. Thus, until relatively recently, cats have not been viewed as companion animals. Rather, their roles in human society have been based either on their utility or on their association with religion.[15]

Anthropomorphism

Attachments between species are more likely to form when each species is familiar with the communication systems of the other. Familiar communication systems create more opportunities for mutual communication, social interaction, and influence on one another's behavior. These conditions potentially increase the degree of mutual attachment. Familiarity occurs when either the communication signals between two species are similar[16] or when humans are very knowledgeable and well informed about the species-typical behaviors and communication signals of another species.

A seeming paradox is suggested by the fact that strong attachments often form between people and companion animals, even though the communication systems of humans do not closely resemble those of dogs, cats, birds, or horses.[13] This apparent contradiction may be explained, in part, by the fact that many pet owners, who are not well-informed about the species-typical or normal behavior patterns of their pets, tend to anthropomorphize their companion animals and thus *perceive* that mutual communication occurs. When people anthropomorphize they give nonhumans or objects humanlike characteristics and traits. Human emotions, thoughts, and behaviors are thus often attributed to animals despite the fact that little or no scientific evidence exists to support the presence of such characteristics (Fig. 1-7). Anthropomorphism may be an important variable in the formation of the human-animal bond.

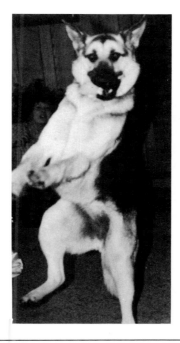

Figure 1-7 Owners anthropomorphize their pets when they attribute human personality traits and physical abilities to companion animals. The german shepherd in this picture, for example, is said to be "dancing."

Let us give some examples of anthropomorphism. A client of the Changes program once told us that her dog was very "polite" because he would only eat when the family sat down to dinner. This behavior, the owner believed, showed that her dog was caring and gentle. Because she found these qualities so endearing, they contributed to her love for and attachment to the animal. In reality, however, species of social animals, including dogs and humans, are likely to do what the rest of their social group is doing. Thus, the dog's eating behavior was socially facilitated by the eating behavior of the other family members and was totally unrelated to the human concept of politeness.

In another instance, a pet owner who had been postponing an out-of-town business trip for weeks was finally forced to leave town. She had been postponing the trip because her elderly cat was seriously ill. Ironically, the cat died the same day she left. She remarked to us later that it was typical of her cat to wait to die until after she had gone. She felt that the cat knew that his death would be easier for her to bear if he waited until she had gone. She spoke of her cat as being considerate of her feelings. In reality, however, no scientific evidence has suggested that animals can choose the time of their deaths. It is more likely that these events were coincidental.

Neoteny

Babies of many species (even humans) possess physical features called "neotenic" or infantile characteristics. These characteristics make all young animals appear "cute" and elicit care-giving responses from at least some human adults. Neotenic characteristics common in puppies, kittens, and other infant animals include large, round eyes; rounded foreheads; and shortened muzzles or noses (Fig. 1-8). For some breeds of adult dogs (Pomeranians or Pekinese) and cats (Persians or Himalayans), neotenic characteristics persist into adulthood. Humans have, either consciously or unconsciously, selectively bred domestic dogs and cats (to some degree) for these neotenic characteristics.

Some animals also possess neotenic behavioral characteristics. Compared to their wild ancestors, for example, domestic dogs are often described as neotenic wolves, in large part because of their easily elicited play behaviors and frequent or relatively high-pitched vocalizations. In adulthood, cats display fewer neotenic characteristics than do dogs, possibly contributing to the widespread, but not altogether accurate, belief that cats can "take care of themselves."

Allelomimetic Behaviors

Many of the species of social animals who live in groups find it advantageous, in some situations, to mimic the behaviors of other group members.

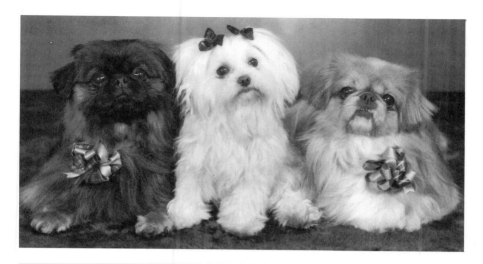

Figure 1-8 Some dogs and cats have been bred selectively for their large, round eyes; rounded foreheads; and shortened muzzles and noses. These "neotenic" or infantile physical features often elicit care-giving responses in human adults. PHOTOGRAPH COURTESY OF CONNIE SWANSON.

For example, if one individual senses danger and begins to flee, another member will probably follow. This behavior frequently occurs even if the animal has not yet become aware of the danger. Because the human family constitutes the domestic dog's social group, dogs sometimes at least ap-

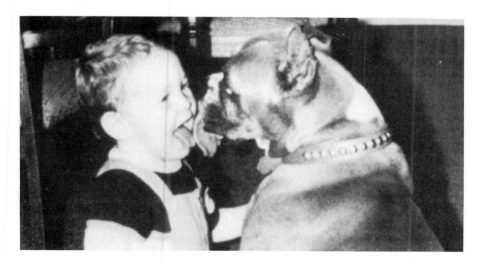

Figure 1-9 Allelomimetic behaviors occur when animals mimic or appear to mimic human behaviors.   PHOTOGRAPH COURTESY OF THE DELTA SOCIETY.

pear to mimic human behavior (Fig. 1-9). When this mimicking occurs, it contributes to people's tendencies to anthropomorphize their companion animals. When pet owners believe that a great deal of mutual communication and understanding is occurring, their attachments are strengthened.

Dogs, much more so than cats, show allelomimetic or mimicking behaviors. Specific examples of allelomimetic behavior are the mimicking of human speech by some species of birds and the facial expressions and physical gestures exhibited by some species of primates.

Social Support

Many factors contributing to the formation of bonds between people and their pets are related to social support. People and their familial pets, as one of our clients said, "eat, sleep, and breathe" together. In other words, like human family members, pets and their owners live and relax in each other's company, a fact substantiated by research. For example, of the pet owners participating in a 1985 survey,[2] 83 percent of dog owners took their dogs with them to run errands, and 72 percent of the same group took their dogs along when they went on trips (Fig. 1-10). In a more recent

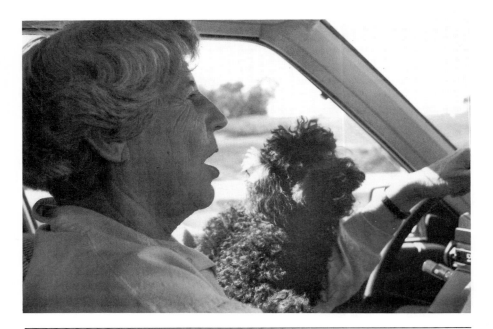

Figure 1-10 Pet owners enjoy the sense of companionship that comes from interacting with their pets during daily routines and leisure time activities.
PHOTOGRAPH BY BARBARA MILLMAN.

study,[17] 70 percent of pet owners said that they exercised their pets daily, with walking and jogging being the two most popular activities for dogs and playing with toys being the most popular activity for cats. Research, in fact, has shown that frequent contact may be the only requirement for the formation of attachments between people and animals.[8]

Just as some pet owners associate their pets with relaxation and the "good times" in life, others feel attached to companion animals based on the "bad times" they have endured together. For example, many pet owners credit their companion animals with getting them through a time of divorce, the death of a friend or family member, or a serious illness. It is common for highly attached pet owners to make comments such as, "I would not have made it without Fluffy," or "Shadow was my reason for getting up in the morning." These comments allow the veterinarian to look into the private lives of clients and to view the historical significance of their human-companion animal relationships.

Many other life circumstances tend to bond animals and people together in significant ways. For example, young adults are often deeply attached to the pets with whom they grew up. They often think of these animals as siblings and "can't remember a time when Max wasn't there." People are also often highly attached to animals whom they believe they have rescued. Examples of rescued pets include strays who have been given homes, seriously ill or injured animals who have been nursed back to health, and unwanted pets who have been saved from death at shelters through timely adoptions. Other highly attached pet owners include people (such as the homebound elderly) who are deprived of contact with others and those who have sole responsibility for the care of their animals.[18]

It is also not uncommon for highly attached pet owners to associate certain companion animals with significant persons or events in their lives. For example, parents often link a child who has died with the family pet who was that child's playmate and protector. After the child's death, the pet becomes a means by which the parents can remain connected to the child. This relationship is called a symbolic attachment. Pet owners also have other kinds of symbolic attachments. For example, pets are often symbolic of spouses or friends who have died or of relationships and lifestyles that have ended.

Consequences of the Formation of a Human-Animal Bond

Pet owners, on average, are much like everybody else. Assessing pet owners' levels of attachment to pets based on stereotypes such as age or gender results in grossly, and probably embarrassingly, incorrect conclusions. The pet owners with whom we have had contact through Changes: The Support for People and Pets Program at Colorado State University's Veterinary

Teaching Hospital (CSU-VTH) have included people of all ages, both sexes, and all walks of life. The highly attached pet owners we have seen run the gamut from a stereotypical elderly woman living alone with several cats to a strongly independent, middle-aged man who not only headed one of the defense branches of the United States military but also considered his 14-year-old dog to be his God-given child. No matter who the pet owners are, you can be sure that the dynamics of their particular human-animal relationships influence both the pets' and the pet owners' lives. Sometimes this influence is positive, and sometimes it has more negative effects.

Consequences from the Human Perspective

The relationship between people and their pets has become a popular subject for scientific study. The work of Boris Levinson, which began in the early 1960s, is often cited as the impetus for serious inquiry into these relationships. In 1961, Dr. Levinson, a child psychiatrist, presented a paper[19] on the benefits of a dog's presence in a counseling setting. He found that several of the more withdrawn children, who had had difficulty communicating with him during counseling sessions, easily made friends with his dog Jingles, to the point of ignoring Levinson during their sessions. After this discovery, Levinson began to make use of Jingles' presence as a social "ice-breaker" and to provide a therapeutic basis for more open communication.

In the ensuing years since Levinson's pioneering work, myriad studies have been conducted. The primary goal of these studies has been to examine the effects of companion animals on various aspects of human psychological and physiological health and well-being. The rewards of this research have been encouraging. The benefits of pet ownership that have been discovered for some human populations include increased survival rates in a group of patients with a previous cardiac arrest,[4] lowered blood pressure among persons in stressful situations,[20] socializing potentials for physically disabled people who are in the presence of service dogs,[21] longer survival rates for elderly retirees with pet birds,[22] lowered rates of depression among elderly persons who are strongly attached to their pets,[23] fewer physical and psychophysiologic symptoms after bereavement in adults,[24] and increases in self-esteem for children and adolescents.[25]

Therefore, the term "human-animal bond" in the literature is most often used to connote a positive, mutually beneficial relationship. It implies that the behaviors of individuals who are bonded to each other are always friendly or affiliative in nature. When attachments form between individuals of different species, however, each individual responds to the other as though it were a member of its own species (a conspecific). Not all interactions between conspecifics are positive or friendly. Conspecifics compete for resources such as food, territory, mates, and social rank and often display aggressive behavior toward each other as a result of this competition. Thus, problems such as dominance, possessiveness, or intermale aggression directed toward humans by animals such as dogs and llamas are also realistic respects of the human-animal bond.

In their studies, Voith[26] and Serpell[27] provide a wide variety of examples in which pet ownership results in negative outcomes for owners. These include the destruction of personal property and severe physical injuries to family members. For pet owners, some of the most common and exasperating negative outcomes of pet ownership are animal behavior problems. Dogs often become destructive, soil the house, or vocalize excessively only when they are left alone. These behaviors are *not* the result of spite or revenge (another example of anthropomorphism) but rather of separation anxiety.

Separation anxiety occurs when social animals are involuntarily separated from the individuals to whom they are attached. During the separation, they show signs of separation distress. This distress is, in fact, one sort of evidence that an attachment exists. Animals who become anxious and distressed when separated from their owners often manifest anxiety in the kinds of previously mentioned problem behaviors.

Cats can also display behaviors symptomatic of separation anxiety but usually do so less frequently than dogs. Separation anxiety in cats is usually in response to prolonged absences (a weekend or longer) from the owner. Problem behaviors are negative consequences of the human-animal bond.

Pet ownership does not guarantee beneficial outcomes. Stallones *et al.*[28] found that people between the ages of 21 and 34 who are strongly attached to their pets are at risk of having fewer human social supports. In the same study, it was found that when strong attachments to pets existed in the absence of human supports for people between the ages of 35 and 44, the attachment was associated with emotional distress. In other studies, Grossberg *et al.*[29] could not reproduce the positive effects on blood pressure in stressful situations that had been reported earlier by Friedman *et al.*[20] in their 1983 article. Miller and Lago[30] found that pet attachment had no effect on the psychological or physical well-being of elderly women. Also, in a sample of elderly women, those who were not attached to their pets were more likely to report being unhappy than were those who were attached to their pets or those who were not pet owners.[31] Although pet ownership can provide various benefits to children, such as an enduring and self-enhancing source of affection, potential costs to children include "getting into trouble" as a result of interactions with, or lack of interactions with, their pets and distress when their pets die or are given away.[32] The ways in which the veterinarian can deal with the potentially negative affects of pet loss on all these populations are discussed in Chapter 12.

In recent years, another tragic consequence of the human-animal bond has come to light. These problems are brought on by "animal collectors." Animal collectors are people who amass more animals than they can properly care for and who then fail to recognize, or refuse to acknowledge, that the animals in their custody are victims of gross neglect. Animal collectors are characterized by a dysfunctional need to own animals and a deeply held belief that any kind of life is far preferrable to a humane death. Thus, they pride themselves on rescuing scores of animals from the shelters and the streets, even though they have neither the physical nor the financial means to care for them. Animal collectors are most often intelligent, articulate people who, when confronted by veterinarians, humane agencies, or law enforcement authorities, have remarkable ability to attract sympathy to themselves and to their plights. Animal collectors are often portrayed as heroes or martyrs by the media and others, yet rebuff any offers of help generated by their own publicity. This is the result of the fact that, unless help comes in the form of monetary assistance, it is viewed as interference and as an attempt to reduce the number of animals involved. Unless psychiatric help is obtained, animal collectors invariably resume their collecting activities even when they are convicted of cruelty to animals (Box 1-1). The human-animal bond can have both positive and negative consequences for animals as well.

Consequences from the Animal Perspective

· The relationships between companion animals and humans are symbiotic, which means that different species of animals live in close association with each other. Clearly, sufficient evidence has indicated that most of these relationships are mutualistic, that is, that both species benefit from the association. Other possible outcomes of the relationships, however, include commensalism, in which one species benefits and the other is unaffected, and parasitism, in which one species benefits and the other is harmed. The emergence of the animal rights and animal welfare movements is forcing closer examination of these types of human-companion animal relationships.

Very little research has been done to identify the effects that the human-animal bond has on our animal companions. Organizations with an interest in this area, such as The Delta Society, have focused their efforts on the effects of human-animal relationships on *human health*. Similarly, animal-oriented groups, such as the American Veterinary Medicine Association (AVMA), have been more interested in the physiological, rather than the psychological, health problems of companion animals and have concentrated their efforts there. Thus, the effects of the human-animal bond on companion animals is an area of research that seems to have "fallen through the cracks" and is in need of further study.

Objective data on the effects of people's strong attachments to their companion animals are not available. Clinical evidence suggests, however,

BOX 1-1

Traits of Animal Collectors

Animal collectors are people who amass more animals than they can properly care for. Such persons generally fail to recognize or refuse to acknowledge that many of the animals in their custody are victims of gross neglect. Animal collectors have:

- an apparent need to have many animals,
- a "love for animals" combined with a failure to care for them responsibly,
- a perception that reverence for life is synonymous with preservation of life, regardless of its quality,
- a hero-martyr complex, often receiving favorable publicity about the personal sacrifices made on behalf of the animals,
- a need to control every aspect of the existence of animals in custody, often denying them veterinary care, exercise, and human companionship,
- a stubborn refusal to part with any of the animals, be it through adoption of the relatively healthy or euthanasia of the sick,
- an apparent inability to see the situation for what is is, often insisting that ill animals are healthy, that animals are perfectly happy in squalid surroundings, *etc.*,
- a high rate of recidivism and a general return to animal collecting even after being convicted of cruelty to animals.

Adapted from a 1990 fact sheet developed by Samantha Mullen, Public Affairs and Programs Administrator for the New York State Humane Association.

that most of these companion animals receive high-quality care. In our work at Colorado State University, for example, we have encountered numerous animal owners who spare no expense in obtaining quality medical care for their animals. This care frequently includes state-of-the-art treatment for cancer and other life-threatening conditions.

However, cases of psychogenic behavioral and physiological problems in companion animals have been documented. Serpell,[27] for example, reported a case in which a pet owner induced an ulcerated colon in her German shepherd by forcing it to sit on a chair at the dinner table while she spoon-fed it. Savishinsky,[33] an anthropologist, stated that having companion animals assume myriad complex roles in families (including that of children, parents, or best friends) and making them be "an all-purpose person . . . in a single household and in a single lifetime" may be stressful for the animal.

We also know that the human-animal bond is not always enduring. Of the 110 million dogs and cats in our country, approximately 5 to 10 million are euthanized[34] each year. Dogs, cats, and small mammals are surrendered to shelters for such diverse reasons as divorce, owner relocation, financial problems, animal behavior problems, and housing codes that restrict pet ownership. In these situations, animals may also be brought to the veterinarian for what is called a euthanasia of "convenience." "Convenience" euthanasias are sure to provoke some moral and ethical dilemmas for the veterinarian and for the members of his or her staff. The ways in which the veterinarian can deal with this client request are discussed in Chapter 14.

THE VETERINARY CLIENT

Who are the pet owners who become highly attached to their companion animals? Over the years, several research and marketing studies have attempted to profile veterinary client characteristics. Many of these studies show that most veterinary clients are women and that women are most often identified as the primary caretakers of pets.[35] One study has indicated that a high percentage of veterinary clients are married, work outside the home, have both children and pets, and have attained some level of higher education. It has also shown that pet owners in upper socioeconomic and occupational levels are more likely than those in the lower socioeconomic classes to view their pets as personal companions.

This same study has shown that clients with four or more children are somewhat less likely to report that pets are personal companions than are those with no children or those with one to three children. Also, married women with children are more likely than any other group to report that pets are personal companions. In this study, people over 50 years of age viewed pets primarily as personal companions rather than as companions to other people within the household.[36] For an easy reference to the key factors forming the basis of your veterinary clients' human-animal bonds, see Box 1-2.

THE VETERINARY PROFESSIONAL

It is apparent from the information presented in this chapter that perspectives in veterinary medicine are changing. Before World War II, veterinarians were viewed primarily as large-animal practitioners.[37] In this climate, the emotional needs of clients were not considered to be the concern of veterinarians. Companion-animal medicine experienced significant growth in the 1950s and, along with this growth, came a parallel growth in the awareness of the emotional needs of the owners of companion animals. Acknowledgment of veterinarians' roles in support of the human-companion animal relationship gained momentum in the 1970s. In the 1980s, several factors worked together to make it clear that, as stated by Kolodny, "practitioners who ignored the message did so at their own peril."[37] These factors included the interest of the AVMA in human-animal issues and the influence of interdisciplinary educational opportunities providing perspec-

BOX 1-2

Keys to Attachment

Human-animal relationships may be perceived as stronger and more important when:

- owners believe that they rescued their companion animals from death or near-death,
- owners believe that their companion animals "got them through" a difficult period in life,
- owners spent their childhoods with their companion animals,
- owners have relied on their companion animals as their most significant source of support,
- owners anthropomorphize their companion animals,
- owners have invested extensive time, effort, or financial resources into their companion animals' long-term medical care,
- owners view their companion animals as symbolic links to significant people who are no longer part of their lives (for example, children who have died or moved away, significant relationships or marriages that have ended) or to significant times in their lives (for example, futures that would be lived in the mountains, past times spent hiking, fishing, camping, etc.).

tives on veterinary medicine from various disciplines within the social sciences.

In 1982, the Executive Board of AVMA recognized the human-animal bond as an emerging discipline within the field, and in 1993, the American Association of Human-Animal Bond Veterinarians was formed. To acknowledge the important roles that animals play in people's lives, they established the Human-Animal Bond Committee. In 1977, three veterinarians, Drs. Stanley Diesch, R.K. Anderson, and William McCulloch, and a psychiatrist, Dr. Michael McCulloch, established the DELTA Foundation in recognition of the human-animal bond. These farsighted professionals had been exploring the interactions between people and animals and, as a way of describing their findings, coined the term "human-animal bond." The Delta Foundation later became The Delta Society. As Dr. Earl O. Strimple, DVM, and former president of The Delta Society, wrote:

> Delta Society was the first group with a mission to study and promote the special relationship that exists between people and animals. Delta began with 12 founding members and has grown to about 2600 members. Approximately a third of the members are veterinarians or human health care professionals, a third are in academia, and a third is made up of humane officers, veterinary technicians, volunteers, and pet owners. Slow and steady growth in the non-veterinary

membership of Delta Society is contrasted with little growth from our own profession. This is surprising and disappointing because we, the veterinarians, are gaining the most from the favorable publicity that appears in the news media and from the new respect for companion animals.[38] (p. 206)

John Albers, DVM, and Executive Director of the American Animal Hospital Association (AAHA) believes that, on a profession-wide level, it is beneficial for veterinary medicine to support and encourage the human-animal bond movement. In Dr. Strimple's 1991 article, Dr. Albers is quoted as saying:

We know that the positive relationships between people and pets are extremely beneficial: in hospitals, prisons, and homes for the aged; for people with visual and hearing disabilities and for many others who are disabled in some way, and significantly, in every pet-owning family . . . caring pet owners are persons who recognize the value of pet ownership and companionship, thus exhibiting a significant bond with their pet. They accept the responsibility of proper care. They promote the benefits of pet ownership to others. They will enable us to provide the high-quality care that we are capable of offering. As the human/animal bond becomes stronger, so too will our profession.[38] (pp. 207–208)

CONCLUSION

The human-animal bond is most often thought of as representing only a slice of the veterinary medicine pie (Fig. 1-11). However, those of us involved in human-animal bond education and clinical practice encourage students to view the relationship between veterinary medicine and the human-animal bond from a new perspective. In the classroom, we alter the "pie" to resemble the diagram in Figure 1-12. In the not so distant future, this representation may not seem unrealistic. An increasing number of veterinary professionals are beginning to agree with Dr. Leo K. Bustad, Dean Emeritus of the Washington State University College of Veterinary Medicine and the first president of The Delta Society, who stated that "the bond between people and animals is the primary basis for our professional existence."[38]

Dr. Bustad also stated, "I firmly believe that your success in life and in the practice of veterinary medicine will in a great part depend on your understanding of the various aspects of the human-animal bond and how you integrate these aspects into your life everyday."[39] We agree wholeheartedly with Dr. Bustad.

Over the last several years, thousands of veterinary students, practicing veterinarians, and animal health technicians have learned about the human-animal bond as it pertains to pet loss and grief among pet owners. Their feedback on this subject has ranged from open acceptance to blatant resistance. Some memorable comments include:

> "I will change the way I practice veterinary medicine based on what I've learned about pet loss and grief."

> "Never before have I realized the importance of the human-animal bond to some of my clients. Now I have much more empathy for some of their strange behaviors!"

> "I was hired as a new veterinarian because the clinic owner was impressed that I knew how to handle situations involving death and euthanasia."

They also include comments such as:

> "I did not become a veterinarian so I could get in touch with my feelings."

> "The task of counseling people who are troubled or in crisis belongs to someone else! I'm not trained in it and I don't want to do it!"

Whether veterinary professionals are enthusiastic supporters or skeptical detractors, concerns about integrating the human-animal bond into the daily practice of veterinary medicine always arise. Your own concerns will arise as you read this book. If cowboys thought of horses solely as a means of transportation or if home owners thought of dogs solely as protectors of property, communication with veterinary clients regarding the human-animal bond and the effects of pet loss would not be so important. The truth, however, is that many sane and respectable people are highly attached to the animals with whom they live. Consequently, they seek out the best *overall* care possible for their animals, and for themselves, when the bonds they share with their companion animals are threatened. Whether the consequences are positive or negative, the power inherent in the human-animal bond makes it a force to be addressed in contemporary veterinary medicine.

The following story illustrates the power of the human-animal bond.

What the Dog Taught Me
Robert Fulghum

A houseboat on our dock was sold, and since we have a "no dogs" rule and the new owners had a dog, the possibility of social conflict was high. However,

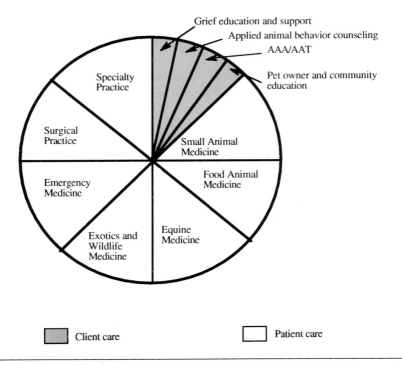

Grief education and support
Applied animal behavior counseling
AAA/AAT
Pet owner and community education

Specialty Practice

Surgical Practice

Emergency Medicine

Small Animal Medicine

Food Animal Medicine

Exotics and Wildlife Medicine

Equine Medicine

Client care   Patient care

Figure 1-11 The field of veterinary medicine, focus A. For many practitioners, the field of veterinary medicine focuses on providing medical care to animal patients. As this pie chart shows, client care constitutes only a small portion of veterinary medicine. The emotional needs of clients, resulting from relationships with their companion animals, are not usually a significant part of everyday practice.

with unexpected sensitivity, the couple went door to door explaining that they understood the rule, but theirs was a very old, very well-behaved dog that did not bark and spent most of its time inside. Besides being old, the dog was not in good health and would probably die soon. They wanted permission to have the dog on the dock on a try-it-and-see reality check. The alternative was to have the dog put away. If the dock tenants voted thumbs down on the dog, then the owners would do what had to be done.

Now, I'm afraid of dogs, if you want to know the truth. Seriously afraid. Having been chewed up by big dogs twice as a child, and having twice gone through the full rabies treatment, I am not enthusiastic about being around dogs.

But what am I supposed to say? "Too bad, lady, but you'll have to kill your dog."

Still, I don't care what they say about their pooch—all dog owners think their

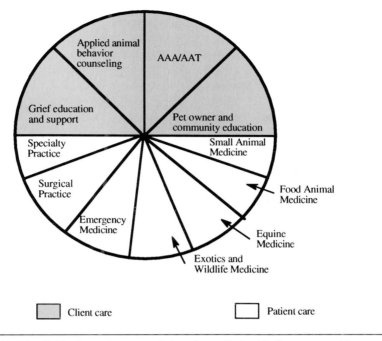

Figure 1-12 The field of veterinary medicine, focus B. In this figure, practitioners are encouraged to change their view of veterinary medicine. With this perspective, a more equal emphasis is placed on meeting the medical needs of patients and the emotional needs of clients that result from the human-animal bond.

dog is an exceptional dog. Ha! I know all canines are hyenas at heart. But I can work around this problem—all I have to do is stay inside for a month and vote no, and the dog is out of my life.

So, here comes the dog.

Big dog. Half German shepherd and half Dalmatian. Stout, black and white, lady dog.

Name is Gyda—a name you would expect for a blond Norwegian bank teller in a bikini on a beach in Spain—but not for a four-legged pet with bad breath.

During the trial month, as I was sitting on the deck of my houseboat each morning, she and her mistress would pass me on their walk. When the pooch would see me, she would stop, sit down, cock her head and look at me. No bark, no whine, no slobber. Just looking. Me? No dog had ever just looked at me like this before. I felt like an antelope must feel when a lion sits down and takes a look. Attack dogs do this just before they go for your throat.

In time, though, my fear turned to curiosity. What's with this dog? Then curiosity became respect. What's with me?

One morning I reached out and petted her on the head.

I know people pet dogs all the time and it's no big deal, but if you were as afraid as I was (notice the past tense), then you'd know this was not an incidental moment. She let me pet her. No hand-licking, no jumping around and barking. Just a solemn acknowledgement of kindness received. With that touch, Gyda and I became connected. Much to my wife's astonishment, I even invited Gyda over to our house as a personal guest on occasion. We sat together on the porch and watched ducks. My wife wanted to know what was going on, and I didn't want to talk about it. It was embarrassing to be wrong about something— humiliating to have to change my mind.

Sometimes I took Gyda along on walks. I talked to her. Me, the man who thinks talking to dogs is dumb. Though she never barked or made a sound that I know of, she would stop and sit down and look at me while I talked. I once explained the difference between the music of B. B. King and Chuck Berry to her, and she never took her eyes off me. That's a cool dog.

The vote never came up on the dock. Gyda took us all in. Everybody had a personal relationship with her. I learned a lot from that dog about the power of keeping your mouth shut and your eyes open. She became a kind of great-aunt figure to us all. So she stayed and became a welcome part of daily life. We needed a classy dog and just didn't know it.

I'll tell you just how far things went. When her owners decided to get married and asked me to perform the wedding, I went along with the idea of Gyda being part of the ceremony. Because she was, after all, the mistress's best friend.

If I could show you the video of the wedding this is what you'd see: You'd see me, the minister, in my black gown, walking into the site of the ceremony in the park with a big old black-and-white dog at my side. The dog is wearing a huge white bow around her neck—white because she was, as far as anyone knows, a virgin. Truly, the maid of honor.

Gyda had cancer all this time. Her mistress went to the vet one morning with Gyda in her arms and came back alone. I cried. The dock was dressed in invisible crepe for a week. Here's the notice I decided to put in everyone's mailbox.

"Nobody is more surprised than I am to be writing this. Everybody knows about me and dogs. On the other hand, there was Gyda. And there is Bob and Blair. Sometimes I am wrong.

"So I write to invite you to a memorial-service kind of occasion on Sunday morning, August 6. Coffee at nine, followed by a celebration of a life well lived, followed by a potluck brunch.

"Gyda became a kind of symbol for the best kinds of relationships that are possible in the close community on our dock. Almost anything can be dealt with if people are of good will and light hearts and strong values. I believe that. Even a dog on the dock can work out. Gyda reminded me as she went by each day that what makes us rich here is not the escalating value of our floating homes, but the careful quality of our ongoing relationships that somehow respect both individual rights and group needs. Gyda's coming increased our humanity in a funny but critical way.

"Gyda's departing leaves a hole in our daily lives. We were more generous to each other because of her.

"I miss that dog a lot."

We did indeed gather on that Sunday morning in August—thirty of us—and told stories that were as much about us as Gyda. We buried her ashes under a rhododendron bush that's planted in a barrel on her owner's back porch. I always nod in her direction when I pass by.

Gyda. The grand old virgin aunt in the dog suit.

My seminary training didn't cover how to perform a dog funeral. It takes a real dog to teach that. And when the pupil is ready, the teacher appears.

From *UH-OH* by Robert Fulghum. Copyright © 1991 by Robert Fulghum. Reprinted by permission of Villard Books, a division of Random House, Inc.

REFERENCES

1. McKey, E., and Payne, K.: APPMA study: Pet ownership soars. Pet Business, *18*:22–23, 1992.
2. Voith, V.L.: Attachment of people to companion animals. *In* Quackenbush, J., and Voith, V.L., eds: Vet. Clin. North Am. [Small Anim. Pract.], *15*:289–296, 1985.
3. American Pet Products Manufacturers Association: Survey of pet ownership in the USA. Pet Business, *14*:4, 1988.
4. Friedmann, E., Katcher, A.H., Lynch, J.J., and Thomas, S.A.: Animal companions and one-year survival of patients after discharge from a coronary care unit. Public Health Rep., *95*:307–312, 1980.
5. Messent, P.R.: Social facilitation of contact with other people by pet dogs. *In* Katcher, A.H., and Beck, A.M., eds.: New Perspectives on Our Lives with Companion Animals, Philadelphia, University of Pennsylvania Press, 1983, pp. 37–46.
6. Bowlby, J.: Separation anxiety. Int. J. Psychoanal., *41*:1–25, 1960.
7. Harlow, H.F., and Harlow, M.K.: Effect of various mother-infant relationships on rhesus monkey behavior. *In* Foss, B.M., ed.: Determinants of Infant Behavior IV, New York, John Wiley and Sons, 1969, pp. 34–60.
8. Cairns, R.B.: Attachment behavior in mammals. Psychol. Rev., *73*:409–429, 1966.
9. Melson, G.F.: Studying children's attachment to their pets: A conceptual and methodological review. Anthrozoos, *4*:91–99, 1990.
10. Miller, M., and Lago, D.: Observed pet-owner in-home interactions: Species differences and associations with the pet relationship scale. Anthrozoos, *4*:49–54, 1990.
11. Ainsworth, M.D., Blehar, M.C., Waters, E., and Wall, S.: Patterns of Attachment, Hillsdale, N.J., Lawrence Erlbaum Associates, 1978.
12. Templer, D.I., Salter, C.A., Dickey, S., Baldwin, R., and Veleber, D.M.: The construction of a pet attitude scale. Psychiat. Rec., *31*:343–348, 1981.
13. Estep, D.Q., and Hetts, S.: Interactions, relationships and bonds: The conceptual basis for scientist-animal relations. *In* Davis, H., and Balfour, D., eds.: The Inevitable Bond: Examining Scientist-Animal Interactions, New York, Cambridge University Press, 1992, 6–26.
14. Zeuner, F.E.: A History of Domesticated Animals, New York, Harper and Row, 1963.
15. Young, M.S.: The evolution of domestic pets and companion animals. *In* Quackenbush, J., and Voith, V.L., eds.: Vet. Clin. North Am. [Small Animal Pract.], *15*:297–310, 1985.
16. Hediger, H.: Man as a social partner of animals and vice versa. *In* Ellis, P.E., ed.: Social

Organization of Animal Communities, London, Symposium of the Zoological Society of London, 1965, pp. 291–300.

17. Survey: Exercise common among pets. J. Am. Vet. Med. Assoc., *199*:1132, 1991.

18. Stallones, L., Johnson, T.P., Garrity, T.F., and Marx, M.B.: Quality of attachment to companion animals among U.S. adults 21–64 years of age. Anthrozoos, *3*:171–176, 1990.

19. Levinson, B.M.: The dog as a "co-therapist." Ment. Hygiene, *46*:59–65, 1961.

20. Friedman, E., Katcher, A.H., Lynch, J.J., and Thomas, S.A.: Social conditions and blood pressure: Influence of animal companions. J. Nerv. Ment. Dis., *171*:461–465, 1983.

21. Hart, L.A., Hart, B.L., and Bergin, B.: Socializing effects of service dogs for people with disabilities. Anthrozoos, *1*:41–44, 1987.

22. Mugford, R.A., and M'Comsky, J.G.: Some recent work on the psychotherapeutic value of cage birds with old people. *In* Anderson, R.S., ed.: Pet Animals and Society, London, Bailliere Tindall, 1975, pp. 54–65.

23. Garrity, T.F., Stallones, L., Marx, M.B., and Johnson, T.P.: Pet ownership and attachment as supportive factors in the health of the elderly. Anthrozoos, *3*:35–44, 1989.

24. Akiyama, H., Holtzman, J.M., and Britz, W.E.: Pet ownership and health status during bereavement. Omega, *17*:187–193, 1986/1987.

25. Covert, A.M., Whiren, A.P., Keith, J., and Nelson, C.: Pets, early adolescents and families. *In* Sussman, M.B., ed.: Pets and the Family. Marriage and Family Review, Vol. 8 (3–4), New York, Haworth Press, 1985, pp. 95–108.

26. Voith, V.: Attachment between people and their pets: Behavior problems of pets that arise from the relationship between pets and people. *In* Fogle, B., ed.: Interrelations Between People and Pets, Springfield, Ill. Charles C. Thomas, 1981, pp. 271–304.

27. Serpell, J.: In the Company of Animals, Oxford, Basil Blackwell, Ltd., 1986.

28. Stallones, L., Marx, M.B., Garrity, T.F., and Johnson, T.P.: Pet ownership and attachment in relation to the health of U.S. adults, 21–64 years of age. Anthrozoos, *4*:100–112, 1990.

29. Grossberg, J.M., Alf, E.F., and Vormborck, J.K.: Does pet dog presence reduce human cardiovascular responses to stress? Anthrozoos, *2*:38–44, 1988.

30. Miller, M., and Lago, D.: The well-being of older women: The importance of pet and human relationships. Anthrozoos, *3*:245–251, 1990.

31. Ory, M.G., and Goldberg, E.H.: Pet possession and life satisfaction in elderly women. *In* Katcher, A.H., and Beck, A.M., eds.: New Perspectives on Our Lives with Companion Animals, Philadelphia, University of Pennsylvania Press, 1983, pp. 303–317.

32. Bryant, B.K.: The richness of the child-pet relationship: A consideration of both benefits and costs of pets to children. Anthrozoos, *3*:253–261, 1990.

33. Savishinsky, J.: Pet ideas: The domestication of animals, human behavior, and human emotions. *In* Katcher, A.H., and Beck, A.M., eds.: New Perspectives on Our Lives with Companion Animals, Philadelphia, University of Pennsylvania Press, 1983, pp. 112–131.

34. Rowan, A.N.: Shelters and pet overpopulation: A statistical black hole. Anthrozoos, *5*:140–143, 1992.

35. Troutman, C.M.: The Veterinary Service Market for Companion Animals. Overland Park, Kan. Charles, Charles Research Group and the American Veterinary Medical Association, 1988.

36. Harris, C.T.: Human-pet relationships among veterinary clients. Comp. Cont. Vet. Med. Ed., *9*:424–430, 1988.

37. Kolodny, S.W.: Companion animal illness and human emotion: Historical overview. *In* Cohen, S.P., and Fudin, C.E., eds.: Problems in Veterinary Medicine, Vol. 3, Philadelphia, J.B. Lippincott, 1991, pp. 1–5.

38. Strimple, E.O.: The human/animal bond: A time for commitment. J. Am. Vet. Med. Assoc., *199*:206–208, 1991.

39. Bustad, L.: Our profession's responsibilities regarding the living bond: People, animals, environment. Intervet, *23*:10–14, 1988.

2

When the Bond Is Broken

The death of a companion animal may be one of the most significant losses we experience throughout our lives. In a recent study conducted by the University of Minnesota's Center for the Study of Human-Animal Relations and Environment, researchers examined the responses of 242 middle-aged couples who reported the death of a pet within the past three years. Couples were asked to rate the stress level associated with 48 events they endured, including death of a spouse, divorce, marriage, loss of children, an arrest, loss of a job, and death of a pet. Researchers found that the death of a pet was the most frequently reported trauma experienced by the couples participating in the study. Survey participants said the deaths of their pets were less stressful than the deaths of human members of their immediate families but more stressful than the deaths of other relatives. Forty percent of wives and 28 percent of husbands reported that the loss of a pet was "quite" or "extremely" disturbing.[1]

Pets who are viewed as sources of emotional and social support and treated as family members are likely to elicit strong feelings of attachment from their owners. Yet, according to researchers at the University of California-Davis, veterinarians characteristically underestimate the importance of their clients' attachments to their animals.[2] Veterinarians who trivialize the human-animal bond can cause damage to the relationships between themselves and their clients, especially when pet owners are experiencing the deaths of their pets and the subsequent feelings of grief.

Pet death is an inevitable part of pet ownership. Because most domestic animals have relatively short life spans, few pets outlive their owners. Some animals die from acute or chronic illnesses. Others are victims of accidents. Many pets die of old age or are euthanized because they have behavior problems or untreatable terminal illnesses.

Companion animal death is also an inevitable part of veterinary medicine. Largely because of the option of euthanasia, it is estimated that veterinarians experience the deaths of their patients five times more often than do their counterparts in human medicine.[3] In fact, one study reported that, over a 1-year period, 3 percent of the companion animals treated by veterinarians died; 66 percent of these deaths were the result of euthanasia.[4] Animals' deaths and euthanasias are therefore issues of central importance to the field of veterinary medicine.

The option of euthanasia puts the veterinarian in a unique position. Like physicians in human medicine, veterinarians are morally and ethically obligated to save lives. Yet, when quality of life ceases to exist for an animal, veterinarians are also morally and ethically obligated to put an end to suffering and pain. Euthanasia allows veterinarians to legally and humanely end the lives they once saved. The client's presence at a pet's euthanasia puts the veterinarian in an even more unique position because, while a pet owner is in the room engaged in the process of saying goodbye to a beloved companion animal, a drug is injected into the animal's vein, causing the animal's death to occur. At this point, the veterinarian witnesses what very few medical professionals ever see—the planned death of a family member. The pet owner's immediate displays of grief are also witnessed (Fig. 2-1).

When euthanasia is skillfully and sensitively performed, the experience is profound. Thus, in the presence of death and grief, the veterinarian is also often moved. Therefore, pets' deaths are often as emotionally challenging for the veterinarian as they are for the clients.

Authors John James and Frank Cherry, in their book *The Grief Recovery Handbook,* write:

> We are far better prepared to deal with minor accidents than we are to deal with the grief caused by death. Simple first aid gets more attention in our world than death and emotional loss. Please don't think we are exaggerating. Stop and consider your own experience. In grade school you took a class on first aid; in high school you took a class on health and safety; the local Red Cross offers classes on first aid in the community. You're probably prepared to take action if an accident occurs in your presence. Nationwide, we have a convenient 911 number to call in case of emergency. At some level we're all prepared to aid an accident victim. How many classes have you taken on how to deal with the grief caused by death or loss? We think it's a little strange that we all know what to do if someone breaks an arm, but no one's prepared to assist grievers, although

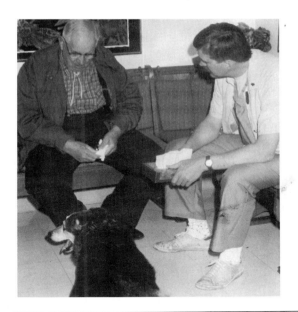

Figure 2-1 As pet owners prepare for euthanasia, they often experience overwhelming feelings of loss. During these times, they may need quiet support from their veterinarians.

there are eight million new ones caused from [human] deaths alone each year.[5]

Despite society's state of denial, it is difficult to ignore the mounting evidence indicating that the grief people feel at the deaths of their pets is real. Recent studies have made the impact of this grief clear. One study, for example, showed that the grief owners feel when pets die is often overwhelming and that the responses to pet loss often parallel the grief responses to the loss of human companions. In this study, 75 percent of pet owners experienced difficulties or disruptions in their lives after pets died. One third of the owners experienced difficulties in their relationships with others or needed to take time off from work because of their feelings of grief.[1]

So, what does the grief triggered by pet loss feel like for pet owners, and how can you, a veterinarian, best offer your help? One of the basic tenets of any helping relationship is that you cannot effectively help others until you have first helped yourself. Therefore, the necessary process of examining personal beliefs and past experiences with loss and grief is discussed in Chapter 11. The first step toward becoming an effective helper, however, is to become well-informed about the normal manifestations and typical processes of grief and about its antecedent event known as loss.

UNDERSTANDING LOSS

When the human-animal bond is broken, owners and veterinarians experience loss. Loss is defined as an ending or as a point of change and transition. Some losses are as traumatic emotionally as an injury or burn is physically.[6] We each determine the impact of loss based on criterion unique to our own lives. These criteria include personal attitudes about, perspectives on, and previous experiences with loss.

The significance of any loss is thus best judged by the individual who is actually involved with and affected by it. Using this guideline, pet owners themselves are the most qualified to define the impact of pet loss on their personal lives. In our experience, most pet owners judge the deaths of their companion animals to be, at the very least, sad and slightly disturbing. However, when others intentionally or unintentionally trivialize, negate, or even ridicule the grief caused by pet loss, slightly disturbing feelings all too often become devastating.

Examples of the trivializing of pet loss abound. It is not uncommon, for example, for people to attempt to comfort grieving pet owners by saying, "I know you feel bad, but it was just a dog. You can get another one" or "Your horse lived a good, long life and you can be happy you had him for as long as you did." Some pet owners unfortunately also hear these comments from well-meaning veterinarians.

Types of Loss

Death is only one type of loss. Experts in grief counseling have identified many others. Four types are especially pertinent to the discussion of pet loss. These are referred to as primary, secondary, ambiguous, and symbolic losses.

Primary and Secondary Loss

For pet owners, primary losses are represented by the actual deaths of their pets; that is, the deaths of their pets are the main cause of their grief. Primary losses often create disruptions in other areas of pet owners' lives. These additional disruptions are referred to as secondary losses.[7] Secondary losses have the greatest impact on those pet owners who share their leisure activities and daily routines with their pets. For example, pet owners who participate in competitive shows lose more than their show partners when their companion animals die. Along with the primary loss of their animals, they also experience the secondary loss of no longer participating in an enjoyable pastime (Fig. 2-2).

When pets play roles in peoples' lives beyond those of confidante and companion, the secondary losses are often more significant. The rancher whose Border Collie rounds up cattle every day, the person with disabilities whose service dog follows over 90 commands, and the self-care or "latch-key" child whose dog provides friendship and protection after school experience more secondary losses than does the person whose cat is sheltered and fed merely to keep the house free of mice.

Another kind of secondary loss common to pet owners is the loss of the supportive relationship that the veterinarian has provided. For many pet owners, this relationship ends with the deaths of their pets. A letter from a former client illustrates this point.

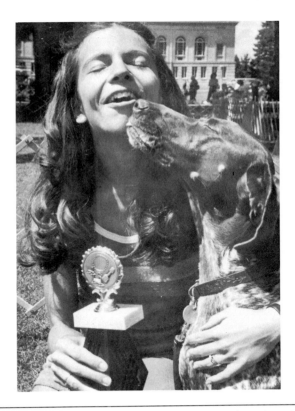

Figure 2-2 Pets play significant roles in their owners' social routines. Therefore, when these pets die, primary and secondary losses are experienced. Owners experience one form of secondary loss when they are no longer able to share leisure activities, such as participating in competitive shows, with their pets.

Over the eighteen months that Tiger and I came to your clinic, we got to know you and most of your staff as well as we have ever known anyone in the veterinary field. During Tiger's treatment, we considered you to be our personal veterinarian and our very special friend. I know you are busy with your work and family. I also know the likelihood of our families seeing each other socially is slim. Still, I hope you will have time to see me if I stop into the clinic to say hello now and again. Once in awhile, I feel I just need to see your bright face and hear your kind, gentle voice. You were a big part of Tiger's last months and, now that I have lost her, the fact that I have also lost contact with you makes me feel doubly sad and grieved.

Ambiguous Loss

Ambiguous losses are those that leave questions and, therefore, stay unfinished in pet owners' minds.[8] In cases of ambiguous losses, the whereabouts of animals or the causes of their deaths are unknown. Examples of ambiguous pet losses are runaway or stolen pets, pets who die unexpectedly or without known cause, and pets whose fates remain unknown after surrender to humane societies or animal shelters.

With ambiguous loss, the course of grief is unclear because information about the loss is missing. In these situations, owners don't know when to give up hope for their pets' safe return, when to stop searching for their pets, when to stop asking questions about their pets' deaths, or when to begin (as well as when to stop) grieving their losses (Fig. 2-3).

After the disappearance of her dog, a young woman wrote:

> I left hurriedly for work on Monday morning. I put my brown Sharpei, Mocha, in the fenced back yard, as usual. I did not check to see if the back gate was latched, even though it was very windy the night before. When I returned home from work that evening, the back gate was open and Mocha was gone. I drove frantically around the neighborhood. I looked everywhere. Over the days, weeks, and months that followed, I placed ads, called shelters, veterinarians, and Sharpei rescue services, but could not locate Mocha. I thought I saw him everywhere. My mind was filled with questions. Was he stolen, hit by a car, injured, dead? Would I ever learn what happened to him? There were no answers.

Symbolic Loss

Symbolic losses, as we define them, are associated with earlier losses in peoples' lives.[9] Pets may represent the last links that pet owners have to

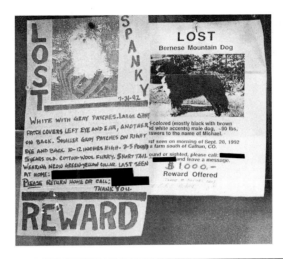

Figure 2-3 Many pet owners go to great lengths trying to find their lost pets. When animals cannot be found, pet owners experience ambiguous loss.

special people, places, things, or times in their lives. The pets' deaths remove those links. Although pet loss is truly a significant loss in its own right, the grief owners feel may be greater when old losses are regrieved in conjunction with their current ones. A symbolic loss is described in this letter from an older client:

> Rowdy was an extra special dog who had a special place in my life. He was a very important link to my husband John who died two years ago. Rowdy grieved for three months and became very sullen when John died. Many times I would find him hiding and hugging John's shoe. He sensed my loss, too, and would not touch his food, nor gather up his balls in the back yard to strike up a game. When Rowdy died last May, it was particularly difficult for me because I felt that I was losing my last living connection to John and the life the three of us shared together. (Fig. 2-4)

Understanding that pet loss is significant for pet owners in many different ways is important to the delivery of bond-centered veterinary care. Understanding, for example, that grief due to a symbolic loss is often more intense or that grief due to a secondary loss may last longer or be reactivated more easily enables the veterinarian to prepare clients to better deal with such losses. It also enables the veterinarian to be a more effective helper, confidently reassuring clients that their feelings of grief are appropriate and to be expected.

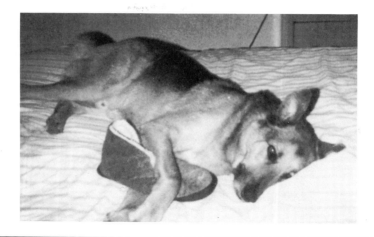

Figure 2-4 Rowdy hugging John's shoe.

UNDERSTANDING GRIEF

In reviewing his experience with pet loss, a 60-year-old client wrote:

> My veterinarian did a beautiful job explaining what was going to happen to Dusty during the euthanasia. He prepared me in great detail for the procedure and for the handling of his body afterwards. But, he didn't tell me what was going to happen to me.
>
> After Dusty died, I couldn't watch a simple 30-minute television program. I couldn't read the Readers' Digest. There were times I even thought about killing myself. I couldn't express these feelings to anyone because I thought I was the only person who had grieved this deeply for a dog. I couldn't call my veterinarian, the person that knew the most about my relationship with Dusty, because I figured he would think I was crazy. I know now that, if he would have given me just five minutes of grief education, it would have helped me make sense of many of the feelings and behaviors I experienced after Dusty died.

Just as it is almost impossible for pet owners to escape the experience of pet loss, it is also impossible for them to escape the experience of grief after their pets have died. As you begin to play a more active role in your clients' experiences with pet loss, you learn that most people know very little about coping with grief. You will also find that what they do know, or think they know, is generally inaccurate.

Research and clinical experience have shown that what people say and do during bereavement is based on the myths and misinformation about grief that are passed along in families from generation to generation.[10] One of the most prominent of these myths is the belief that the best way to handle loss is to be strong and composed during grief. Another is the belief that staying busy and keeping one's mind off the loss is the best way to feel better and to recover more quickly.

These methods of grieving, however, can actually prolong the process of grief and cause grief to become complicated and even pathologic. To avoid reinforcing the myths and misinformation, veterinarians need to become knowledgeable about the normal, healthy grieving process.

Types of Grief

Leaders in the fields of grief education and grief counseling have developed numerous theories to explain people's typical responses to loss. Drs. Therese Rando, J. William Worden, John Bowlby, and Elisabeth Kubler-Ross are four of the best known grief theorists and therapists. Each of these professionals describes the progression of grief in slightly different ways, but all of their theories and interventions have three common components. These commonalities include an initial phase of shock or denial, one or more middle phases of emotional pain and suffering, and a final phase of recovery. Kubler-Ross, for example, delineates five "stages" of grief. She labels them denial, anger, bargaining, depression, and acceptance.[11] Kubler-Ross' work with grief has been discussed frequently in magazines, journals, and books aimed at veterinary professionals. Knowledge of her model has helped many veterinarians gain a greater understanding of the feelings and behaviors involved with pet loss.

The field of grief counseling has evolved a great deal, however, since Kubler-Ross' pioneering work in the late 1960s and early 1970s. For example, we know today that the "stages" of grief are not concrete and sequential and that each griever experiences denial, anger, bargaining, depression, and acceptance differently. Some grievers, for example, get "stuck" in one phase and rarely experience the other four.

We believe it is more useful for veterinarians to have a basic working knowledge of the normal manifestations and the normal progression of grief than to have a great deal of theoretical knowledge about the various models because veterinarians are more likely to respond to grief in its early, acute phases than in its middle or final stages. In the practice of medicine, the veterinarian first must know what "normal" is before being able to diagnose or assess grief as "abnormal."

Normal Grief

Loss and grief are two of the most common human experiences. All people experience loss and grief repeatedly during their lives. However, loss and grief are also the two normal life processes about which we probably know the least. This gap in our knowledge exists because, until recently, conversations about loss, death, and grief have been viewed as morbid, morose, and even taboo. Let us begin our examination of normal grief with a discussion of what we *do* know about it.

We know that grief is the natural and spontaneous response to loss. We also know that it is the normal way to adjust to endings and to change. Grief is the necessary process for healing the emotional wounds caused by loss. Grief is a *process*, not an event, and, because grief often begins with the anticipation of loss, we may not always realize when grieving actually begins.

The end of the grief process is as unclear as the beginning. The progression of normal grief is not limited to a specific time frame. In fact, normal grief may last for days, weeks, months, or even years, depending on the significance of the loss.

During the process of normal grieving, the level of emotional intensity ranges on a continuum from no reactions at all to thoughts of suicide. The intensity of a person's grief response is based on several factors, including the nature of the loss; the circumstances surrounding the loss; the griever's "preloss" emotional status; and the availability of emotional support before, during, and after the loss. If progressing in a healthy manner, grief lessens in intensity over time.

The grief response is unique to each individual. There is no right or wrong way to grieve. Grief also varies among groups, societies, and cultures. In most cases, the variables of age, gender, and developmental status greatly affect people's expressions of grief. For example, research has conclusively confirmed that women shed more tears and cry more often during grief than do men.[12] This is probably because men are socialized to maintain their composure during emotional times, whereas women are socially conditioned to express their feelings more openly.

Research has also confirmed that children grieve as deeply as adults. Because they have shorter attention spans, however, they grieve more sporadically. Children most often express their grief through behaviors rather than through words. They act out their grief through artwork, play behaviors, or expressions of anger and irritability (Fig. 2-5). Such acting out is due in large part to the fact that, until children reach the ages of 8 or 9 years, they do not possess the cognitive development and language capabilities necessary to express grief verbally.[13] Children and their grief responses are explored further in Chapter 12.

Clinical experience has shown that, when the expression of grief is in some way restricted, the healing time for recovery is prolonged. Similarly, when grief is freely expressed, the healing time for recovery from loss is generally greatly reduced. Veterinarians can help their clients by encouraging them to openly express their grief-related thoughts and feelings. The

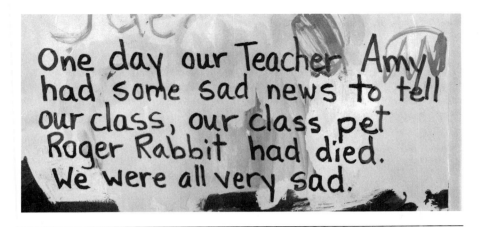

One day our Teacher Amy had some sad news to tell our class, our class pet Roger Rabbit had died. We were all very sad.

Figure 2-5 Children benefit from participating in activities that give them opportunities to express feelings of loss. They can be supported in this process by parents and teachers.

veterinarian can give clients permission to grieve by encouraging them to cry, to ask questions, to view their companion animals' bodies, and to reminisce about their pets' lives.

Permission from the veterinarian, as an authority figure, reassures them that grief over the death of a pet is not immature, overly sentimental, or crazy. As Dusty's owner said in his essay about pet loss, a veterinarian's encouragement, along with 5 minutes of grief education, can save clients months and even years of emotional pain, worry, and embarrassment after pet loss.

To provide clients with 5 minutes of education about normal grief, you must understand how normal grievers generally think, feel, and behave. As noted grief expert Murray Colin Parkes[14] suggested, "It is important for those who attempt to help the bereaved to know what is normal." Box 2-1 provides an overview of the normal manifestations of grief. Box 2-2 provides a model of grief that can aid in predicting the normal course of grief for pet owners.

Toward the natural end point of a normal grief process, many grievers find meaning in their pets' deaths. Finding meaning in death is important for many pet owners because it helps them believe that their companion animals did not die in vain. As a young, divorced woman said when writing about her pet's death:

> My dog Bubba helped me through a difficult divorce seven years
> ago. Last year, he was diagnosed with a malignant tumor and died
> one month later. The death was initially devastating for me, but later

BOX 2-1

Manifestations of Grief

Although grief responses generally differ from one person to another, many predictable manifestations of grief do exist. These manifestations occur on physical, intellectual, emotional, social, and spiritual levels. Before, during, and after loss, grief may appear in several of the following forms.

Physical

Crying, sobbing, wailing, shock and numbness, dry mouth, a lump in the throat, shortness of breath, stomachache or nausea, tightness in the chest, restlessness, fatigue, exhaustion, sleep disturbance, appetite disturbance, body aches, stiffness of joint or muscles, dizziness or fainting

Intellectual

Denial, sense of unreality, confusion, inability to concentrate, feeling preoccupied by the loss, experiencing hallucinations concerning the loss (visual, auditory, and olfactory), a need to reminisce about the loved one and to talk about the circumstances of the loss, a sense that time is passing very slowly, a desire to rationalize or intellectualize feelings about the loss, thoughts or fantasies about suicide (not accompanied by concrete plans or behaviors)

Emotional

Sadness, anger, depression, guilt, anxiety, relief, loneliness, irritability, a desire to blame others for the loss, resentment, embarrassment, self-doubt, lowered self-esteem, feelings of being overwhelmed or out of control, feelings of hopelessness and helplessness, feelings of victimization, giddiness, affect that is inappropriate for the situation (nervous smiles and laughter)

Social

Feelings of withdrawal, isolation and alienation, a greater dependency on others, a rejection of others, rejection by others, a reluctance to ask others for help, change in friends or in living arrangements, a desire to relocate or move, a need to find distractions from the intensity of grief (to say busy or to overcommit to activities)

Spiritual

Bargaining with God in an attempt to prevent loss, feeling angry at God when loss occurs, renewed or shaken religious beliefs, feelings of being either blessed or punished, searching for a meaningful interpretation of a loved one's death, paranormal visions or dreams concerning a dead loved one, questioning whether or not souls exist and wondering what happens to loved ones after death, the need to "finish business" with a purposeful ending or closure to the relationship (a funeral, memorial service, last rites ceremony, goodbye ritual)

BOX 2-2

Growth from Grief: A Model for Recovery from Pet Loss

Initial Awareness of Loss

In this early phase of grief, pet owners acknowledge that pets' deaths are imminent. Veterinarians probably see clients in this phase during emergency situations
or during the delivery of terminal diagnoses or worsening prognoses. Clients
dealing with the initial awareness of loss often show signs of shock or denial. It is
therefore important for veterinarians to remember that, during veterinarian-client
interactions, their clients' abilities to concentrate, to take in information, and to
make decisions about their pets' care may be greatly diminished.

Coping with Loss

During this phase of grief, clients experience their pets' dying processes or
deaths. Here, the dying process may refer to a period of minutes, days, weeks,
months, or even years, depending on the individual situation. Veterinarians can
effectively help clients cope with loss by answering questions, assisting with
important decisions, preparing clients for their pets' deaths or euthanasias, informing them about options regarding body care, and by continuing to support
and to validate their feelings of grief.

Saying Goodbye

Many pet owners want to say goodbye to their pets before, during, and after their
pets die. For this reason, clients should be allowed to participate in their pets'
deaths in ways that are meaningful to them. For example, clients may wish to be
present during their pets' euthanasias or to view their pets' bodies after death.

Veterinarians should give clients permission to say goodbye in their own ways
and provide them with ideas for drawing closure to their human-companion
animal relationships. Suggestions for drawing closure might include funeral ceremonies after burial or cremation, symbolic gestures like dedicating scrapbooks to
pets' memorabilia, or memorial rituals like planting trees each Memorial Day.
Veterinarians should support clients' methods of saying goodbye by encouraging
their open expressions of grief and by remaining nonjudgmental about the
choices clients make.

Painful Awareness of Loss

In this phase of grief, many pet owners realize that no way exists to avoid grief
and, thus, allow themselves to experience the full extent of their painful emotions. The numbness that accompanies shock and denial seems to lift and can
leave, among other grief manifestations, deep feelings of sadness, depression,
loneliness, and guilt. The changes and adjustments that pet owners make in their
day-to-day, companion animal-centered routines are common catalysts for the
onset of painful feelings. The phase can occur and last for days, weeks, or even
months after death, depending on the individual situation. Veterinarians can
acknowledge their client's pain by sending condolence cards, following-up with

Box 2-2 continued on following page

telephone calls, or making referrals to pet loss support groups and grief counselors, when appropriate.

Recovery from Loss

Pet owners who reach the recovery phase of grief focus their energy back into normal life activities. Often, they let go of attachments to deceased pets enough to reinvest emotionally in other companion animals. Thus, pet owners are able to have new pets in their lives without feeling disloyal to the ones who have died. For some feelings of sadness still surface at times, but happier memories again gain prominence.

Veterinarians most often encounter clients in this phase of grief when contact is re-established with new pets. During these veterinarian-client interactions, it is important for veterinarians to remember that, even though clients have new pets, they still welcome opportunities to reminisce about their pets who have died.

Personal Growth through Grief

Many pet owners who progress through normal, healthy processes of grief find meaning in their pets' deaths. They realize that their pets' deaths taught them important lessons or helped them change old, outdated habits and attitudes. Some clients are eager to relate their personal growth experiences to their veterinarians. It is important for veterinarians to listen to these clients' stories with patience and acceptance. Nonjudgmental listening often helps pet owners to finally reconcile their pets' deaths.

It should be emphasized that the phases of this model are not discrete; therefore, most grievers move back and forth among them. Models are useful only as reference guides and should not be used as prescriptions for how and when grief should proceed.

Adapted to pet loss from Schneider, J. *Stress, Loss, and Grief*. Aspen Publications, Gaithersburg, Md., 1984. Used with permission.

> I was able to accept the loss by acknowledging that it was time for me to move on. I came to believe that, through his death, Bubba was telling me that my years of "hibernation" were behind me and that it was time to get out of the house and begin to meet people again.

Meaning is sometimes harder to find when the death of a pet occurs suddenly, leaving no time to anticipate the feelings stimulated by it.

Sometimes the grief process begins before death actually occurs. At other times, it does not progress in a timely fashion or it deviates from the usual range of normal expression. Because grief is unique and encompasses a wide range of feelings and behaviors, it may be difficult for the veterinarian to determine whether or not a client's expressions of grief are normal. Thus, for the purposes of assessment, the types of grief discussed here are all considered normal, with the exception of pathological grief. Other types of grief with which veterinarians should be familiar are anticipatory, discrepant, complicated, and unresolved grief. Brief descriptions of each follow.

Anticipatory Grief

Anticipatory grief occurs before an actual death.[7] For pet owners, it begins whenever they sense that they may potentially lose their relationships with their companion animals (Figs. 2-6 and 2-7). Examples of owners who experience anticipatory grief include those with aging pets, those with pets who have been seriously injured, those with pets with chronic disease, and those whose pets are terminally ill. The symptoms of anticipatory grief include any or all of the manifestations of normal grief shown in Box 2-1.

As pets' conditions deteriorate, owners adjust to the changes that have occurred in their pets' appearances, personalities, and physical capabilities resulting from treatments or surgeries. As they adjust, many experience a sense of loss as they give up knowing their pets in the ways in which they used to know them. During this period of anticipatory grief, pet owners begin the process of saying goodbye to their pets and many, either consciously or subconsciously, become detached from their pets, investing emotional energy into other aspects of their lives. For the most part, emotional detachment is healthy and represents pet owners' attempts to prepare for their pets' deaths.

As one of our teenage clients who experienced the unexpected death of his cat wrote:

> I knew the minute the vet came into the room that Samson was going to die. Even though he lived for three more days after that, I really lost him the day he was hit by the car. He was never the same after that and it was hard for me to be around him for very long at any one time. I knew right away he was going to die and I felt just as lousy the day he got hit as I did the day I actually lost him. I miss him.

Discrepant Grief

Because each individual feels loss in a personal way, each also responds to loss in a unique way. Thus, discrepancies in people's coping styles often cause further anguish for grievers. For example, a husband who has experienced the death of his dog may regard the experience as private and feel reluctant to share his thoughts with anyone. His wife, however, may wish to express her feelings more openly and frequently. The asymmetry of the couple's grief responses therefore causes further stress and often creates discord within their relationship. Gender differences are discussed in more detail in Chapter 12.

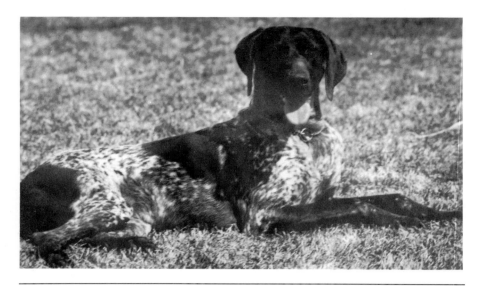

Figure 2-6 Brandy in her youth.

The discord caused by discrepant grief often arises when a spouse, friend, or family member becomes angry at another because of a perceived lack of understanding or needed support.[15] In terms of pet loss, the discord that arises from discrepant grief may have a basis in fact. It is not unusual for one family member to be highly attached to a pet whereas another may feel little attachment or even dislike the animal.

Veterinarians often find themselves in the middle of their clients' discrepant grieving styles. In these situations, it is important to ascertain whether the discord can be resolved by grief education or whether it can only be alleviated by matching the highly attached owner with a better source of emotional support.

An example typical of discrepant grief is described in this excerpt from a client letter:

> When my dog Fred died, I was devastated. However, my wife was never attached to Fred and had always wanted a cat instead. When Fred was euthanized, Wanda expressed very little grief while I cried openly for several days. Also, before Fred's death, Wanda had been adamant about spending no more than $200.00 on our dog's medical care.
>
> I reluctantly agreed to adopt a cat the day after Fred died. Now, two weeks later, Wanda interacts affectionately with the new cat and seems to have forgotten all about Fred. I, on the other hand, dislike

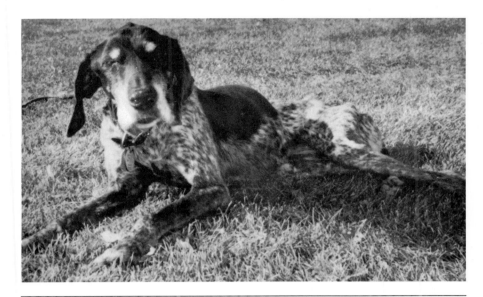

Figure 2-7 Brandy in her old age. Although anticipatory grief is often acutely felt at the time of diagnosis, it is also experienced as animals grow old.

> this cat intensely and feel tremendously guilty that I didn't spend more money on Fred's treatment. How can my own wife be so insensitive and feel so differently about Fred's death?

Complicated Grief

Sometimes the circumstances of a pet's death make grieving more difficult than usual. The fact that companion animals' deaths are often trivialized or ignored by others complicates the grief process and, ultimately, affects pet owners' abilities to fully resolve their feelings about their losses. The factors that most often contribute to the complication of grief for pet owners are listed in Box 2-3. You can probably recall cases in which several of the factors in Box 2-3 complicated grief for your clients. Ways in which to help prevent complicated grief and to assess it when it occurs are further discussed throughout the text.

Here is an example of complicated grief as described by Suzanne:

> Amos died completely unexpectedly. My husband found him dead on the living room floor the day after I left town on a business trip. He was only 13 years old; not terribly old for a cat. I expected him to be with me for much, much longer as he seemed to have been completely healthy. I didn't get to say goodbye, to tell him how much I

BOX 2-3

Factors That Can Complicate Grief

- No previous experience with significant loss, death, or grief
- Other recent losses
- A personal history involving multiple losses
- Little or no support from friends or family
- Societal norms that trivialize and negate the loss
- Insensitive comments from others about the loss
- Generally poor personal coping skills
- Feelings of guilt or responsibility for a death
- Untimely deaths like those of children, young adults, or young companion animals
- Deaths that happen suddenly, without warning
- Deaths that occur after long, lingering illnesses
- Deaths that have no known cause or that could have been prevented
- An unexplained disappearance
- Not being present at a death
- Not viewing the body after death
- Witnessing a painful or a traumatic death
- Deaths that occur in conjunction with other significant life events like birthdays, holidays, or a divorce
- After-death anniversary dates and holidays
- Stories in the media that misrepresent or cast doubt on medical treatment procedures
- Advice based on others' negative experiences with death or on inaccurate information about normal grief

---

loved him, or to be there with him when he died as he had always been there for me when I needed cheering up or someone to hug. My veterinarian understood that I still needed that chance to say goodbye, to see him one last time. She agreed to keep Amos' body frozen for me so I could see him when I returned. Her understanding of my feelings and her willingness to provide me with the opportunity to say goodbye made the difference in how I was able to cope with his death.

In addition to being so unexpected, there were other reasons why Amos' death was so hard to recover from. My mother had died about a year before Amos, in much the same way. A neighbor found her body on the living room floor. I didn't have a chance to say goodbye to her either. When Amos died, I was out of town on a two-week trip. I didn't get to see his body for two weeks after his death. I don't think I really believed he was dead until I got home and he wasn't there. Going into the house knowing he wouldn't be there was one of the hardest things I've ever done. If it hadn't been for my veterinarian who agreed to do a cosmetic necropsy and to save Amos' body so that I could take him myself to be cremated, I don't think I could have coped.

Unresolved Grief

Unresolved grief occurs when normal grief is not given free expression or when the normal grief process is arrested or blocked.[13] We believe that most people in Western society carry some remnants of unresolved grief. We also believe that the vast majority of pet owners whom we have encountered have issues of unresolved grief that underlie their responses to pet loss. These unresolved or unfinished issues are frequently restimulated while pet owners are experiencing pet loss. Thus, when pet owners express thoughts and feelings about their recent pet losses, they usually talk also about past losses. You will undoubtedly have these conversations with your clients. Therefore, it is important for you to understand unresolved grief.

Unresolved grief is manifested in various forms. Three primary forms are absence, prolongation, or distortion of grief.[7] Examples of absence or prolongation are persons who either refuse to grieve or grieve with great intensity for much longer than is either normal or healthy. Examples of distortions of grief are pet owners who make elaborate arrangements in their lives to avoid any reminders of their dead pets. These arrangements may include the use of circuitous routes when driving to avoid passing former veterinarians' clinics and the avoidance of parks, portions of their yards, or rooms in their homes because those are the places in which they spent the last days with their pets.

In terms of the frequency with which it occurs in society, unresolved grief can be considered normal. It does not, however, represent a healthy grief response.

Sometimes unresolved grief from a previous loss is reconciled as owners find the courage to grieve for their pets. The following comments from a client provide an example of how a current pet loss can affect long-standing unresolved grief:

> My mother died when I was seven and I was never allowed to cry about her when I was a child. When my dog Angel died, it was the first time in my life that I was allowed, and even encouraged, to cry. At first, it felt wrong, but, as I let it go, it felt wonderful and I felt free of something old and overwhelmingly burdensome.
>
> Angel's loss has stirred my older, still incomplete loss so much that the grief I feel has become a symbol for me. Her time is over

just as my time of holding back my feelings for my mother is over. Angel has served her purpose—letting me know that the shackles of unresolved grief are gone. Before Angel, I was afraid to receive love because I feared it would only be taken away. Now, I am not so much afraid. What she helped me do was a small step, but it was a foundational step. I will always be grateful to her.

Pathological Grief

One of the most disturbing forms of grief is called pathological grief. Although the terms "pathological" and "unresolved" are sometimes used interchangeably in the literature, we refer to pathological grief as an intense form of either complicated or unresolved grief that does not progress to resolution.

For our purposes, an assessment of pathological grief is made if the deterioration in a person's ability to function causes the onset of suicidal or homicidal threats or acts. A primary indicator of pathological grief is suicide-gesturing. Suicide gestures involve the creation of suicide plans, the gathering of the means necessary to carry through with plans, or actual suicidal attempts. *Thoughts* of suicide are normal and acceptable during grief; however, *taking action* based on those thoughts is considered pathological.

In his book *In the Company of Animals,* James Serpell[16] relates a number of examples of pathological grief occurring after the death of a pet. One of these is about a 55-year-old woman whose symptoms of listlessness, insomnia, weight loss, and anorexia dated from the death of her 14-year-old poodle 18 months earlier. We have observed several cases involving pathological grief during the years the Changes Program has been in existence. They have included several clients who were suicidal and two who were potentially homicidal. One of the homicidal cases involved the display of a gun and the other involved a threat to the life of the counselor's child. However, most veterinarians do not commonly encounter many clients who are experiencing pathological grief reactions. You may see only one or two such cases within a lifetime of medical practice. If a client exhibits symptoms of pathological grief or talks about suicide, it is important for you to be able to determine whether it is a normal manifestation of grief or a pathological grief reaction. In either case, it is important to know what, if anything, can be done. The role of the veterinarian is extremely limited when it comes to pathological grief or suicide. Because clients who express abnormal or pathological manifestations of grief are prime candidates for referrals to professional grief counselors, it is best, under most circumstances, to refer them to a qualified human service professional. Referrals to grief counselors and coping with suicidal threats are examined further in Chapters 10 and 13, respectively.

Conclusion

Advances in veterinary medicine now make it possible for many animals to live well into old age. As a result, chronic diseases and diseases of the aged such as cancer, heart disease, and kidney disease are encountered more often. As pets age, it is not unusual for them to require more and more care from their owners and from their veterinarians. Extended caregiving requires pet owners to invest significant amounts of time, energy, and money in caregiving for older pets. Similarly, it requires them to invest proportionate amounts of emotional trust in their veterinarians. When pets die, owners do not want that trust to be betrayed. They want (and deserve) at least some reassuring words and overtures of support in acknowledgment of their companion animals' deaths.

As Patsy Mich, one of our former veterinary students, wrote in an assignment for class, "As veterinary professionals, we have the choice to treat bonds, as well as bodies." We believe that the simultaneous treatment of bodies and bonds is a satisfying way to practice veterinary medicine on a day-by-day, case-by-case basis. The veterinarian's role in the simultaneous treatment of bodies and bonds is therefore the subject of the next chapter.

The following story illustrates the grief that can occur when a companion animal dies.

Death of a Friend
Stuart Heller

I lay in bed, staring into the darkness just barely lit by the green glow of the digital numbers on the clock radio. I listened to the tiny gurgles in the humidifier and the faint pings as the window panes contracted against the cold, the agonizing twenty-below-zero cold that had thundered into Colorado on the Arctic Express the week before and had set up camp in Boulder. Cold that penetrated my old dog's body, constricting his chest, knotting his belly, stiffening his hips so that he could barely walk, much less run.

How he had once loved to run, radiating joy with every bristle of his gray-black-tan, wire-haired, Schnauzer-mix coat, with every atom of his compact, 35 lb. body.

He'd run at my side, just by my left heel. Perfectly. The leash between us totally slack, nothing more than a concession to my paranoia and to the laws of Boulder County.

In 12 years we ran more than 30,000 miles. Along the mountain trails to the west of town, or the rolling country roads to the east or just the city streets. And in the spring of 1985, our longest single run together: all 26 miles, 385 yards of the Denver Marathon.

I lay in bed and thought about my dog so silent in some other part of the house. My dog, Fido. Fido. A rather silly name for an actual dog, and one that still embarrassed me from time to time. When we brought him home from the Denver Humane society in the summer of 1974 I started it as a small joke, but my son, who was five at the time, thought it was terrific, so I let it ride. A couple of weeks later, when he saw our puppy's shiny new name tag with F-I-D-O on it and not F-I-G-H-T-O as he'd expected, he didn't think it was so terrific. By then though, Fido was already Fido.

6:03 a.m. Saturday. February 4, 1989. Electronic, green blink. 6:04.

I heard a kitchen chair scrape across the linoleum and a thump. My heart lurched in my chest. Not from fear, but from pain. My heart already knew that this was Fido's last day.

Naked, I scrambled out of bed and hurried to the kitchen. Fido was on his side, breathing fast and shallow. He didn't even raise his head and look at me with that mute plea I'd seen a thousand times before whenever he was hurt or sick, and that I'd seen so much of for the last three days; now even his eyes were sick, oscillating rapidly in a desperate back-and-forth twitch. Guilt whispered that I'd already delayed his final trip to the vet too long, then slid an icy fist into my solar plexus.

Kneeling, I put my hand on his side and crooned softly. His breathing seemed to ease as the nonsense syllables freighted with love that I'd always used to talk with him poured from my lips just as the tears flowed from my eyes. His eyes, however, continued their mindless tic.

How long I stayed like that I don't know, but I suddenly realized I was beginning to shiver, so I covered Fido with an old beach towel we'd been using as a blanket and returned to the bedroom.

My wife Barbara looked at me, her eyes like fractured mirrors reflecting my breaking heart. We'd been discussing euthanasia for the past week and now I said, "It's time."

Barely able to see through my tears, I struggled into my sweats and then Barbara and I went to our dying dog. We stayed with him on the floor, weeping, comforting him, comforting each other. I held his head and chanted nonsense syllables of gentleness and support. Huddled on the floor together, we said our goodbyes over and over, and contemplated the hole opening in our lives.

At 8:00 a.m. the vet's office opened. At 8:01 I called. Heidi, the "receptionist," answered. She's actually the head and heart of Boulder Veterinary Hospital, and over the years of itches and rashes, of injections, and physicals, we'd become friends. I blurted, "Oh, Heidi, Fido's real bad. We'd . . . we'd like to bring him in . . . and put him to sleep."

Sympathy filled her voice as she said she'd "clear the decks" and to bring him right over.

Barbara drove. I carried Fido, wrapped in his colorful towel. Craig, the younger of the vets and the one I'd dealt with the most, was there. He explained the procedure and asked if we wanted to be present. We both said yes.

In the exam room we put Fido on the metal table. I held him as Craig clipped some fur from his foreleg and slipped the needle into the large vein there. As clear fluid in the syringe was injected I felt my dog's trembling body go soft. Completely soft. Completely still.

Craig listened to Fido's chest with his stethescope. "He's gone," he said. "There might still be some movement, but that's only reflex." There was a long, gentle pause as he looked at us both, then he quietly left us alone.

I put my dog on his side, straightened his legs, closed his eyes, made him comfortable. We stood over the small, quiet form, crying quietly for several minutes.

Suddenly, Fido's chest moved, his lip curled and a tiny, moaning sigh whispered through the room.

Startled, Barbara said, "What was that?"

"That was just his little spirit leaving," I heard myself say. Something deep in me knew this was no mere reflex, but was some essential transformation.

Now it was time to let go.

I bent and gently bit my dog's neck, a gesture of greeting and farewell I'd used many times before, then I turned my back on that now empty body lying peacefully on the cool, stainless steel table he'd always dreaded so much.

Over the next several weeks I cried when I came home to silence, when I awoke in the middle of the night to silence, when I got out of bed in the morning to silence. No barking. No skittering toenails on linoleum. No imperious scratching at the door. My warm tears gradually dissolved the spikey chunk of ice lodged high in my belly, until I found at its glacial core the frozen wails, the hidden agony I still felt about the death of my first dog, killed by a truck when I was 11.

I found myself, finally, crying tears that were 40 years old.

Fido would have been 15 had he seen the spring.

I loved him.

From Nexus (magazine), September/October, 1991, p. 15. Reprinted with the author's permission.

REFERENCES

1. Gage, G., and Holcomb, R.: Couples' perceptions of the stressfulness of the death of the family pet. Family Relations, *40*:103–105, 1991.
2. Hart, L.A., Hart, B.L., and Mader, B.: Humane euthanasia and companion animal death: Caring for the animal, the client, and the veterinarian. Special commentary. J. Am. Vet. Med. Assoc., *197*:1292–1299, 1990.
3. Hart, L.A., and Hart, B.L.: Grief and stress from so many animal deaths. Companion Animal Practice, *1*:20–21, 1987.
4. Harris, J.: A study of client grief responses to death or loss in a companion animal veterinary practice. *In* Katcher, A.H., and Beck, A.M., eds.: New Perspectives on Our Lives with Companion Animals. Philadelphia, University of Pennsylvania Press, 1983, pp. 370–376.
5. James, J., and Cherry, F.: The Grief Recovery Handbook. New York, Harper & Row, 1988, p. 12.

6. Hetts, S., and Lagoni, L.: The owner of the pet with cancer. *In* Couto, C.G., ed.: Vet. Clin. North Am. [Small Anim. Pract.] *20*,879–896, 1990.

7. Rando, T.A.: Grief, Dying and Death: Clinical Interventions for Caregivers. Champaign, Ill., Research Press, 1984.

8. Boss, P.: Family Stress Management. Beverly Hills, Calif., Sage Publications, 1988.

9. Lagoni, L., and Hetts, S.: Bereavement. *In* McCurnin, D.M., ed.: Clinical Textbook for Veterinary Technicians, 2nd ed. Philadelphia, W.B. Saunders Company, 1990, pp. 546–559.

10. Anonymous: Loss: An interview with University of Chicago's Froma Walsh. Psychology Today, *25*:64–94, 1992.

11. Kubler-Ross, E.: On Death and Dying. New York, Collier Books/Macmillan, 1969.

12. Frey, W. H. and Lanseth, M.: Crying: The Mystery of Tears. Minneapolis, Winston Press, 1985.

13. Cook, A.S., and Dworkin, D.S.: Helping the Bereaved: Therapeutic Interventions for Children, Adolescents, and Adults. New York, Basic Books (HarperCollins), 1992.

14. Parkes, M.: Bereavement: Studies of Grief in Adult Life. New York, International University Press, 1972.

15. Cook, A.S., and Oltjenbruns, K.A.: Dying and Grieving. New York, Holt, Rinehart and Winston, 1989.

16. Serpell, J.: In the Company of Animals. Oxford, Basil Blackwell, Ltd., 1986.

3

Responding to the Human-Animal Bond:
How Veterinarians Help Clients

After reading Chapters 1 and 2, you now have a great deal of theoretical knowledge regarding the human-animal bond, pet loss, and the grief response. You also, we suspect, have some basic questions rumbling around in your head. The first question probably is, "How do I actually apply this information to the day-to-day practice of veterinary medicine?" The second probably is, "Why *should* I?" We will address the first question in this chapter and the second question in Chapter 4.

APPLYING INFORMATION ABOUT THE HUMAN-ANIMAL BOND TO DAILY PRACTICE

Some human-animal interactions evolve into deep, mutually beneficial relationships. The strong attachments that develop as a result of these relationships often acquire qualities that resemble human-human relationships. The essence of these human-animal relationships are more easily understood through use of terms that most often identify and quantify human-human relationships. These terms include friendships, kinships, partnerships, and, on a more spiritual level, the concept of soul-mate relationships. With varying degrees of importance and intensity, the human-like relationships that develop between people and animals are significant. They form the basis of what is referred to as the human-animal bond.

BOX 3-1

A Brief Description of a Bond-Centered Practice

In a bond-centered practice, veterinary care is focused where the medical needs of animals and the emotional needs of humans coincide. This conjunction, this point of attachment, is referred to as the human-animal bond. In a bond-centered practice, the unique significance of each human-animal relationship is assessed and respectfully acknowledged.

Veterinarians understand that the levels of attachment between companion animals and their owners translate into various human behaviors, needs, and expectations, especially when the bonds are threatened by illness, injury, misbehavior, or death. This correlation often causes the medical needs of patients and the emotional needs of clients to arise concurrently. In a bond-centered practice, the needs of animal patients and human clients are addressed simultaneously. This is accomplished by providing both quality medical-based and support-based services, thus extending veterinary care beyond the medical treatment of companion animals.

The term "bond-centered veterinary practice" was developed at Colorado State University by Laurel Lagoni, M.S., Carolyn Butler, M.S., and Suzanne Hetts, Ph.D. The concept forms the basis of Changes: The Support for People and Pets Program's clinical work and is also taught within the professional veterinary curriculum.

When the stability of the human-animal bond is in jeopardy, sensitive veterinarians know they must deliver at least two kinds of care simultaneously. They must attend to the patients' medical needs and, at the same time, show compassion for their clients' emotional needs. We know from experience that veterinarians who recognize the valuable roles that animals play in their own lives most readily respect the important role of the human-animal bond in their professional lives. Thus, they are the ones who understand that, when companion animals are in need of medical attention, owners often also need care. As Jacob Antelyes said, "We have to express the sincerest kind of dual guardianship while administering the highest level of state-of-the-art medicine that we can."[1] This concurrent approach to the delivery of both medicine-based and support-based veterinary services is the basis for what we call a bond-centered practice (Box 3-1).

The establishment of a bond-centered practice conveys a message of care and understanding to clients and indicates the veterinarian's willingness to help (Box 3-2). In a bond-centered practice, help is provided directly by the veterinarian and more indirectly through several support-based services designed to extend the veterinarian's care beyond the medical treatment of animals. These services create a continuum of care (Fig. 3-1) because they provide clients with access to a variety of nonmedical support and help. Let us define the elements of a bond-centered practice more specifically.

BOX 3-2

A Description of Helping

Helping is defined as giving aid or assistance to others. It is also defined as providing others with the means toward what is needed or sought, as being of use or service to others, and as contributing to the alleviation of others' pain or difficulties. Helping takes many forms. It can range from listening informally to someone in need to providing a service from within a formalized, established agency or private counseling practice.

Helpers and clients usually enter helping relationships by mutual agreement. In effective helping relationships, helpers understand that they cannot control how clients respond to their problems. They can, however, control how their clients' responses are handled.

When helpers assist clients as they cope with loss and grief, the helping relationship guides clients toward the healthy integration of loss into their personal lives. Helpers provide emotional palliative care as they soothe and comfort clients. Ultimately, helpers assist clients in finding ways to feel enriched, rather than diminished, by their losses. When helping grievers:

It is NOT helpful to:

- Offer sympathy or cliches
- Compare one griever's loss to another
- Shift the focus of conversation to yourself
- Attempt to distract grievers by keeping them busy
- Attempt to cheer up grievers by encouraging them to take vacations, move, go shopping, etc.
- Discount grievers' thoughts and feelings
- Give advice or reinterpret grievers' beliefs
- Scold, lecture, or give pep talks
- Encourage grievers to medicate their pain
- Encourage loss replacement

It IS helpful to:

- Offer empathy and genuine feelings
- Talk and ask openly about the current loss
- Encourage the griever to talk and engage in emotional catharsis
- Encourage grievers to slow their lives down and take time to grieve
- Be there for grievers, offer to help with everyday tasks, lend support and simple companionship
- Acknowledge and validate grievers
- Listen, be silent
- Help grievers prepare, plan, and make decisions
- Offer therapeutic hugs and touches
- Encourage use of transitional objects

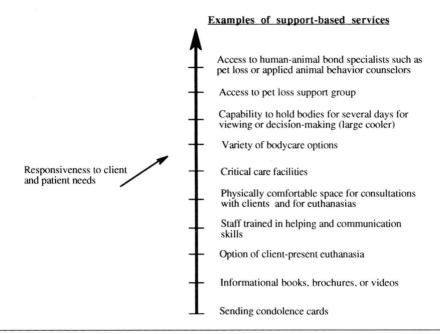

Examples of support-based services

Access to human-animal bond specialists such as pet loss or applied animal behavior counselors

Access to pet loss support group

Capability to hold bodies for several days for viewing or decision-making (large cooler)

Variety of bodycare options

Responsiveness to client and patient needs

Critical care facilities

Physically comfortable space for consultations with clients and for euthanasias

Staff trained in helping and communication skills

Option of client-present euthanasia

Informational books, brochures, or videos

Sending condolence cards

Figure 3-1 Veterinary support services continuum of care. In a veterinary practice, a correlation exists between the availability of support-based services and the level of responsiveness to both patient and client needs. This graph illustrates responsiveness in the area of grief education and support, but similar figures could be done for other areas of client care based on the human-animal bond. The service elements offered in the continuum vary from practice to practice as they are affected by time, money, and geographic location. In general, the more services that are provided, the greater the degree of responsiveness.

CLIENT CARE IN A BOND-CENTERED PRACTICE

In a bond-centered practice, veterinarians and members of the veterinary staff understand that the human-animal bond plays an important role in creating "good will" and positive client relations. The unique significance, as well as the unique needs, of each patient-client relationship are always assessed and respectfully acknowledged.

In addition, veterinarians understand that the levels of attachment between companion animals and their owners translate into various human behaviors, needs, and expectations, especially when bonds are threatened by illness, injury, misbehavior, or death. Thus, this correlation often causes the medical needs of patients and the emotional needs of clients to arise simultaneously, and, in a bond-centered practice, the veterinarian addresses these needs concurrently.

Inherent in the concurrent delivery of medical-based and support-based veterinary services is the development of a helping relationship. In a bond-centered practice, the goal of a helping relationship is to extend the veterinary practice's services beyond the medical treatment of companion animals. The techniques used to accomplish this goal range on a continuum from the use of simple, supportive communication techniques—the kind most veterinarians use everyday—to in-depth, structured counseling sessions. Typically, in-depth consultations are not offered by the veterinarian; rather, they occur in conjunction with programs that offer specialized veterinary-related services. These services are designed to help clients in the areas of pet owner education, animal-assisted activities and therapies, applied animal behavior counseling, and pet loss education and support. Although well-qualified human service professionals often facilitate one or more of these programs on behalf of a veterinarian, the veterinarian who seeks further education, training, and certification in a human-animal bond-related field can become sufficiently knowledgeable and skilled to intervene directly with clients.

The concept of a bond-centered practice is an idea we developed at Colorado State University (CSU) to help students and veterinarians understand that they can respond to the human-animal bond in relevant ways. We realize that this approach personifies the human-animal bond and implies that, when attachments are strong, the bonds between people and companion animals are tangible, observable, and measurable. This personification is intentional. Although as professionals we know that the human-animal bond is a theoretical concept and not a tangible object, we believe that, in terms of learning to create effective helping relationships with clients, the personification of "the bond" is a useful teaching tool. Our rationale for this approach is based on our personal experiences and on two lessons we have learned through direct interventions with bereaved pet owners.

The first lesson is that a vast gap exists between pet owners and veterinarians in terms of how they view human-animal relationships. Because veterinarians have some knowledge of animal behavior, they tend to interpret relationships more objectively. Because most pet owners know very little about animal behavior, their perspective tends to be more subjective and emotion-based. These relationships, viewed by pet owners to be the result of mutual care and love, have meaning and influence in pet owners' lives. For them, the human-animal bond is palpable. It is capable of being touched or felt. They anthropomorphize their pets and, therefore, anthropomorphize the bonds they share with their pets. They generally want the veterinarian to address these bonds in the same way.

The second lesson is that, during times of loss and grief, it is useless, pointless, and definitely not helpful to try to transform the client's relationship with his or her companion animal into anything other than that which the client perceives it to be. Thus, it is important for you, as a helper, to remember that, when a pet owner arrives with her dog who has been hit by a car, she doesn't want or need a philosophical discussion about why Pepper can't possibly be angry with her or blame her for the accident. What she does need is acknowledgment of the very special relationship that she shares with Pepper and reassurance that you will do your best to care for her and her "baby" during this precarious time.

In other words, during loss, clients need the veterinarian to respond to their human-animal bonds in terms of the way *they* see them, not in terms of the way the veterinarian sees them. This method of meeting clients at "their model of the world" is one of the basic tenets of helping relationships. This and other communication techniques designed to help you sensitively respond to the bond are more fully discussed in Section II.

When human-companion animal relationships are in jeopardy, pet owners present you with much more than mere animals in need of medical care. They bring you the shards of their damaged or lost relationships and ask (and expect) you to put them back together again. When repair is impossible, and when the client's loss cannot be prevented, the result of a broken human-animal bond is often immediately personified in the form of intense human grief. When you come face-to-face with grief, you also come face-to-face with human beings who are in great need of help and compassion.

This is the time when it may be necessary for you to create special opportunities to meet clients' needs. For example, you may need to help owners view their pets' bodies, be present at their pets' euthanasias, or say personal goodbyes to their pets, before, during, and after their deaths. Yet, how far should the veterinarian go toward creating these opportunities? What role do you play in your clients' grief processes? Let us further examine the veterinarian's role in pet loss and grief.

DEFINING AND LIMITING THE VETERINARIAN'S ROLE IN GRIEF

After the veterinarian has embraced the philosophy of a bond-centered practice, it is helpful to know how, when, and to what extent to use it. Although it is important to acknowledge the significance of the human-animal bond throughout the entire lifespans of animals, five situations exist in which intense emotions are most prevalent for clients: a medical emergency, the delivery of a diagnosis, the process of decision-making, the failure of treatment, and the death or euthanasia of an animal. These situations all involve loss or the threat of loss. During these times, it is vital to respond to the bonds between clients and their companion animals because these situations represent the times during which clients feel especially stressed and vulnerable.

In situations of loss, veterinarians often feel stressed and vulnerable too. When veterinarians genuinely care about patients and clients, they often find themselves struggling to balance their personal responses to their patients' deaths with their professional identities. When trust, rapport, and respect develop between veterinarians and their clients, the boundaries of their relationships are easily blurred. Because role ambiguity correlates with job tension, job satisfaction, self-esteem, and depression,[2] it is important to clearly define the veterinarian's helping role during pet loss and grief. In terms of intervening in pet loss and grief, it might be easier to define what a veterinarian's helping role is by first defining what it is not.

A veterinarian who assumes a helping role with clients during times of pet loss and grief is not:

- a psychiatrist, psychologist, social worker, or therapist,
- a member of the clergy,
- a suicide prevention counselor.

Veterinarians who are compassionate want to help their clients in any way possible. It's tempting for them to practice "armchair psychology" in attempts to "fix" or take away their clients' feelings of grief. Unfortunately, however, without advanced training in the principles of grief therapy, helping often takes the form of problem-solving, advice-giving, rationalizing, or rescuing, none of which are helpful or appropriate when dealing with another person's emotions. Effective helping techniques do exist, however, and are introduced in Section II.

Clients sometimes begin to question their religious beliefs during the grieving process. They may feel that God betrayed or abandoned them by letting their pets die. Other clients may renew their religious beliefs during pet loss. They may promise to go to church every day or to donate great sums of money to religious causes in return for their pets' recoveries. Some pet owners bargain with their God (and with their veterinarian) for their pets' lives. When pets die, despite owners' pleas to a "Higher Power," they may be consumed with guilt and feelings of failure. Without a spiritual source of strength, grieving clients may turn to their veterinarians for help. Veterinarians may attempt to help clients by trying to convince them to reaffirm their faith or by engaging them in a lengthy discourse based on their own personal religious convictions. This is not part of the veterinarian's job. In most cases, it is more helpful to grievers when others refrain from religious instruction and refer them to ministers, priests, or rabbis who are empathetic to pet loss and who know how to comfort people regarding death and the afterlife.

Occasionally, clients hint at suicide or designate the end of their pets' lives as the end of their own. Although it is very important to take these threats seriously and to ask clients outright whether or not they are considering suicide, the veterinarian's role in suicide prevention is extremely limited. As far as we know, actual suicides resulting from pet loss are rare; however, in case of suicidal threats, it is imperative for veterinarians to know what to do. For example, every veterinarian should know which local professionals to contact to report a potential or attempted suicide. Suicide resource networks (such as hotlines, emergency clinics, and therapists) should be researched with referral telephone numbers made available to everyone on staff. If veterinarians find themselves making pacts or contracts with suicidal clients (for example, "Promise to call me, day or night, if you think you're going to hurt yourself") or if they try to stop suicide attempts without police assistance, they are overly involved. Professional ethics dictate that a veterinarian must keep the boundaries between treating animals and treating humans clear. Further suggestions for dealing with suicidal clients are made in Chapter 13.

Based on our clinical experience and on what the grief literature says about effective helping before, during, and after loss, we suggest that veterinarians add four specific, helping-oriented roles to that of their previously established role of medical expert. These four additional roles are those of educator, facilitator, source of support, and resource and referral guide. Adherence to these roles enables veterinarians to teach clients about normal grief, to assist them in their processes of decision-making, to calm them during their crises, and to prepare them for the deaths or euthanasias of their companion animals. A delicate balance exists between educating (primarily talking), supporting (primarily listening), guiding (primarily suggesting), and facilitating (primarily acting). When this balance is achieved, grief is usually addressed, and helping is usually effective.

The Role of Educator

Death education is a controversial subject. Opinions range from the belief that people should be educated formally about death to the belief that learning should take place only during "teachable moments" as part of the natural progression of grief. In terms of veterinary medicine, where companion animal death is a nearly inevitable part of pet ownership, a case can be made for both forms of education. Veterinarians who recognize the impact of pet loss take steps to formally educate themselves, their staffs, and their clients about loss and grief. They make books, pamphlets, videotapes, and grief counselors available to clients, and they sponsor educational workshops, trainings, and support groups for clients and veterinary colleagues.

As educators, veterinarians also take advantage of the informal opportunities they have to teach clients about grief. Thus, they observe, ask questions, and offer information when they feel pet owners need it. The most important thing to remember about the role of educator is that educators provide information to clients when the clients themselves are ready and willing to receive it.

The Role of Support Person

Lending support to grieving clients means listening to their nonmedical concerns without taking action to solve their problems. Supporting clients also means normalizing loss, giving permission to express thoughts and emotions, and listening to their painful as well as to their pleasant memories. Listening is an overlooked skill in veterinary medicine. Veterinarians often feel they cannot be of help unless they know the "right" thing to say or the "right" thing to do. Yet, grieving people often find that it is infinitely more comforting simply to sit with someone in understanding silence than to try to carry on a conversation.

Much support is nonverbal. Veterinarians show support by holding a client's hand or by allowing their own tears to fall when they participate in or learn of a pet's death. Nonverbal support is especially important and can be communicated in several ways. These techniques are explained in Chapter 6.

The Role of Facilitator

Elisabeth Kubler-Ross has called death "the final stage of growth."[3] She advocates planning and preparing for it during healthy times so the difficult decisions surrounding it do not have to be made during emotional crises. Veterinarians spend much time facilitating death-related decisions for their clients. As facilitators, they ask questions, make suggestions, review pertinent medical information, and attempt to gain family consensus on decisions. Facilitators remain neutral, nonjudgmental, and respectful of pet owners' individual wishes. Facilitators never "take charge," but rather provide just enough structure to prevent emotions from interfering with the tasks to be accomplished. Through skillful facilitation, veterinarians can help clients face the inevitability of their pet's death and can help them prepare and plan for it. Communication techniques related to effective facilitation are described throughout Section II.

The Role of Resource and Referral Guide

Resources are qualities, assets, or supplies that can be drawn on during times of need. The people and programs offering expertise in particular areas of human-related and animal-related services certainly qualify as resources. These resources exist so that those in need can be directed or referred to them. Guiding clients toward referral resources means leading

BOX 3-3

Four Areas of the Human-Animal Bond

The human-animal bond field is comprised of four basic areas. Work in these areas involves professionals and lay people from many walks of life. Veterinarians can offer extended support-based services to clients in one or more of these areas.

- Animal-assisted activities (AAA) or animal-assisted therapy (AAT)
- Pet owner and community education
- Applied animal behavior counseling
- Pet loss education and support

or showing them the way. Guides inform clients about available resources and sometimes make recommendations about which are most appropriate for clients to contact. The general rule about making referrals is to give clients information about how to contact resources, but to let them do the "leg work." In reality, the more clients do for themselves, the more control they feel over their situations.

Extended Services

In a bond-centered practice, extended services are offered to clients in four basic human-animal bond-related areas (Box 3-3). These areas are animal-assisted activity (AAA) or animal-assisted therapy (AAT), pet owner/community education, applied animal behavior counseling, and pet loss education and support. We feel it is important to have an understanding of how you might refer clients to or become involved with each of these areas. Making a conscious decision about ways in which to get involved with human-animal bond services helps you focus additional education and training in areas of specific interest. A brief overview of each service area follows.

Animal-Assisted Activities and Therapy

The idea that interactions with animals often result in physiological, psychological, emotional, social, and spiritual benefits for humans is the basis of many innovative programs designed to help people with disabilities or special needs. These programs have a long, multicultural history.[4] For example, the early Greeks used horseback riding to raise the spirits of people who were terminally ill. Records also indicate that the ninth-century community of Gheel, Belgium, encouraged its residents to accept animals into their homes to help the handicapped people who lived with them. Medical literature from the 17th century contains occasional references to horseback riding as beneficial for gout, neurological disorders, and low morale. In the late 18th century, the York Retreat in England included animals in the facility in which mentally disturbed persons lived. About 75 years later, at Bethel in Bielefeld, Germany, animals were integral components of the community for disadvantaged and disabled persons.

In the 1940s, the American Red Cross and the Army Air Corps set up a program for recuperating patients at the Pawling New York Convalescent Hospital. The program involved encouraging patients to associate with a wide variety of animals in a farm situation. Beginning in Europe and spreading to the United States during the 1960s, numerous programs used horses as partners in the treatment and rehabilitation of persons with disabilities. Horseback riding (more commonly called hippotherapy) programs now exist all across North America.[5] These programs enable persons with a wide range of disabilities to ride horses for recreation, sport, therapy, and the simple sensation of movement (Fig. 3-2).

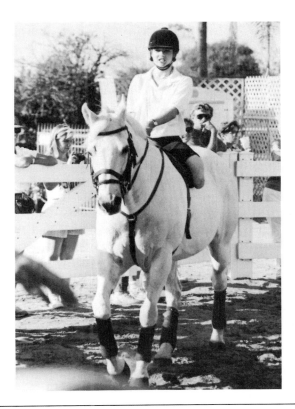

Figure 3-2 Horses provide disabled persons with physical therapy. Horseback riding as a form of rehabilitation is called hippotherapy.

Florence Nightingale, the famous nurse, wrote, "A small pet animal is often an excellent companion for the sick, for long chronic cases especially. A pet bird in a cage is sometimes the only pleasure of an invalid confined for years to the same room."[6] One hundred and twelve years later, Boris Levinson elaborated on nurse Nightingale's comments. In his pioneering book entitled *Pets and Human Development*, Levinson wrote:

> Pets are not a panacea for all the ills of society or for the pain in-
> volved in growing up and growing old. . . . However, pets are both
> an aid in that they help to fill needs which are not being met in
> other, perhaps better ways, because society makes inadequate provi-
> sion for meeting them. . . . In the meantime, animals can provide
> some relief, give much pleasure, and remind us of our origins.[7]
> (p. 7)

Today, animal-assisted activity and therapy programs abound. Some programs train and provide assistance animals for persons who are sight- or hearing-impaired. Others certify therapy animals to work in schools, hospitals, nursing homes, and shelters for battered women. A dog's eyes enable a person who is blind to see, and a horse's legs enable a person who is wheelchair-bound to walk and run. The outcomes of AAA and AAT programs are often moving and dramatic.

The result of one animal's visit to a hospitalized patient was prominently featured in the national media. In this case, an 11-year-old boy who was in a coma for 2 weeks as the result of a car accident regained consciousness after his dog Rusty jumped up onto his hospital bed. Coming out of his coma, the boy clearly said, "Bad, Rusty." Rusty's visit, it seems, provided the impetus for the boy's recovery and; within a few days, he regained many of his normal functions. Thousands of similar stories substantiate the potentially positive effects of personal experience with the human-animal bond.

The veterinarian can, in many ways, become involved in and make use of the AAA and AAT programs available in the community. For example, you could serve as a consultant to these groups, helping them find and certify therapy animals. You might also sponsor one or more organizations by supporting their efforts financially or by providing them with meeting space. You might also become an active member of such an organization. If other commitments do not allow leisure-time involvement with animal-assisted activities, you might oversee the therapy animals' health care or provide them with medical treatment at a reduced rate.

Involvement with local AAA and AAT programs benefits the veterinarian professionally in that these programs offer opportunities to gain valu- able animal-related publicity within the community. High visibility is an important practice builder for veterinarians because animal enthusiasts know other animal enthusiasts, and all are potential clients and friends to a veterinarian's practice.

Involvement also offers personal benefits. Along with creating opportunities to meet people with common interests, they create opportunities for you to know your colleagues in new and different ways. As veterinarian Guy Hancock said in his 1988 article in *DVM Newsmagazine,*

> Your staff can participate in any of these which gives you the opportunity to work side-by-side with them outside of your employer/employee relationship. Your staff's personal growth and development, not to mention your own, is enhanced by these mutual activities outside the office.[8] (p. 49)

The Delta Society offers informational packets and resource guides covering most aspects of AAA and AAT programs. They also help set the criteria and standards for certification of therapy animals. Their address is included in the resource section located at the end of this book. Contact them for further information.

Pet Owner and Community Education

Everyone in a community benefits from educational programs that concern the humane care of animals. Proper nutrition, breed selection, responsible pet ownership, and pet overpopulation are just some of the topics that must be covered in greater depth and detail with the pet-owning public. Staff and volunteers from local organizations such as humane societies often give presentations to school children, but companion animal care and welfare are seldom included in the public school curriculum (Fig. 3-3).

The rise in AAA programs has created a corresponding rise in public awareness and interest in animal-related issues. Currently, for example, even non-pet owners show an interest in learning more about the animals with whom they share the planet. In Fort Collins, The Raptor Program at CSU (Fig. 3-4), an organization that rescues, rehabilitates, and releases wild birds of prey, has one of the largest volunteer pools of any nonprofit agency in the city. The program brings in several thousand dollars in donations each year and, in turn, provides information and education about raptors to the general public. Volunteers with the program visit schools, club meetings, fairs, and shopping malls. The strong public support shown for their program is evidence of the growing interest in animal- and pet-related education.

There are many ways the veterinarian can provide animal-related education in the community, even without thousands of dollars and hundreds of volunteers with which to work. For example, you can offer Saturday semi-

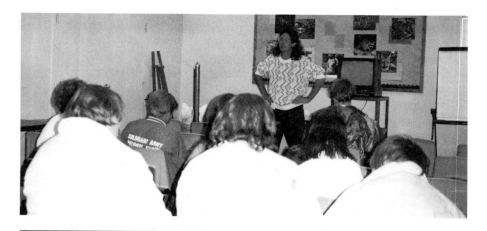

Figure 3-3 Some local humane organizations give presentations on basic pet care and fill an important role in pet owner and community education.

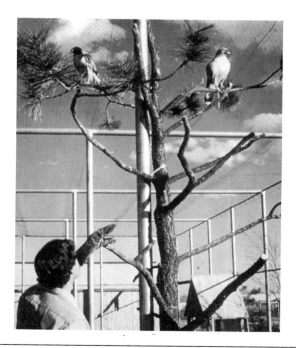

Figure 3-4 The Raptor Program volunteers educate the public about the birds they rescue, rehabilitate, and release. Birds that cannot be rehabilitated and returned to their natural habitats are used in educational settings like this one.

nars on various topics of interest to pet owners. These might include seminars on pet safety (topics could include the dangers of antifreeze, off-leash walking, or poisonous plants) or breed selection (the group could discuss which breeds of dogs make good playmates for young children or which breeds of horses offer the best fit for recreational riding). You might also offer to write a column for a local newspaper, offer to provide pet care spots to a weekly radio show, speak at community club meetings, or teach within the public or private school systems. Offering to donate health care services to local humane organizations is also an appreciated community service. Veterinarians in rural communities could get involved with the local 4-H clubs or the Extension Service programs.

Several organizations may already be in existence to assist in these educational efforts. In Fort Collins and at CSU, we have 3 such organizations. They are the Larimer Animal-People Partnership (LAPP), Human-Animal Bond in Colorado (HABIC), and the Students for Human-Animal Relationship Education (SHARE) programs. For the most part, all are staffed by volunteers. SHARE's volunteers are a cross-section of CSU's preveterinary and veterinary students. HABIC's and LAPP's are a sampling of the community's teachers, breeders, trainers, pet owners, human service and veterinary professionals. Members of these groups organize and participate in animal-assisted activity or therapy programs and in community education programs. They also encourage and appreciate interactions with veterinarians (Figs. 3-5 and 3-6).

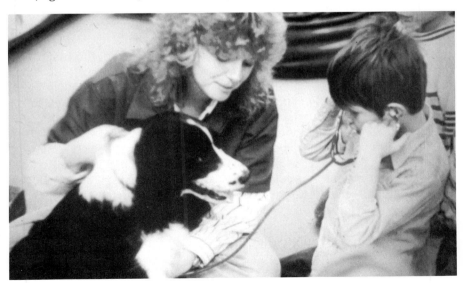

Figure 3-5 A senior veterinary student and SHARE volunteer helps an elementary school child listen to a dog's heartbeat.

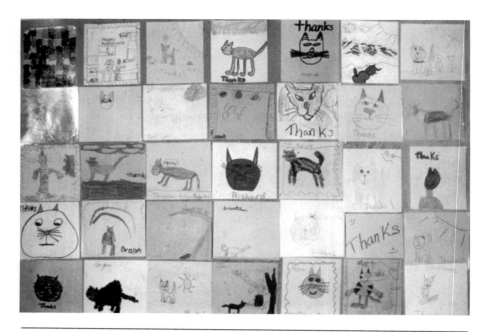

Figure 3-6 Children learn about pet care from SHARE volunteers. They often express their thanks by writing letters or drawing pictures.

The Delta Society distributes a series of lessons designed to be used with children from kindergarten through the sixth grade. This series was developed by Leo Bustad, Professor Emeritus with the Washington State University College of Veterinary Medicine, along with a group of educators with 10 years of experience in pet education. The handbook is called *Learning and Living Together: Building the Human-Animal Bond.* It is 137 pages long, includes carefully outlined methods of presentation, resources for teachers, and grade-specific lessons and information.

Owner education programs cement the relationships that veterinarians already enjoy with their loyal, dedicated clients. The benefits of involvement with pet owner and community education programs are much the same as those related to involvement with AAA or AAT programs. Through public education, veterinarians reap the additional reward of knowing that they are responsible for making useful, accurate information available to the pet-owning public. In the current era of information overload, this public service has value beyond measure.

Applied Animal Behavior Counseling

Applied animal behavior counseling is the process of working with pet owners to assist them in modifying the problem behaviors displayed by their pets. It is important to emphasize that the owners define what behaviors are problems for them. In the behavior counseling process, it is also the owners who act as agents of change in behavior modification. Most behavior problems reported represent normal behavior for animals but unacceptable behavior for owners.[9] For example, dogs who urine-mark in the house are displaying normal behavior for their species, but this behavior is classified as "problem behavior" by most owners.

The techniques used to resolve behavior problems are based on scientific knowledge of animal behavior. Veterinarians who have not received formal training in animal behavior may feel comfortable giving basic behavioral information to clients, but may best serve their clients and patients by referring problem behavior cases to behavior specialists.

The most qualified behavior specialists are either board certified veterinary behaviorists or certified applied animal behaviorists. Applied animal behaviorists are certified by the Animal Behavior Society (ABS). They have Master's degrees or Ph.D.s in animal behavior, animal psychology, or a related behavioral science. Veterinarians with post-graduate training in behavior are also eligible for certification. Certification requires 2 to 5 years of professional experience, letters of recommendation from professional peers, review and approval by the board of certification of 3 case histories, and course work in ethology and animal learning. The Veterinary Behavior College has recently received provisional approval from the AVMA and, as of this writing, standards for board certification for veterinary behaviorists are being developed. Because animal behavior counselors spend much of their time working directly with animal owners, many also have some level of training in the human service field. This experience may include course work in the areas of crisis intervention, basic helping skills, social work, or family therapy.

The process of animal behavior counseling involves determining the cause of behavior problems, recommending techniques for resolving the problems, and following up on clients' progress toward resolution. Determining the cause of the problem requires the taking of detailed histories and often direct observations of animals (Fig. 3-7). Such evaluations may require anywhere from 30 minutes to 2 hours or more, depending on the nature of the problem. History-taking and counseling sessions can take place in a client's home, in veterinary clinics, or, in some cases, over the telephone.[10] Medical problems should be evaluated first.

The success of behavior counseling depends not only on the ability to correctly diagnose problems and devise the most appropriate techniques to resolve them, but also on the ability to facilitate, encourage, and convince the members of families to implement and follow through with their programs. Veterinarians can become involved with this process on many levels. At minimum, clients can be referred to certified veterinary behaviorists or applied animal behaviorists. If a more direct involvement with pet owners' cases is desired, the veterinarian can financially subsidize the cost of

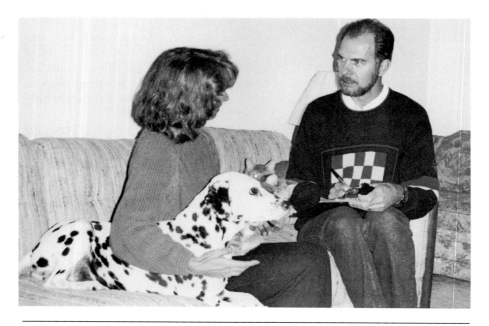

Figure 3-7 An applied animal behaviorist begins by taking a detailed history from the owner regarding the animal's problem behavior.

clients' consultations with a behaviorist by paying all or part of the counselor's fee. The veterinarian can also allow the behaviorist to meet clients at the clinic and, if experienced and trained in this field, the veterinarian can even provide such consultations.

Animal behavior counseling requires time, effort, and commitment from both behaviorists and animal owners. Because behavior problems cannot be solved in 100 words or less, they are, in fact, sometimes made worse by offering "tips" or uninformed advice. Veterinarians should not attempt to "wing it" by offering popular solutions that have no basis in theory. Even well-meaning attempts at behavior modification can backfire, causing harm to clients' pet-pet owner relationships as well as to the veterinarian's reputation and credibility. For a list of certified applied or veterinary animal behaviorists, contact the Animal Behavior Society's Board of Certification, the current president of either the Behavior College, or the American Veterinary Society of Animal Behavior. Their addresses are listed in the Resource Appendix at the back of this book.

Pet Loss Education and Support

Many veterinarians are comfortable providing their own grief support to pet owners. Sometimes, however, even the most compassionate veterinarians are either unable or unwilling to intervene further with clients. When the needs of clients exceed the capabilities or time available to veterinarians, it is good to have a pet loss counselor or support group to whom to refer.

In the last 5 to 10 years, pet loss support groups have sprung up all over the country. Many are led by human service professionals with credentials in psychology, social work, or family therapy. Others are led by lay volunteers, usually former pet owners who have themselves experienced pet loss and grief (Fig. 3-8).

Veterinarians can become involved with pet loss support groups on many levels. At minimum, you can refer your grieving clients to them. If you desire more involvement, you can sponsor a group financially by paying all or part of the counselor's fee for facilitating it. The support group can also meet at your clinic and, if you are experienced with veterinary work in this area, you can even cofacilitate a group with a therapist.

Ideally, pet loss support groups are designed to emphasize the positive aspects of grieving.[11] Many combine grief education with relatively informal counseling sessions. In general, support groups are not substitutes for grief therapy. Rather, they are safe environments wherein pet owners are able to share stories about their pets and openly express their grief. The effectiveness of any self-help or support group is derived from the willingness of people with similar experiences to come together on a regular basis to reflect on the meaning of those events with one another.

As a rule, support services target people experiencing "uncomplicated" grief processes. This means that the people attending have no significant blocks to the accomplishment of the tasks of grieving. In general, grievers

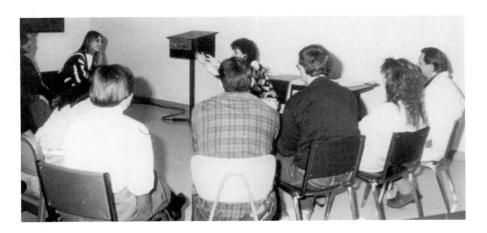

Figure 3-8 Pet loss support groups provide pet owners with opportunities to vent emotions in a safe environment. Support groups also help validate the normal grieving process.

who benefit from support groups have successfully coped with stress in the past and, although they may be experiencing some difficulty with the process, can be expected to work through the current crisis gradually, even without professional help. Group support acts as a preventative measure in that it increases the likelihood that if difficulties occur, they will be identified and addressed in some forum.

Although support services are helpful components of any referral network, complicated grieving requires the advanced interventions of grief therapy. The need for therapy means that a need exists for significant emotional and cognitive change. Complicated grief usually indicates the presence of unresolved issues, multiple or current losses, or unusual circumstances surrounding loss. Although the goal of grief support is to maintain the momentum of the grieving process, the goal of a therapeutic process is to prod grief that is "stuck" to move toward healthy resolution.[11]

The Delta Society offers a nationwide directory of pet loss counselors, therapists, and pet loss support groups (Fig. 3-9). If a group is not available in your community, you can start one yourself by teaming with competent,

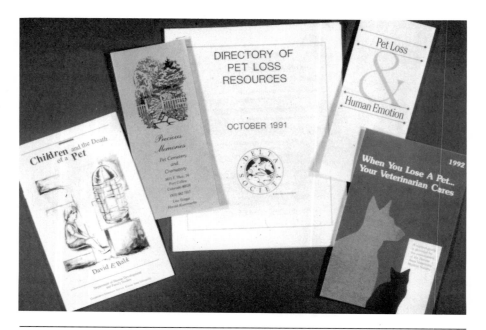

Figure 3-9 Various brochures and pamphlets are available to help pet owners during pet loss. Helping children during pet loss, locating information about cremation, the specifics of euthanasia decision-making, and making referral to support groups are some of the topics addressed in this format.

BOX 3-4

The Mission, Goals, and Objectives for Establishing a Bond-Centered Veterinary Practice

Mission

To promote an awareness of the significance of the human-animal bond and to provide concurrent medical and emotional care to animal patients and human clients, respectively.

Goals

1. To provide leadership and facilitation for the creation of services that meet the needs created by the bond itself (for example, the need for owner education, animal assistance training, animal behavior modification, or grief counseling).

2. To build and maintain a caring clientele (for example, people who value their pets and their veterinarian's skills and talents).

3. To treat your staff and yourself with the same care and respect that you give to clients (for example, plans to provide staff members and yourself with grief counseling, peer support, and methods of stress management).

Objectives

1. Demonstrate an acknowledgement of and respect for the human-animal bond.

2. Commit to delivering concurrent medical and emotional care to humans and animals.

3. Develop a philosophic foundation and method of case management based on the concept of bond-centered practice.

4. Develop a team approach to client care that can be agreed on and used by the entire veterinary staff. Train staff members in the theories and techniques useful for establishing helping relationships.

5. Create a physical structure and working environment that caters to human emotional needs as well as to the medical needs of animals.

6. Make one or more human-animal bond-related, support-based services available for clients. Learn how to assess and refer clients to them.

7. Plan protocols for helping clients during emotionally vulnerable times such as emergencies, diagnoses, unexpected deaths, treatment failures, euthanasias, and behavior problems that require immediate attention.

8. Develop the ability to work with persons of all ages (especially children) and lifestyles.

9. Create standardized procedures regarding case follow-ups.

10. Create standardized plans for individual and staff debriefings.

local human service professionals. Be sure that whomever you choose to work with holds credentials in one or more areas of advanced study related to human services. Also, be sure they are experienced in grief counseling or therapy and that they view the deaths of companion animals as significant losses. Pet loss support groups are discussed in more detail in Chapter 10.

Offering one or more of these services to clients is important because the acknowledgment of the human-animal bond and the simultaneous care of patients and clients begins long before the bonds between people and pets are broken by death. In fact, helping relationships build all through animals' lifespans as the veterinarian answers questions about puppy care and nutrition or assists owners with their animals' behavior problems. A lifespan approach to helping clients lets them know that the veterinarian can be counted on for help whenever and for whatever reason they may need it. It is far easier for clients to trust you and to allow you to help them during grief when they have already experienced your help during other, less emotional times.

When preparing a bond-centered practice, set up a referral network comprising professionals and paraprofessionals who offer services that are related, in some way, to those of the practice. These services might include (along with those already described) breeders, trainers, pet-sitters, and animal rescue groups. Together, these services comprise a human-animal bond-related network and create a continuum of care for clients and patients.

Veterinarians who believe it is in their best interests to remain detached from clients tend to, consciously or unconsciously, ignore and avoid pet owners' emotional needs. Such attitudes, however, benefit no one. Numerous, more effective alternatives to detachment exist. The concept of a bond-centered practice provides an overall framework from which to implement these alternatives (Box 3-4).

By encouraging the establishment of a bond-centered practice, we urge that attention be paid to the needs of the bond that are often the most obvious. We are, in effect, saying, "Choose *how* you want to be involved with human-companion animal relationships, but *choose* to be involved!"

CONCLUSION

In an interview with *DVM Newsmagazine*, Kathy Mitchener, a member of the Human-Animal Bond Committee of the AVMA, said, "Unless practitioners look at the human-animal bond at work in our daily lives, we're going to miss the boat. Veterinarians need to begin to visualize the human-animal bond in every relationship they see in their practice."[12]

We believe that bond-centered veterinary practices represent the future of veterinary medicine. Therefore, it is important to realize that the effec-

BOX 3-5

Evaluating the Effectiveness of a Bond-Centered Practice

To evaluate the effectiveness of a bond-centered practice, first establish baselines in the areas of profits, staff turnover, number of client complaints or lawsuits, levels of personal and staff stress, and personal satisfaction with work. Then, observe and, if possible, measure the:

1. Increase in positive feedback from clients
2. Higher rate of client retention
3. Increase in personal satisfaction with work
4. Increase in profits
5. Lowered rate of staff turnover
6. Lowered levels of personal and staff stress

In a bond-centered practice that is operating effectively, all these factors may be positively affected; however, benefits cannot necessarily be measured and do not necessarily occur in this order.

tiveness of a bond-centered practice does not lie in the simple proliferation of support-based services. Rather, it lies in the daily work of medically competent *and* emotionally supportive veterinarians (Box 3-5). Repeated interactions between clients and consistently sensitive veterinarians infuse the basic principles of care into the mainstream of veterinary medicine itself. In turn, the enriched quality of veterinarian-client relationships improves the image of veterinary medicine overall. As a contemporary practitioner, a veterinarian's willingness to learn how to help clients during times of loss will have a significant impact on the direction of future growth and development in veterinary medicine (Box 3-6).

Client Grief Support: A Clinician's Point of View

Mike Lee, Senior Veterinary Student

As part of a 1992 senior clinical rotation, Dr. Greg Ogilvie was interviewed on his views concerning the support of clients who are grief-stricken over the loss of a pet. Dr. Ogilvie has extensive experience in this matter, having been an oncology specialist at Colorado State University for many years. The following is the transcript of the interview with Dr. Ogilvie.

Mike: How often—on the average week—do you provide grief support to clients?

Dr. Ogilvie: To some degree, I provide support between 5 to 10 times per week, with around 1 to 2 "really tough cases" per week. This is with a case load of about 20 per week. When I was in private practice, I would say I provided

BOX 3-6

How to Describe a Bond-Centered Practice to Pet Owners

Clients can be informed about a bond-centered practice in many ways. One of the most effective ways is through the use of a brochure. The following statements represent an example of how to begin such a brochure.

The All-Pets Clinic is a Bond-Centered Veterinary Practice. This means that, along with paying attention to the medical needs of your companion animals, we pay attention to your needs as well. You have a relationship with your pet that is unique and special. This relationship is referred to as a human-animal bond. In a bond-centered veterinary practice, the bond you share with your companion animal is always acknowledged and respected.

Because we strive to meet the various needs created by human-animal relationships, we offer you a range of support-based services, extending our care beyond the medical treatment of animals. These services include: (You may then continue with a list and brief description of your support-based services and special practice features.)

support around 1 to 2 times a week, with an average caseload of 20 per day (of course, many more of these were of the routine kind, the type that did not require grief support).

Mike: In your experience, are there any particular scenarios that are most difficult for a client to handle?

Dr. Ogilvie: There are two situations that seem to be the most difficult for clients to handle. The first of these are the sudden, unexpected deaths. The second are ones where there is a history of tragedy in the family. In these cases, the animal's death can prove to be a "lightning rod," a floodgate for all of these past, unresolved tragedies.

Mike: Are there any situations that push your buttons, triggering any grief-connected emotions in your past?

Dr. Ogilvie: Any animals that resemble my own animals, past and present, trigger deeper emotions. Also, there is a fine line between caring and getting "hooked" with a client. You want to maintain some degree of buffer between yourself and your client, or else you can really get over-involved.

Mike: What signals from a client do you interpret as important in determining how you should handle them or their grief?

Dr. Ogilvie: A lack of willingness to recognize their grief or show signs of emotion. The people who are more open about their emotions are showing healthier signs. People who have divorced recently are really vulnerable, as often their pet represents a tie to their past. Finally, it is always difficult when parents try to protect their children.

Mike: Have you noticed any age/gender patterns in the way clients tend to act through their grief?

Dr. Ogilvie: "Yuppie" groups are more open and willing to recognize their attachment. Older people tend to seal that up more. Location is very important. For example, people from progressive, urban areas tend to be very open, sometimes to an unusual pattern; rural people—farmers, ranchers—are often embarrassed about showing grief and emotion about their pets.

Mike: Do clients often try to get you to make their tough decisions for them?

Dr. Ogilvie: All of the time.

Mike: How do you handle this?

Dr. Ogilvie: Recognize that it's difficult for them; gently "lob the ball back in their court," without being invasive. Also, it's important to allow owners to recognize that it's o.k. for them to have trouble making decisions. Finally, make sure that they use their *own* values and not worry about what the clinician thinks.

Mike: Are there any situations in which you simply cannot honor a client's wishes or requests?

Dr. Ogilvie: There are two settings. The first, which has only occurred about three times in my career, is when the quality of the animal's life is so bad, and when the owners demand continued care when the probability of restoring quality of life to the animal is small. At this point, I feel I must maintain the animal's rights. In this case, I do try and direct the client with information about the case and by exploring why they are so intent about progressing despite poor odds. Almost always, these people have underlying emotions that are not being dealt with and openly recognized. If the client refuses euthanasia, I help them find someone else who can work with them along their lines.

The second setting, which has happened once, is when the situation is very destructive to the owner. We once had an owner who sold her house, her car, and most of her possessions to fund her animal's care. The animal's case had a poor outlook, in terms of prognosis, and she was literally living in the streets and was suicidal. When we found this out, we knew we had to get help for her and for her to make a decision. I believe that you do have to recognize how powerful your opinion is to a client, and be careful of that.

Mike: Is there any program here where clinicians, students, and other workers can come to talk their feelings connected with difficult cases?

Dr. Ogilvie: Besides the Changes Program, no; that's why the program is so important. There have been times when we have had to deal with deaths, not only of patients, but of students and residents.

Mike: So then do you see the need for a special program, and do you think other clinicians would be interested in and supportive of such a program?

Dr. Ogilvie: Definitely; I also do think others would support a program. In the old days, no one besides oncology used the grief counselors. Now everybody is using them. Such a program has also had a vast teaching impact on the students. I think it really provides a positive influence on them as practitioners, aside from the medical aspect.

Mike: Well, thank you for your time, Dr. Ogilvie. Is there anything else you'd like to add?

Dr. Ogilvie: I want to point out how the Changes Program helps the sanity of the workers so much. People often wonder how even a half hour with the grief counselors can make a difference, but especially for the people in oncology week after week, just having half hour rounds each week helps so much. Just having an arena to discuss concerns is life-saving for us all.

REFERENCES

1. Antelyes, J.: Caring in veterinary practice. J. Am. Vet. Med. Assoc., *195*:904–905, 1989.
2. Kahn, R.L., Wolfe, D.M., Quinn, R.P., Snock, J.D., and Rosenthal, R.A.: Organizational Stress: Studies in Role Conflict and Ambiguity. New York, John Wiley and Sons, 1964.
3. Kubler-Ross, E.: Death: The Final Stage of Growth. Englewood Cliffs, N.J., Prentice-Hall, 1975.
4. Hines, L.M., and Bustad, L.K.: Historical perspectives on human-animal interactions. Phi Kappa Phi Journal, *66*:4–6, 1986.
5. De Pauw, K.P.: Therapeutic horseback riding in Europe and North America. *In* Anderson, R.K., Hart, B.L., and Hart, L.A., eds.: The Pet Connection. Minneapolis, CENSHARE, 1984, pp. 141–153.
6. Nightingale, F.: Notes on Nursing: What It Is, and What It Is Not. London, Harrison, 1859.
7. Levinson, B.L.: Pets and Human Development. Springfield, Ill., Charles C. Thomas, 1972.
8. Hancock, G.: Let human/animal bond help build practice and offer client support. DVM Newsmagazine, *19*:49–50, 1988.
9. Borchelt, P.L., and Voith, V.L.: Classification of animal behavior problems. *In* Voith, V.L., and Borchelt, P.L., eds.: Vet. Clin. North Am. [Small Animal Pract.], *12*:571–585, 1982.
10. Hetts, S.: Animal behavior. *In* McCurnin, D.M., ed.: Clinical Textbook for Veterinary Technicians, 2nd ed. Philadelphia, W.B. Saunders Company, 1990, pp. 560–573.
11. Cook, A.S., and Oltjenbruns, K.A.: Dying and Grieving. New York, Holt, Rinehart and Winston, 1989.
12. Anonymous: Practioners can do their part to foster human-animal bond. DVM Newsmagazine, *23*:23, 43, 1992.

4

Why Veterinarians Help Clients

Now that we have established a better understanding about how to apply human-animal bond information to the practice of veterinary medicine, let us talk about *why* you might want to apply this knowledge. Why should you—a highly educated, busy medical professional—concern yourself with the psychosocial and emotional aspects of your cases? Why should you strive to establish a bond-centered practice? Why shouldn't you limit your role to that of medical expert and let your technicians or, better yet, your clients' families and friends help them deal with pet loss and their resultant grief? As we see it, three main reasons can explain why you should actively work to build helping relationships with your clients and be personally involved with them during loss and grief:

1. Doing so benefits your clients because their needs and expectations are more consistently and sensitively met.
2. Doing so benefits you personally and benefits your practice financially, thus increasing the level of satisfaction you feel for your job.
3. Doing so is your professional and ethical responsibility.

Let us examine these points individually.

MEETING CLIENTS' NEEDS AND EXPECTATIONS

Why are you a veterinarian? The classic answer is, of course, that you love animals and have a deep concern for their health and well-being. Beyond your devotion to animals, you probably chose to become a veterinarian because you are fascinated with the field of medicine, dedicated to eradicating disease, and committed to maintaining and improving a high standard of public health.

Speaking as veterinary educators and counselors who have worked within your profession for the last 10 years, however, we suspect that you chose a career in veterinary medicine for yet another important reason: because you like and respect people and have a strong, internal need to be of service to them. The drive to serve humanity is a compelling force for many of the veterinarians we know and work with personally, although their caring and compassion are rarely discussed openly.

In medicine, caring and compassion are sometimes viewed with suspicion. It is believed that the facts regarding diagnosis, treatment, and even death are most effectively delivered when offered with objectivity and with a certain degree of detachment. When facts are offered otherwise—with concern and empathy for patients and clients—it is often thought that the veterinarian has lost perspective on his or her case.

Yet, today's clients want more than quality medical care from their veterinarians. In studies examining patient satisfaction with human medicine, patients have reported that caring is a more valuable component of their doctor-patient relationship than is curing.[1] Surveys have also shown that, along with patients' long-standing wishes for courtesy, respect, sincerity, and honesty, they also want medical professionals who acknowledge their emotions and truly listen to their concerns.[2] It has been said that physicians in human medicine interrupt their patients within the first few seconds of conversation and that physicians who don't listen to their patients commonly lose them to other doctors. We are quite certain these principles also apply to the relationships between veterinarians and their clients.

Clients want you to be a competent doctor *and* a compassionate confidante. They want to know that you are committed to helping them, that you will not abandon them, and that you will "stick it out" with them, even when the going gets rough. In short, they want to trust you.

According to marketing studies, pet owners do trust veterinarians in a special way. In fact, they most often compare the trust they place in veterinarians to the trust that they place in their childrens' pediatricians. Like the pediatrician, the veterinarian is viewed by pet owners as caring for the most vulnerable members of their families—those who cannot speak or make decisions for themselves.[3]

According to our clinical experience, pet owners also see the veterinarian as an authority figure. Therefore, although they are often quite intimidated by you, they also depend on you for guidance and emotional reassurance. Your role as a medical professional is an influential one, and this influence makes clients' expectations of you extremely high. During loss, based on how you are viewed, it is you from whom clients draw strength and you to whom they look for guidance and leadership.

When clients' feelings are not acknowledged with sincerity and respect, many become dissatisfied, disillusioned, and even angry with their veterinarians. In fact, the results of one survey showed that 68 percent of survey participants stopped going to a veterinary practice due to the indifferent attitudes of one or more of its employees.[4] Thus, a lack of compassionate care, even when it is unintentional, can prompt some grieving pet owners to take their business to other practices.

PERSONAL AND PRACTICE BENEFITS

There are two ways you are likely to benefit when you help clients. The first is the increased probability that you will retain a greater number of your clients over time and thus create a more caring clientele. The second is that you will develop a deeper feeling of satisfaction based on your work and enjoy an increase in happiness among the members of your staff. Other benefits, such as lowered stress levels and higher profit margins, are discussed in Chapter 11. For the purpose of this discussion, however, it is appropriate to elaborate on the two previously mentioned items.

Retaining Clients

If veterinarians are not prepared to deal with the deaths of companion animals, they are often caught off guard by the intensity of their clients' emotions. Similarly, when veterinarians are not prepared to deal with the various manifestations of grief, they commonly misinterpret them. Confusion, anxiety, anger, and defensiveness are often dismissed as symptoms of psychologic disorders, rather than recognized as symptoms of normal grief. When clients' feelings and behaviors are misinterpreted, they feel misunderstood. Misunderstandings lead to breakdowns in communication, and, when communication breaks down, clients often view veterinarians as insensitive, instead of caring. Regrettably, the reverse is also true, and pet owners who are in need of emotional support are viewed by veterinarians as difficult or problem clients.

Twenty years ago, a practitioner survey on the subject of problem clients was conducted.[5] The practitioners who responded to the survey described their most difficult clients as those who asked unending questions, attacked their doctors' medical competencies, demanded unreasonable telephone time, or questioned their doctors' diagnoses and treatment recommendations. Specific examples of these difficult clients were given by practitioners. These included "peculiar, nervous people," "overprotective clients who drop in without appointments," "clients who come in or call with hostility," and "nuisance clients who insist on calling four times a day or more to find out how their pets are doing."

The veterinarians surveyed had various ways of dealing with their difficult clients, ranging from charging problem clients higher than normal fees to asking clients not to come back to their practices. Whatever the methods, veterinarians' widespread rejection of difficult clients indicated that most practitioners preferred to cut off communications rather than to negotiate more positive relationships. Yet, even though rejection of clients was the norm in the survey, very few veterinarians seemed satisfied with the tactic.

In some ways, things haven't changed much during the last 20 years. Despite an extremely competitive marketplace and the rising costs of wooing business, "firing" and referring clients are still common practices in the 1990s. In fact, a survey conducted in 1990 showed that today's veterinarians continue to deal with difficult clients through methods similar to those mentioned in the 1972 survey.[6]

In an article, entitled "Difficult Clients in the Next Decade," Jacob Antelyes wrote:

> We have to develop a strategy calculated to retain, rather than relinquish, clients, even testy ones. If the arguments emphasizing improved human relations and practice satisfaction are not convincing, then the economic outlook should be more persuasive.
>
> I am positive that some difficult clients, even if correctly categorized as such, are retainable. They are therefore worth at least a moderate amount of personal investment on the part of practitioners and their staff.[7] (p. 551)

We agree with Antelyes. Many so-called "problem" clients are retainable and worth a great deal of personal investment. We believe this is true because we also believe that most of these so-called "problem" clients are actually pet owners in the midst of their struggles with grief.

As discussed in Chapter 3, loss is pervasive in our society. We all experience it, on some level, every day of our lives. Loss occurs when we perceive that we have been hurt or damaged in some way. It occurs when we change our lifestyle, argue with friends, or misplace items of importance or value. With most small losses, recovery is fairly fast and easy. With significant losses, such as the deaths of companion animals, however, recovery is often a long and arduous process.

As we pointed out in Chapter 2, grief is the normal response to loss and is a universal and spontaneous process. In some situations, the symptoms of grief begin to appear long before the actual death occurs. Anticipatory grief is often characterized by anxiety, worry, guilt, shock, confusion, and indecision. Grief is disturbing to all who are in its presence. Grief potentially distorts people's personalities, making otherwise calm persons rave

Table 4-1
Characteristics of "Problem" Clients in Terms of Grief

Characteristics	Normal Manifestations of Grief
Clients who "ask unending questions."	Disbelief, denial, confusion, shock, the inability to focus or to concentrate, fear, preoccupation with the loss, possible lack of a support system, possible anticipatory grief
Clients who "attack veterinarians' medical competencies," who "question diagnoses and treatment recommendations," who "come in or call with hostility."	Anger, blame, guilt, the lack of trust, fear, irritability, miscommunication, possible unresolved grief
Clients who "demand unreasonable telephone time," who "drop in without appointments," and who "insist on calling four times a day or more to find out how their pets are doing."	Helplessness, paranoia, alienation, loss of control, need for reassurance, feelings of isolation, a preoccupation with loss, anxiety and panic, possible lack of support system
"Peculiar, nervous people."	Anxiety, fear, sadness, depression, stress, withdrawal, restlessness, preoccupation with loss, paranoia, insecurity, fear of losing control

in anger and otherwise tough persons weep with despair. Everyone feels grief, yet, due to individual personalities, belief systems, and coping styles, everyone grieves slightly differently. The ways in which grief manifests itself, therefore, are somewhat unpredictable. Each of us expresses grief in unique and varied ways. Some of the most common manifestations of grief are present in the descriptions that the veterinarians who participated in the 1972 survey gave of difficult clients. Table 4-1 presents the characteristics of these "problem" clients again, this time in terms of grief.

We believe that by reframing pet owners' comments and behaviors into a context of the "grieving client" rather than into one of the "problem client" we can establish the foundation of the "strategy calculated to retain, rather than relinquish clients" called for in the article written by Dr. Antelyes. We also believe that, with practice, veterinarians can transform even their most challenging clients into loyal, cooperative consumers of their veterinary services.

Time spent on this endeavor is financially worthwhile. Statistics have shown that it is five times more expensive to solicit business from new clients than to maintain the loyalties of existing ones.[8] Statistics have also shown that word-of-mouth is often a powerful form of advertising. Marketing studies have shown that a satisfied client will tell an average of five other persons about you and your practice. Dissatisfied clients, on the other hand, can tell up to 11 persons,[9] and, sooner or later, one of these persons is bound to be a lawyer! Thus, treating your clients with sensitivity and respect is not only compassionate, but also pragmatic.

Satisfaction with Work

Each of us has a comfort zone, an area within which we find it easy to operate. When you push yourself past your personal comfort zone, you gain greater knowledge and develop more skill. The more knowledge and skill you possess, the more empowered and comfortable you feel while guiding your clients through times of loss. The more you challenge yourself to push the boundaries of your comfort zone, the more mastery you develop over your job. Thus, a higher comfort level and a deepening sense of mastery over grief pays off in a higher commitment to your work.

Your newfound confidence also has ramifications for the people you work with. Your comfort with grief allows the members of your staff to also feel less intimidated by death and less often caught off guard by the intensity of clients' emotions. As a team, your trust in each other deepens and the belief that "whatever happens; together, you'll be able to handle it" grows. Confidence in your abilities as a team reduces everyone's stress levels (Fig. 4-1).

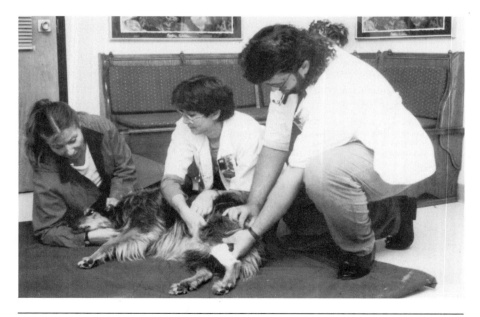

Figure 4-1 When veterinariany professionals approach difficult cases with a "teamwork" philosophy, they ensure that pets and pet owners receive full attention. Simultaneously, they also reduce their own stress levels.

Clients can sense the comfort and confidence levels that exist in veterinary practices. It is important to remember that most pet owners have little or no medical knowledge or training and thus have no criteria with which to judge the veterinarian's medical abilities. They do, however, know about communication and about how they like to see people interact. In most cases, pet owners want to take their business to veterinarians who are friendly and kind and who seem genuinely to like their work. The practice of veterinary medicine is more profitable and enjoyable when you and the members of your staff have lowered stress levels and a more loyal, caring clientele with whom to work.

A recent research study has shown that an added bonus may exist for veterinarians who are willing to help their clients during times of need. This bonus comes in the form of a phenomena known as the "helper's high." A recent study surveyed 3296 volunteers who work with patients with the acquired immunodeficiency syndrome (AIDS), homeless families, crime victims, runaway adolescents, and other human service programs.[10] Participants consistently reported feeling better physically and emotionally when they helped other people on a regular and frequent basis. The benefits reported by the volunteer helpers included increased energy levels, a reduction in symptoms of stress, a heightened sense of emotional well-being and calm, feelings of increased self-worth, and gains in such areas as happiness and optimism. Helpers also reported decreases in feelings of helplessness and depression (Box 4-1).

Apparently, emotional intensity is not required for one to benefit from the act of helping others. Participants in this study reported that they experienced "helper's high" while performing simple kindnesses like opening doors for people in need of assistance or helping children learn skills. Thus, even simple acts of helping seem to be powerful antidotes to the stresses and strains of daily life.

PROFESSIONAL AND ETHICAL RESPONSIBILITY

There are two reasons why it is your responsibility to at least minimally intervene in your clients' grief. The first is the option you have to conduct client-present euthanasias, and the second is the oath and ethical principles by which you abide that instruct you to promote the public health. Ethical issues relevant to responding to animal death, client grief, and to your level of responsibility are discussed in more depth in Chapter 14.

Euthanasia

As a medical professional with the right to end life, it is your responsibility to facilitate the deaths and euthanasias of companion animals in ways that

BOX 4-1

Tips for Achieving "Helper's High"

In a 1987 survey, Allen Luks, executive director of Big Brothers/Big Sisters, and Howard Andrews, senior research scientist at the New York State Psychiatric Institute, found a cause-effect relation between helping others and improvement of helpers' physical and psychologic health. Survey results clearly showed that, through helping, helpers not only assist others but that they also improve their own health. They suggest the following activities to maximize the health benefits of helping.

- **Make personal contact.** Meeting the person whom you are helping increases your satisfaction. It leaves a more long-lasting impression on you than a less personal task such as donating money or clothing to a nonprofit organization.
- **Help others frequently.** One of the most crucial factors in creating health benefits for yourself is the frequency of your helping. According to the survey, helpers who most frequently help others are the least likely to report health problems. The ideal frequency of helping is about 2 hours per week.
- **Help a stranger.** Survey respondents reported that they were more likely to experience helper's high when helping strangers rather than family members. This finding is attributed to the fact that, without the obligations that accompany family ties, helping becomes a choice, and you can decide for yourself whether and in what way to help.
- **Find a shared problem.** Helpers who assist others with problems that they have experienced (for example, alcoholism, cancer, poverty) are more likely to experience helper's high and to feel increased empathy for the person's struggle.
- **Work with an organization.** Helpers report that, when they feel a sense of teamwork and connection with other helpers, they are more likely to help others and to help with regularity. Helping others without such a structure appears to be more sporadic in nature.
- **Use your skills.** To experience helper's high, your abilities should be appropriate to the level of challenge, thus insuring that helping produces positive results for your client and reassures you that you have made a positive contribution.
- **Let go of results.** Health-enhancing emotions come from participating in the helping process itself, not from concentrating on producing certain outcomes or results. This philosophy of helping is also more beneficial for those who are being helped.

are beneficial for your animal patients, for your human clients, for the members of your staff, and for yourself. This responsibility requires you to become an advocate of client-choice when it comes to client-presence during euthanasias. It also requires you to attend to, rather than to avoid, your clients' grief responses during euthanasias.

Although euthanasia is often thought of as an emotional burden, it can also be thought of as a gift. We need look no further than human medicine to see the truth of this statement. Each day thousands of people suffer with incurable diseases, irreversible injuries, untreatable disabilities, and unrelenting pain. Legally and ethically, however, neither the doctors nor the patients possess the right to humanely end their lives. Thus, in most cases, friends and family members stand by, helpless to do anything to help except watch and wait for death. Many veterinarians feel that their right to bestow a peaceful, dignified death on a suffering animal is a privilege beyond value. From this perspective, therefore, timely euthanasia is more than an overwhelming responsibility—it is a noble service (Fig. 4-2).

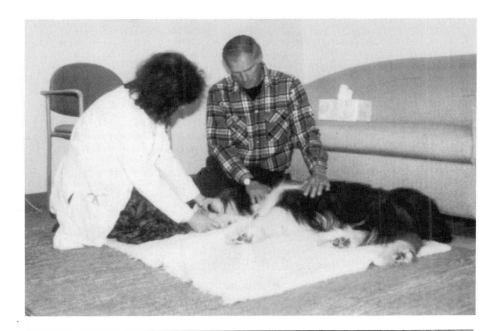

Figure 4-2 When animals must be euthanized, veterinarians cannot and should not keep pet owners from grieving their losses. Veterinarians can, however, keep pet owners from grieving for the "wrong reasons" by helping animals to die with dignity and without pain. Thus, with euthanasia, veterinarians provide a noble service to pets and to pet owners.

Yet, the option of euthanasia, particularly client-present euthanasia, puts the veterinarian squarely in the path of grief. Because you play an integral role during euthanasia, you also unavoidably play a vital role during grief. Because the deaths of companion animals are often trivialized, clients encounter people who do not believe that the deaths of animals are worthy of grief and who will ridicule them if they openly express their sadness and pain. They will expect a more sensitive response from you, and, in some cases, you will be the only one who will provide them with true comfort.

No sanctioned rituals, such as funerals or memorial services, exist to help pet owners draw closure to their companion animals' lives. Many pet owners are not allowed to take time off from their jobs when their pets die, even though the deaths of their animals are very distressing. The time they take to grieve during and immediately after their pets' deaths may be all they have, and you may be the only one with whom they can share their grief.

The Veterinarian's Oath and the Principles of Veterinary Medical Ethics

As a veterinarian, you know from experience that pet owners are emotional about their companion animals. Each day in practice, you witness open displays of love and devotion between pet owners and their pets. When medical problems arise, you also see the manifestations of clients' fears and anxieties. If you are like most veterinarians currently in practice, you may want to reach out to worried clients but may feel helpless to assuage their fears. You may also feel unsure about the kind of help you can appropriately provide for clients. When clients whom you barely know are in the midst of emotional crises, it is difficult for you to know what to say or to do that will comfort rather than offend them. This feeling of helplessness has been illustrated by research. For example, in one study, 80 percent of women and 74 percent of men reported feeling sympathetic and indicated that they would like to respond in a supportive manner when someone else cries.[11] Yet, most of these persons said that they typically don't respond because they simply don't know what to say or do.

We understand people's feelings of resistance when it comes to helping others, but we do not cater to them. We believe that it is everyone's responsibility to move beyond the feelings of awkwardness and self-consciousness and to learn how to communicate with our fellow human beings so we can truly provide them with comfort during times of crisis and loss. This is especially true for professionals such as veterinarians who, due to the circumstances of their jobs, find themselves consistently thrust into the role of helper. Thus, it is your responsibility to learn to assess and intervene in pet loss-related crises, to facilitate treatment decisions, to prepare clients for their pets' deaths and euthanasias, to normalize clients' feelings of grief, and to provide clients with short-term, direct support or referrals to pet loss counselors or other qualified human service professionals.

These interventions may sound like the functions of medical social workers but are, in fact, the interventions on which any paraprofessional helping relationship is based. Helping clients with these simple interventions is also the direction in which many experts believe veterinary medicine is heading. For example, in the 1989 report entitled Future Directions for Veterinary Medicine, the study panel for the Pew National Veterinary Education Program wrote:

> In the future, the veterinarian will play an important role in bereavement following the death of an animal companion. Veterinarians must learn to recognize and appreciate the importance of dealing effectively with client symptoms and signs of grief, anxiety, depression, and behaviors associated with the loss of a pet. They can be useful in helping a bereaved owner cope with his-[or]-her loss and by helping identify those cases in which additional professional assistance is needed. Increasingly, veterinarians, either individually or as local associations, offer pet loss support services for their clients. By sharing the client's grief, the veterinarian is less likely to find that the client avoids returning to the practice in the future. The veterinarian's role in coping with bereavement plus the growing understanding of the importance of companion animals to good mental health and well-being, suggests that veterinarians might have a place in the structured social and mental health services of the country.[12] (p. 35)

When it comes to pet loss and client grief, some veterinarians resist roles that resemble those of "counselors" or "social workers." They adamantly declare that, because veterinarians take oaths to serve animals, the medical needs of animals are their *first and only* priority. We know hundreds of other veterinarians, however, who disagree. These veterinarians have no problem with simply helping their clients on an emotional level. Most believe that both the Veterinarian's Oath (Box 4-2) and the Principles of Veterinary Medical Ethics by which they abide are human-oriented, as well as animal-oriented, because each charges veterinarians with promoting and safeguarding the public health and with contributing to the communities in which they live. They feel therefore that they are just as obligated to prioritize and attend to their clients' needs. William McCulloch, for example, commented:

> In addition to caring for animal patients, today's veterinarian is responsible, directly or indirectly, for maintaining and improving the

BOX 4-2

The Veterinarian's Oath

Being admitted to the profession of veterinary medicine,

I solemnly swear to use my scientific knowledge and skills
for the benefit of society through the protection
of animal health, the relief of animal suffering,
the conservation of livestock resources, the
promotion of public health, and the
advancement of medical knowledge.

I will practice my profession conscientiously, with dignity,
and in keeping with the principles
of veterinary medical ethics.

I accept as a lifelong obligation the continual improvement
of my professional knowledge and competence.

The Veterinarian's Oath was designed by the American Veterinary Medicine Association (AVMA) Judicial Council and adopted by the 1969 AVMA House of Delegates. From: LaFrana, J., ed. Schaumburg, Ill., AVMA Directory, 1992.

physical, mental, and emotional well-being of his or her clients. Society has only recently begun to realize that veterinarians in companion animal practice are more than "luxury" practitioners serving those who can afford pets. They are increasingly applying their veterinary skills, knowledge, and resources to the protection and improvement of human health.[13] (p. 423)

In reality, however, the argument over whose needs should take precedence in the practice of veterinary medicine is moot. Most veterinarians do not practice medicine with an exclusive focus on either animals' or clients' needs. In fact, a recent survey conducted at Tufts University asked veterinary students, among other questions, "Do you see yourself first serving clients or animals?" On a 10-point scale in which 1 represented clients and 10 represented animals, the students placed themselves, on average, at 7 on the scale.[14] Most veterinarians attempt to strike a balance between the medical care they provide for animal patients and the emotional help they give to human clients.

As a veterinarian, you take an oath to use your scientific knowledge and skills for, among other things, "the benefit of society" and the "promotion of public health." According to the terms of the oath, you also promise to accept as your "lifelong obligation" the continual improvement of your "professional knowledge and competence." You also agree to abide by the

Principles of Veterinary Medical Ethics. Within the Principles, one of the stated Guidelines for Professional Behavior states:

> Veterinarians should seek for themselves and their profession the respect of their colleagues, their clients, and the public through courteous verbal interchange, considerate treatment, professional appearances, professionally acceptable procedures, and the utilization of current professional and scientific knowledge. Veterinarians should be concerned with the affairs and welfare of their communities, including the public health.

Research has suggested that a correlation exists between social support and the quality of people's physical and mental health.[15] Thus, if people's mental and emotional well-being is included in the definition of public health, it becomes your responsibility to support your clients during grief so that the adverse affects of their losses can be minimized or prevented.

CONCLUSION

If you want to assist pet owners during their experiences with pet loss, you and the members of your staff must first examine your own beliefs about death and grief. For example, if you all believe that patient death represents failure and marks the end of your abilities to effectively intervene in cases, your own beliefs limit your abilities to be successful helpers. It is important for you to expand your thinking and to realize that, even when you can no longer do anything medically to help companion animals, you can do a great deal emotionally to help the owners of companion animals. The following unsolicited letter was written in response to the bond-centered care delivered by a CSU alumnus formerly in practice in Brainerd, Minnesota. It is a good example of how the simultaneous care of patients and clients is appreciated. It is not unusual to receive thank-you letters from clients when you are in a bond-centered practice.

> Dear Dr. Piepgras,
>
> Words cannot express how happy we are to be clients at the Lakeland Veterinary Hospital. We have always been very pleased with the staff and services provided by the clinic. However, we want you to know how delighted we are with Michael Hargrove.
>
> During the July 4th weekend, our cat Sheeba was seriously ill. Dr. Hargrove provided care above and beyond the call of duty. We are so impressed with his "bedside manner." He treated the "patient" as well as the patient's owners. His professional, yet warm, caring approach was exceptional. He is incredibly knowledgeable, compassionate, and gentle.

The Brainerd area and Lakeland Veterinary Hospital are truly fortunate to have someone of the caliber of Dr. Hargrove! Thanks again for providing top notch personal care. You are all very much appreciated.

Sincerely,

Deb and Gary Tastad

When your helping philosophies expand to include emotional support for clients, you realize that, in most cases, patient death is not the worst that can happen. Rather, the worst outcome is that the people who survive their loved ones' deaths fail to learn and to grow from their experiences, thus living lives tainted by melancholy, depression, anger, or unresolved grief.

When developing helping relationships, the question you and the members of your staff must answer is "When a companion animal's life has ended, how do you keep that event from marring the self-esteem and sense of well-being for those who are touched by the loss?" In other words, how do you facilitate your clients' expressions of normal grief so that you can minimize the chances that their grief will become complicated? The answer is simply to help, however and whenever you can.

REFERENCES

1. Peters, R.: Practical Intelligence. New York: Harper and Row, 1987, p. 96.
2. Antelyes, J.: Client hopes—client expectations. J. Am. Vet. Med. Assoc., 197:1596–1597, 1990.
3. Troutman, C.M.: The Veterinary Services Market for Companion Animals. Overland Park, Kan., Charles, Charles Research Group and the American Veterinary Medical Association, 1988.
4. Anonymous.: Good communication keeps clients coming back. DVM Management Consultants Reports, 20:1, 1989.
5. Antelyes, J.: The difficult client. DVM Management, 4:2, 1973.
6. Whitford, R.: Marketing for the 1990s [Abstract]. AVMA 127th Meeting, Convention Program, 1990, p. 140.
7. Antelyes, J.: Difficult clients in the next decade. J. Am. Vet. Med. Assoc., 198:550–552, 1991.
8. Anonymous.: The five most common reasons for unhappy clients. Marketing and Practice Strategies for Food Animal Practioners, 2:7, 1989.
9. McCurnin, D.M.: Vocal minority: Difficult clients and how to deal with them. Topics Vet. Med., 1:4–12, 1990.
10. Luks, A.: The healing power of doing good. New York, Ballantine Books, 1993.
11. Frey, W.H., and Lanseth, M.: Crying: The Mystery of Tears. Minneapolis, Winston Press, 1985.
12. Pritchard, W.R., ed.: Future Directions for Veterinary Medicine. Durham, N.C., Pew National Veterinary Education Program, 1989.

13. McCulloch, W.F.: The veterinarian's education about the human-animal bond and animal facilitated therapy. *In* Quackenbush, J., and Voith, V.L., eds. Vet. Clin. North Am. [Small Animal Pract.], *15:*423–430, 1985.
14. Proceedings, Animals in Society. Tufts University School of Veterinary Medicine. Center for Animals and Public Policy, Curriculum Workshop. New Grafton, Mass., Aug. 5–9, 1991.
15. Whittaker, J.K., and Garbarino, J.: Social Support Networks: Informal Helping in the Human Services. New York, Aldine de Gruyter, 1983.

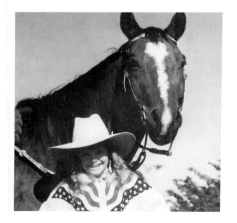

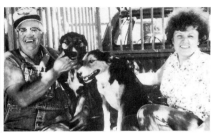

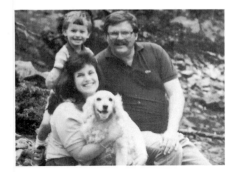

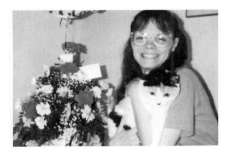

II

The Components of Effective Helping Relationships

5

A Model for Helping Based on Communication

What are the basic components of a helping relationship? What are the foundational interventions and techniques on which helping, as an effective endeavor, is based? We will explore the answers to these questions throughout the next several chapters, but let us first lay the groundwork for successful helping relationships.

Effective helping relationships are based on an attitude of respect for others and on an awareness of the limits and boundaries of personal responsibility. We all possess the knowledge and skills we need to heal our own emotional wounds and to solve our own problems. Respect for others' abilities to do so allows you to *share* the responsibility of problem solving rather than feel you are responsible for solving other peoples' problems. It is *not* helpful to rush in with your own ideas and agendas and take control of someone else's situation. Rather, it *is* helpful to facilitate the process of problem resolution by offering others guidance, structure, and honest information.

Several other tenets are basic to establishing successful helping relationships. These are listed in Box 5-1.

It is necessary, at this point, to impart a few words of caution about dealing with peoples' feelings. It is not an effective helping technique to try to take someone's feelings away in an attempt to make them "feel better." People have a right to their feelings, whether or not you believe that they are justified. The following is a case in point. Ms. Townsend is guilt-ridden for leaving the gate to her yard open because her dog left the yard and was subsequently hit by a car. Ms. Townsend was, in fact, negligent and there-

BOX 5-1

Basic Tenets of Helping Relationships

1. Helpers realize that, in general, the person seeking help is in a less powerful position than the helper. Helpers always keep this in mind when they offer their services to others. Humility and wisdom on the part of the helper is required. Helpers approach clients democratically, with respect, dignity, and nonjudgmental attitudes.

2. Helpers and clients enter into helping relationships by mutual agreement. Helpers use the client's "model of the world" as their therapeutic context and allow clients to move at their own pace and to set their own goals and agendas.

3. Helpers abide by a code of ethics. They convey information according to ethical guidelines in honest and truthful ways. They realize that censoring or withholding information under the pretext of protecting clients is unethical and, ultimately, not helpful.

4. Helpers abide by a code of confidentiality and do not repeat the details of what clients tell them unless they have verbal or written permission from the client. With the exception of situations that involve "harm to self or others," they do not discuss their clients' names or identifying information. Confidentiality also extends to colleagues.

5. Helpers are never the focus of the experience. Helpers' roles, along with the boundaries of their helping relationships, are well-defined and clearly understood by both helpers and clients. Helpers know their limits and view their jobs as the equivalent of medical triage, where the goal is to stabilize people and refer them to the proper resources.

6. Helpers are responsible *to* their clients, not *for* their clients. Helpers insure that they are physically, mentally, and emotionally present while they interact with clients but know how to detach themselves from their clients' case outcomes.

7. Helpers sincerely examine their own values, beliefs, attitudes, and experiences, especially those that relate to the persons with whom they are involved. Personal values, beliefs, attitudes, and experiences are reconciled, or if need be, set aside so as not to interfere with the development of effective helping relationships.

8. Helpers do not necessarily pursue credentials from formal, accredited counseling programs. They do, however, seek education and training from credentialed counseling professionals in subjects pertinent to the areas in which they plan to intervene.

9. Helpers seek feedback from qualified supervisors and knowledgeable peers regarding their helping styles and intervention skills. They also attend regularly scheduled case debriefing sessions during which they receive further guidance and stress management support.

fore responsible for placing the dog in danger. It would be inappropriate to minimize her role in her pet's injury by saying:

> "Don't feel bad, Ms. Townsend. Spot had a good life, and accidents happen. Next time, you'll know better."

Rather than trying to talk her out of her guilt, it is more appropriate and helpful to simply acknowledge her feelings. Compare the following statement with the previous example.

> "Ms. Townsend, I sense your tremendous feelings of guilt about Spot's injury. I know you would do anything to turn back the hands of time."

Note that this example lets the client know you have empathy for her pain, but it doesn't attempt to change or negate her feeling. It also does not sound like you are scolding her for doing something wrong.

As a veterinarian, you can acknowledge your clients' feelings and then respond further with additional facts. Here is an example:

> "Mr. Lawson, I sense that you are blaming yourself for Tuffy's condition because his water ran out while you were at work yesterday. It is a very natural reaction to take on blame when a pet suffers. In Tuffy's case, I want you to know that his condition was not triggered by temporary dehydration."

This brings up the subject of "empathy." Empathy is having an intellectual and emotional comprehension of another's condition without actually experiencing the other person's feelings. The concept of "putting yourself in someone else's shoes" applies here. Empathy is not sympathy. Sympathy is "feeling sorry for" someone. Being the recipient of someone's pity is not helpful when dealing with grief. Feeling like they are pitied by others often immobilizes people and is, therefore, counter-productive to the motivation needed for healthy grief resolution. Remember that one goal of helping is to show empathy, not sympathy, and to convey understanding, not pity.

Most helping relationships begin with empathy and understanding, as well as with an exchange of information. Relationships grow, develop, and become well-established when information is communicated in a warm, direct, clear, and honest way. Some of the techniques used to create this form of communication make use of the spoken word. Others involve using nonverbal techniques. Thus, to be an effective helper, you must also be an effective communicator. You must lay both the verbal and nonverbal foundations on which useful helping relationships are built. Let us begin to build this foundation by gaining a better understanding of the communication process itself.

UNDERSTANDING COMMUNICATION

The word *communication* comes from the Latin word *communis,* meaning "common." When you attempt to communicate with another person, you try to find common language, common experiences, and common attitudes. Your goal when communicating with others is to create a common ground.

Finding common ground is not always easy. For example, although experts[1] report that we spend 70 to 80 percent of our waking time communicating, they also say that, as listeners, we remember only 50 percent of what we have heard, read, or said. Apparently, our memories get worse rather than better, because the same experts tell us that, after 48 hours, we remember only 25 percent of the information we received initially.

What makes it so hard for us to retain information? One old saying offers this theory:[2]

> We hear only half of what is said to us, understand only half of that, believe only half of that, and remember only half of that. (p. 58)

For example, of a 1-hour lecture or program, we simply don't hear half of what is said, possibly because of daydreaming, poor listening skills, or even acoustical interference. Whatever the problem, 30 minutes of the hour are lost. Of the 30 minutes remaining in the hour, we do not understand 15 minutes' worth of that. Of the remaining 15 minutes in the hour, we lose another 7½ minutes because we don't believe half of what we do hear and understand. That leaves 7½ minutes of the original hour. Of this, we lose another 3¾ minutes because we remember only half of what we hear, understand, and believe. Therefore, there are only 3¾ minutes of productive communication during a 1-hour program. If we are only getting 3¾ minutes of value from an hour, we are probably not relating well with the important people around us.

When we are preoccupied, uncomfortable, emotional, intoxicated, medicated, or under stress, we hear, understand, believe, and remember even less than the averages stated here. Therefore, when participating in important interchanges with others, it is important to be focused, comfortable, calm, reassured, and drug- and alcohol-free. Effective communication creates an ambience of trust, friendship, intimacy, and mutual respect. Although it is not always used to its maximum advantage, communication is a powerful tool and should not be underestimated. Clear, direct, warm communication can turn almost any distressing situation around. In fact, communication may be the most important outcome determinant in any personal interchange.

Any communication process has three basic elements.[3] The first is the sender: the person who speaks or conveys the message that is intended to be sent. The second element is the message itself. This is usually an idea,

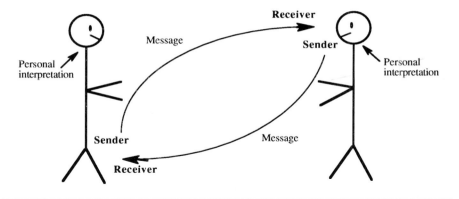

Figure 5-1 The process of communication. During communication, a feedback loop is created. The roles of receiver and sender alternate, and the message sent from one influences the message from the other.

thought, emotion, or piece of information. The third element is the receiver: the person for whom the message is intended, the listener or observer. When the three elements of sender-message-receiver are interrelating effectively, a feedback loop is created. In a feedback loop, the roles of sender and receiver alternate, and information is passed back and forth successfully.

Interpretation also plays an important role in communication.[4] Therefore, the messages received may or may not be those that are intended. Messages are interpreted by receivers who determine what meaning or significance to attach to a word, sentence, gesture, or event and how to respond to that message. Messages may also be influenced by the nature of the relationship between communicators, personal historical information, time, or environmental factors. As information is transmitted and exchanged, a communication process occurs.[5] This process occurs over time and helps individuals gather information about the environment and others around them (Fig. 5-1).

COMMUNICATION IN VETERINARY MEDICINE

Communication plays a significant role in veterinary medicine; in fact, it is impossible to practice without it. According to Cecilia Soares, DVM, MFT, and coordinator of client relations courses at the University of California-Davis, inadequate communication between veterinary professionals and clients is one of the leading causes of client dissatisfaction.[6] Supporting this claim, David McConnell, Trust Representative for the AVMA Professional

Liability Insurance Trust, reports that failure to communicate triggers a significant number of malpractice claims against veterinarians.[7] Specifically, he says, many claims are filed because of inadequate rapport between veterinarians and clients.

In another aspect of communication, Soares notes that many established veterinarians complain that new graduates are deficient in their abilities to communicate with clients.[6] Jacob Antelyes voices this same thought:

> We were and still are so forward looking, so intent on bettering our technical skills, that we have neglected to consider the importance in our work of human relations aptitudes and communications capabilities.
>
> To answer the deniers and the demurrers, I only need to point to many of the help-wanted ads in the Journal. What qualities do the 'progressive' practitioners in every state seek? They want to employ veterinarians who are 'compassionate,' 'caring,' 'client-oriented,' and 'friendly' and 'who possess communication skills.' Obviously, employers feel the need [for] (and the lack) of these qualities in contemporary veterinary medicine.[8] (p. 1534)

Clearly, a focus on communication in the professional veterinary curriculum and in day-to-day veterinary practice is needed.

HELPING MODELS

One of the primary rules governing effective communication is that the techniques used to convey a message should be constructed according to a plan or to a model.[9] The communication techniques used to establish helping relationships with others are no exception to this rule. The human services field contains many models of helping. All vary in depth, structure, and style but have commonalities in that they are goal-oriented and have a beginning, a middle, and an end.

Helping models are designed to provide clients with education, guidance, and support so that they can move toward problem resolution. They are not designed to change people's values, personalities, or basic ways of thinking. Helping models are also designed as guides for those who are doing the helping. They provide helpers with a philosophical orientation on which to base their responses. When used in medical settings, helping models also act as case management tools, providing ways for veterinarians to move clients from problem onset to problem resolution.

A helping model is an extremely useful tool for veterinarians who want to provide grief support to their clients. It is important, however, to remember that the main point of using a helping model is simply to help people cope during loss situations by returning them to their "preloss"

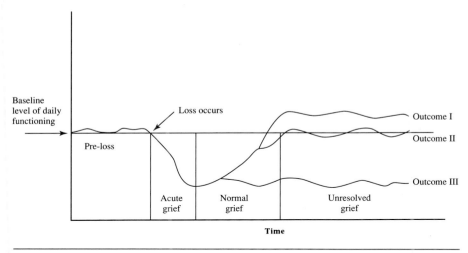

Figure 5-2 Three responses to loss. People operate daily at normal levels of functioning unique to themselves. Because losses are perceived differently by each person, the degree that the individual's normal functioning decreases during acute and normal grief is also unique. As people move through the grief process, they deal with loss with varying degrees of competency. Some grow through grief and achieve higher levels of functioning (Outcome I), some return to previous functioning levels (Outcome II), whereas others remain in unresolved grief and function below their previous normal level (Outcome III).

levels of functioning. Look at the diagram in Figure 5-2. The straight line represents a normal baseline level of functioning. When losses (like serious illness or unexpected death) arise, most clients' abilities to think, reason, and function decrease dramatically. Your goal, when helping your clients during times of grief, is to restore them to their preloss levels of functioning. If you try somehow to improve or enrich their lives by attempting to elevate their functioning beyond their baseline level (Outcome 1), you are operating in the realm of therapy. That is not your goal and you should not strive for it. In fact, attempting to achieve therapeutic results using an approach based only on a helping model would be unethical. You need much more experience, training, and knowledge of more sophisticated intervention strategies to ethically tackle the rigors of therapy.

Now you have a rudimentary idea of what is entailed by a helping model. Let us move on to a detailed explanation of an actual helping model. The helping model described is the one we use and teach at Colorado State University. It is called the TEAM model. TEAM stands for "Trust and Rapport," "Evaluation of Problems and Feelings," "Alternatives and Resources," and "Meeting Needs with a Plan of Action." This acronym has two meanings. Ideally, TEAM implies that several members

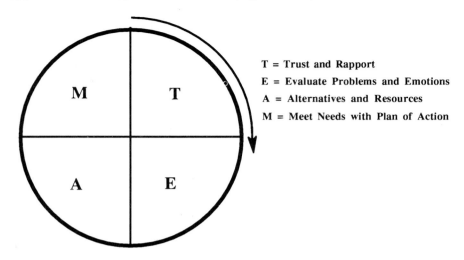

Figure 5-3 The TEAM model of a helping relationship consists of four parts. Usually, the model is implemented clockwise, in order. Although all parts on this model are represented equally, each case is individual. Parts of the TEAM model may vary from one situation to another. For example, with some clients, it will be very easy to establish trust and rapport, and more time will be spent on the other three parts of the model.

of an interdisciplinary team interact with clients when issues of pet loss and grief arise. It also implies that veterinarians and clients work as a cooperative team to implement the elements of a case-management plan.

The TEAM model is composed of four phases. These phases are labeled in Figure 5-3. The TEAM model was adapted from the one developed by the training staff of the Crisis and Information Helpline of Larimer County in Fort Collins, Colorado. This organization is a 24-hour crisis intervention service using paraprofessional volunteers who, like yourselves, have no previous counseling training or experience. These volunteers receive about 70 hours of training and, in return, handle about 24,000 client contacts, both in person and on the telephone, annually. This helping model has proven its effectiveness as it has been used by many diverse groups including medical staffs, social service receptionists, police chaplains, and human service professionals.

THE TEAM MODEL OF HELPING

Phase One: Trust and Rapport

The first phase of the TEAM model is called Trust and Rapport. Trust and rapport are the cornerstones of any helping relationship. They are essential. Without them, you cannot successfully move communication to deeper levels and engage in the other parts of a helping relationship.

Clients internalize their trust in you in many different ways. For example, some clients trust you immediately, simply because you are accredited by a state licensing board and have a diploma hanging on your wall. Others withhold their trust, despite your credentials, until you have proven your competence by successfully treating their animals. Still other clients need to feel a comfortable rapport with you before they allow themselves to trust you. By rapport, we mean that these clients want you to show a personal interest in them. They want to be assured that they are more than statistics in your busy practice. Here are some examples of what you might say to show your interest in an individual client:

> "Mary, last time you were in with Fluffy you were job-hunting. How is your search going?"

> "Mary, Fluffy has lost weight since last time I've seen her! I remember we talked at length about a special diet and the dangers of feeding her table scraps. You told me how hard it was for you to say 'no' to her begging, but you've done an excellent job following my recommendations! Congratulations!"

During times of pet loss, trust and rapport are established through the use of comforting behaviors and gentle, softly-spoken words. For example, as you look directly into Mary's eyes, you might say:

> "Mary, I can see how much Fluffy means to you. I know that, from now on, the decisions we make are based on the love you have for her. I want you to know that, no matter what happens, we'll get through this together."

You must judge, on a case-by-case basis, exactly how much effort you need to expend to establish a solid rapport and trust with each of your clients. Each situation and each client is unique. With some, establishing trust and rapport takes 5 minutes. With others, it takes 5 hours or 5 visits to your veterinary facility. Unfortunately, some clients will never be won over. If you make sincere efforts, however, their unwillingness to trust you will say more about them as individuals than about your personal communication skills.

Phase Two: Evaluation of Problems and Feelings

Phase Two of the TEAM model is Evaluation of Problems and Feelings. This phase of helping consists of getting people to describe their feelings, conveying your own understanding of their feelings, and, refraining from taking away their feelings. While engaged in this phase of the TEAM model, you focus primarily on the thoughts, feelings, and emotions related to your clients' problems.

In part, because of our social and cultural conditioning, we often concentrate on the "hows," "wheres," and "whats" of emotionally difficult situations. Think of the once popular television show "Dragnet" and its main character Sergeant Friday. His claim to fame was the way in which he asked for "Just the facts ma'am," in complete deadpan expression. It is important for you to realize that understanding the full extent of the feelings involved with problems is as important as gathering the complete facts of the situation. Most people, particularly those in the medical professions, are more comfortable, however, avoiding feelings and dealing strictly with facts.

Problem Evaluation

The term "evaluation" implies the need for assessment. In Phase Two the overall goal of assessment is to gather information about the medical needs of pets and the emotional needs of pet owners. We assume that you know how to ascertain medical problems. If not, numerous texts and instructors can help you learn to do so effectively. To assess whatever emotional problems your clients might have, you must examine several areas of each loss-related case. Many of these areas were identified in Box 1-2, Keys to Attachment, and Box 2-3, Keys to Complicated Grief. Let us go back to our example of Mary and Fluffy and examine some of the questions you might ask to assess and evaluate these areas:

1. The relationship between the pet and the pet owner:

> "Mary, how long have you had Fluffy?"
> "What do you and Fluffy usually do together?"
> "How would you describe your relationship with Fluffy?"
> "What does Fluffy mean to you?"

2. The presenting problem—especially from an emotional point of view:

> "Mary, what concerns you the most about Fluffy today?"
> "What is your greatest fear?"
> "What was your goal in coming to see me today?"
> "How is Fluffy's condition affecting your relationship with her?"

3. The pet owner's ability and willingness to cope with the situation:

> "Mary, do you have friends and family members who understand how you feel about Fluffy?"
> "Have you been through an experience like this before with any one else?"

"How do you typically care for yourself during times of loss or stress?"

4. Your own ability and willingness to cope with the situation. Ask yourself:

"Is this a problem to which I am qualified to respond?"

"Do I know of other resources that would be more appropriate for Mary to use?"

"Do I really have the time, energy, and interest it takes to follow this aspect of Mary's case through to resolution?"

When gathering information about loss and grief, you must be direct and concrete with clients, and, in turn, you must encourage them to provide you with information that is delivered in the same vein. The factual segment of assessment, therefore, involves ascertaining such things as the circumstances of a pet's death, the significance of the relationship between the client and their pet, the age and gender of the client, the strength of the client's support system, and the nature of any other current problems affecting the client's life. In certain cases, the impact of any possible secondary losses and the potential for suicide must also be assessed. Suicide assessment is discussed in Chapter 13.

As in medicine, if your assessment of a client's overall situation is too narrow in scope, your interventions will probably be ineffective. Thus, when assessing loss-related situations, it is important to evaluate as many sets of variables as possible. In addition to information-gathering, you must also use your powers of observation and collect information through nonverbal means. Thus, you must evaluate the more subtle information you receive through intuition and impressions. Evaluation based on intuition involves putting aside your intellectual screening devices to *feel* what it is like to be with a client. You must be careful about how you use this information, however, because initial feeling-based experiences are often misleading. Coping strategies used by clients during acute grief may include exaggerated feelings of emotional distress, minimized feelings of grief, or the complete suppression of normal and expected grief responses. When people are in need, they are often unattractive and hard to be around; therefore, you may feel yourself rejecting them and avoiding interactions with them. Assessments based on intuition should therefore take place over several encounters because grieving clients often soften when others pay attention to their feelings.

Evaluating Feelings

After you feel sure you have obtained the pertinent facts and made an overall assessment about the status of the case, addressing the client's feelings is always your next priority. Ask about the client's feelings. *Explore* their feelings! Notice that the word explore is emphasized. Explore means much more than simple identification. Consider this simple identification statement: "Mr. Rogers, I can see you are upset by Ollie's illness." Try to learn more about the feeling of "upset." Ask the client to tell you more about that feeling. In this scenario, you may find that in addition to "upset," Mr. Rogers feels devastated because he is plagued by guilt for not noticing his pet's cancer sooner. In addition, he is feeling persecuted because his wife is heaping all the blame for the advanced state of the disease on him. Recognition of these additional feelings gives you a clearer picture of the problem as it exists for Mr. Rogers. It also tells you that Mr. Rogers probably needs some education about the probable cause of the dog's condition and a referral to a professional in dealing with his guilt and sense of persecution. You would not have this information regarding your precise helping role if you simply accepted the feeling of "upset" at face value.

When you concentrate on discovering people's feelings, you will always find out more about their problems. It would be very difficult to tell someone your feelings without providing a context, some factual account, in which to place those feelings. On the other hand, you can easily relate a problem and omit your personal feelings regarding it. Your job, when responding to grief, is to help your clients examine and address their feelings.

Phase Three: Alternatives and Resources

Phase Three of the TEAM model focuses on an exploration of the available solutions for your clients' problems. This part of the model is called Alternatives and Resources. Exploring your clients' alternatives and available resources is basically an exercise in brainstorming. Brainstorming, in its purest form, means generating a full range of ideas without constraint. It does not attempt to eliminate any of the ideas by restricting them only to the plausible or to the mainstream. Brainstorming, at its best, is creative thinking.

The reason you need to help clients think through their alternatives is that, during grief, people's traditional support systems often fail to function normally. This may be due to the fact that the client's close friends and family members are also affected by the loss and, in the midst of their own grief, are unable to offer effective help to your client. Friends and family members, however, may not understand the significance of pet loss and, feeling unsympathetic toward the situation, may discourage and even ridicule your client.

Alternatives

Let us apply this third phase of the TEAM model to a scenario common in veterinary practice.

Imagine you have a client who has a sick cat. The cat's illness can be treated with a reasonable success rate, however, the procedure is expensive. The client is very attached to the animal but doesn't have enough money to pay for treatment. The client is beside herself with grief and in a mild state of shock. Remember, a client experiencing anticipatory grief may not think clearly, may have difficulty focusing her thoughts, and may tend to forget about her available resources.

Because veterinary medicine is your livelihood, you must resist the urge to give your services away for free. At first glance, there may appear to be only two alternatives—euthanize the cat or donate your time and effort to her medical care. At second glance, however, many more options may become apparent, and, with your help, she may be able to calm down enough to think of them.

One of your goals in Phase Three, therefore, is to help your client generate a list of options and alternatives. You need to start this list by stating the range of medical options, including euthanasia, that are available to your client. You may also need to offer a suggestion or two regarding emotional and financial alternatives to get the client headed in the right direction. Aside from the medical content pertinent to this conversation, most of the brainstorming work, however, should be done by the client. At the end of the activity, you may provide some additional ideas and ask your client to also consider them. Try to encourage your client to think of all of his or her possible options before narrowing them down to those that are truly plausible.

In actual practice, you may want to leave clients alone in a quiet room of your clinic to work on this activity. People often need time alone to collect their thoughts and to sort through their options. If the idea of time alone does not sound appealing to clients, you might encourage them to call friends or family members who might be able to assist them in their decision-making process. Thus, you can proceed with duties and not fall behind in your schedule. Coming and going, checking in periodically with clients, is an effective way to facilitate their decision-making processes. When you gently explain to clients that you have tasks to attend to and will check back with them in 10 or 15 minutes, they know what to expect from you. Providing them with paper and pen is also a helpful and considerate touch. If the situation is not an emergency, send the clients home and relieve as many time barriers as possible.

Sometimes, after brainstorming about alternatives, you may need to remind clients that it is often necessary to choose the "lesser of two evils," admitting that, although no solution is perfect, one is usually the least objectionable. Gently reminding the client of this dilemma may be helpful. Also conveying that you understand there is pain inherent in this kind of dilemma provides comfort and builds rapport.

Resources

After clients have chosen their best option or alternative, they also need to choose the resource that is most appropriate to implementing their choice. Let us talk about people and programs as resources. When we give this lecture to veterinary students, we ask them to identify the most important resource to a client. The answer we generally get is that you, the client's veterinarian, is most important. That answer is incorrect. The most important resource to the client is *the client*! No one else is more accessible or knows the situation better than the client. Wherever you go, you take yourself with you! In diagram form (Fig. 5-4), the client is at the center of concentric rings, illustrating the gradations in the availability of resources.

The next resource from which a client can draw for support is *family and friends.* These persons are the next most important and appropriate sources of help for clients because they are generally available night and day, during crises, and are usually personally committed to both the client's and the patient's well-being.

The next resource consists of *professionals who are personally known to the client.* These include, among others, a client's therapist, doctor, or religious leader. As the client's veterinarian, you most often fit into this category.

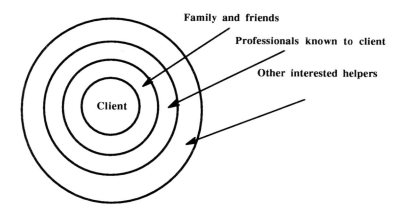

Figure 5-4 A resource model. The most important resource to the client during times of crisis, grief, and loss is the client. Veterinarians are examples of professionals who are known to clients, whereas pet loss support groups may be offered by other interested helpers.

Along with the aforementioned professionals, you have chosen a career that makes you a resource to be considered as part of the resolution to a pet loss-related problem. Although you and most other professionals are not available 24 hours a day, you do, in many cases, have pre-existing relationships with your clients.

The final group of resources is *professionals and other people trained in establishing helping relationships.* Examples include members of pet loss support groups, human service agencies, church groups, and other animal-oriented organizations. Most often these persons have no prior knowledge of the client and are usually only available during specific times. Each category of available resources is useful in its own way. It may be helpful to encourage your clients to identify and use at least one resource at each level.

As a veterinarian helping clients in need, you can guide clients to look at "people" resources that they can enlist for aid and support. You may want to be prepared to make referrals to local support groups or to therapists who are sensitive to human-animal bond issues. As we said in Chapter 3, the general rule about making referrals is to give clients information about how to contact resources, but to let them do the "leg work." In reality, the more clients do for themselves, the more control they feel over their situations. It is important to remember that you are most often a third-level resource, and as such, it is your job to help your client identify more appropriate long-term resources. It is ill-advised for you to become your client's main or sole source of emotional support. Maintaining that type of relationship with every client is impractical because it is time-consuming, emotionally draining, and detracts from your primary medical function.

Phase Four: Meeting Needs with a Plan of Action

Finally, we come to the last stage of the TEAM model. Phase Four calls for action. As its name indicates, this phase involves the integration of information from all the previous parts of the model and setting a course dedicated to problem resolution. Remember that Meeting Needs was drawn as the smallest piece of the TEAM model pie. If you have moved through all the preceding steps, taking action in order to meet clients' needs takes relatively little time and energy. After you have established trust and rapport, come to fully understand the problem and the feelings that accompany it, and assisted clients in examining their alternatives and resources, the way for clients to meet their needs often becomes apparent. In most cases, it falls into place with very little effort on your part.

We have said this before, but it is so important that we are going to say it again: Actual plans regarding how clients will best get their needs met *must* come from the clients themselves. You may believe that you know the right path for your clients to take or that you have the perfect solutions for their problems; however, it is vital for clients to generate and adopt their own plans to ensure their success. For several reasons, it is best for clients to devise their own action plans. First, clients will have more invested in the outcome if theirs is a personal plan. Second, if their plans fail, they cannot blame the veterinarian. And third, although you may think you know what is best in any given situation, *no one knows what is best for the client except the client*! Remember, you are a member of the team, and, unless it is morally, ethically, or professionally impossible, you must support the decisions of your clients.

CAUTIONS ON USING THE TEAM MODEL

Now you know the basics of the TEAM model. When you use it, be careful that you do not go through the phases checking them off as you would the items on a grocery list. Moving through the phases of the TEAM model is not exactly a linear process. Although you generally start at Phase One and proceed through to Phase Four, it is often necessary to backtrack and expend some time and energy on previous phases.

In general, as was depicted by the TEAM model diagram, you proceed through the phases in a clockwise fashion. In some instances, however, the model is used out of sequence. One example is during an emergency in which the client enters your reception area with a seriously injured animal that requires immediate medical attention. It would be impractical, as well as unethical, to start building rapport with this client before attending to the pressing medical needs of the pet. As a veterinarian, you need to quickly assess the health of the animal and determine an appropriate course of medical treatment. You may have to leap to Phase Four, Meeting Needs with a Plan of Action, without discussion of alternatives or resources. However, after the pet has been examined, stabilized, or after it has died, it is time to attend to the client. At this point, you start back at Phase One and work through the other phases of the TEAM model.

By way of another example, let us imagine that a veterinarian has said something that has unintentionally offended a client. After making the statement, he or she intuitively feels the client bristle and become more distant and guarded. A defensive client attitude is incompatible with developing a successful helping relationship. It is then the veterinarian's responsibility to take a quick step back to Phase One, Trust and Rapport, and attempt to heal the bruised relationship. The doctor might say something like:

> "I am aware that my last statement offended you. It certainly was not my intention. Let me try again to better explain myself."

By making this type of statement, the veterinarian acknowledges the client's feelings during the interaction and makes obvious attempts to repair the breach in their rapport. After the rough spot has been successfully addressed, the doctor can continue with the other parts of the TEAM model.

Another example of needing to return to previous phases of the model is evident when a client is working on an action plan and suddenly remembers another resource. For a short time, you return to Phase Three to examine this additional information, determine whether the resource is a good one, and then continue with the development of the plan.

As a final caution, do not think that you are finished helping a client simply because you have gone through the TEAM model once. Loss involves a complex set of circumstances, often with several intertwining problems. In cases where more than one problem exists, it is recommended to look at each problem separately and not to lump them together in a mass of confusion. In this case, establish problem priorities based on patient and client needs, and start there. You may need to apply the TEAM model method of intervention two or three times during a single grief-laden encounter to address each component problem.

We have described the mechanics of the TEAM model in a nutshell. Using the model need not require a large amount of your time. In fact, using these tools to deal effectively with grieving clients may actually reduce the amount of time you spend on cases. When clients feel you are attentive and caring, they are more likely to feel that you served them to the best of your ability. They also realize that you helped put them back in charge, find their own answers to problems, and mobilize their own resources. All these factors help combat the out-of-control feelings that are characteristic when clients experience pet loss.

IMPLEMENTING THE TEAM MODEL

Developing helping relationships does not end with learning to use the TEAM model. You must also prepare yourself to deal with the rigors of facing loss on a daily basis, and you must train your staff so that they can effectively support you in your helping efforts. Creating a team approach to helping clients takes more of your time at first, but it saves you time in the long-run. It also tells pet owners that not only you, but all the members of your staff, are serious about acknowledging the human-animal bond and are available to help when the bond is threatened.

Preparing Yourself

With or without the assistance of the TEAM model, before you can help others during grief it is necessary for you to develop an awareness of yourself and of your own loss-related issues. Your personal experiences with grief, and the person you have become due to your experiences, affect the ways in which you interact with clients. Discussions of death are often highly emotional because they are likely to touch on your own feelings about previous losses, as well as stimulate fear about your own mortality and the potential deaths of your own loved ones. If you are not aware of your own reactions to this subject, your efforts to help clients are often seriously compromised. For example, open displays of grief might intimidate you, and you may discourage client-present euthanasias based on your own reactions to intense emotion.

An awareness of your own fears and anxieties about discussions of death, as well as an awareness of your personal skills and strengths, often have positive effects on your emotional work with clients. Awareness allows you to feel fear, doubt, and apprehension but to intervene anyway. When helping someone through a hard time, the courage you muster and the risks you take often make a significant difference in someone's experience with loss and grief. Personal preparation and ways to manage loss-related stress are discussed in Chapter 11.

Preparing Your Staff

Along with your own awareness, it is important for your staff to develop an awareness of how they, as members of your helping team, interact with clients during their experiences with pet loss and client grief. Just as it is important for you to understand where your responses originate, it is important for them to understand their own personal influences as well.

As with your clients, you can educate, facilitate, and support staff members through their experiences with patient loss and client grief. You can do so by ensuring that they are as well-trained as you are in the topics of human-animal bond, grief, helping relationships, the TEAM model, and effective communication techniques (Fig. 5-5). Efficient teams operate from a shared philosophy and function according to well-defined, individualized roles that are agreed on and understood by everyone. It is your responsibility to let your staff members know what role you envision for each of them and exactly how you want their roles to be implemented.

Working as a team promotes professional growth and development. When two or more professionals participate in emotional interactions, deeper and more refined perspectives of the situations can be gained. A team approach to helping provides veterinary professionals with opportunities to review their words and behaviors with colleagues who witnessed their interactions with clients. Direct observation of each other's skills allows staff members to make suggestions for improvement and to offer reassurance and support to one another. It also allows them to exchange pertinent information about their cases. For example, it is not unusual for

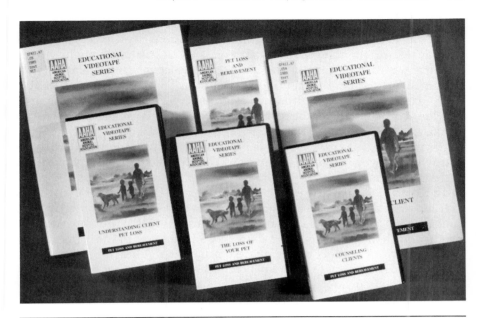

Figure 5-5 The American Animal Hospital Association (AAHA) offers a videotaped educational series on pet loss, grief, and staff communication.

clients to talk more openly about their problems and feelings with receptionists or technicians. In general, clients feel staff members are more approachable than veterinarians and, therefore, are not as intimidated by them. They also feel staff members may have more time to listen than do veterinarians.

It is important, then, for all who are involved with a case to create an opportunity to discuss it. These opportunities are often called debriefing sessions. Debriefing sessions are geared toward staying abreast of ongoing case assessments and evolving treatment plans. They are also designed to help you and your staff gain perspective on emotional cases. Debriefing sessions are most effective when they are held as soon after actual interactions with clients and patients as is possible. They are also most helpful when all of the key players are present for the discussion. These meetings enable everyone to gain from each other's experiences as feelings about clients and patients are shared and effective, as well as ineffective, helping techniques are discussed and evaluated. Debriefing sessions are further reviewed in Chapter 11.

Knowing how, when, and whose responsibility it is to respond to situations involving pet loss and grief helps to change potentially negative experiences with companion animal death into comforting and meaningful ones both for pet owners and for veterinary professionals. A team approach to helping allows veterinarians, technicians, and receptionists to play an important role in client support and in case facilitation. As an employer, it is important to use your team effectively by capitalizing on each member's strengths and interests and by allowing them to grow and to develop professionally. It is also important, however, to guard against overburdening team members, particularly when it comes to dealing with pet loss.

For example, you may have a technician who is very good with people and who is always willing to step in to comfort them or even to perform euthanasia. It is not fair, however, for you and the rest of your staff to label him or her as "the pet loss person." As you have learned, experiences with loss and grief build on one another and can become overwhelming for even well-trained professionals. Therefore, cases involving euthanasia, pet death, and client grief should be shared by all members of the team. If each member of your team is well-prepared to handle pet loss and client grief, your practice will benefit with lowered stress levels; higher commitments to veterinary medicine; and grateful, loyal clients.

CONCLUSION

In *Veterinary Economics,* Cecelia Soares says:

> Every veterinarian should learn how to facilitate the healthy resolution of loss. It is critical in the contemporary practice that veterinarians know how to communicate effectively with clients who have had a loss, and how to assess when a client may be self-destructive or suicidal in his or her grief reaction.[10] (p. 65)

To communicate effectively with clients, especially during times of high anxiety and intense grief, you need to have the proper tools available to you. You would not begin surgery without knowledge of anatomy and access to proper instruments and equipment. Similarly, you should not begin to help clients without knowledge of a helping model and access to proper communication techniques. The next two chapters provide you with knowledge of these techniques.

REFERENCES

1. Steil, L.K., Summerfield, J., and deMare, G.: Listening, It Can Change Your Life: A Handbook for Scientists and Engineers. New York, McGraw-Hill Book Company, 1983.
2. McLaughlin, M.: The Complete Neurotic's Notebook. Seacaucus, N.J., Castle Books, 1981.
3. Schramm, W.: How communication works. *In* Schramm, W., ed.: The Process and Effects of Mass Communication. Urbana, Ill., University of Illinois Press, 1954, pp. 3–4.

4. Berlo, D.K.: The Process of Communication: An Introduction to Theory 〈Practice. New York, Holt, 1960.
5. Watzlawick, P., Beavin, J.H., and Jackson, D.D.: Pragmatics of Human Com A Study of Interactional Patterns, Pathologies and Paradoxes. New York, N〈cation: 1967.
6. Soares, C., Mader, B., and Carmack, B.: Effective responses to the stress of ath. [Abstract]. *In* the Proceedings of the Delta Society Annual Conference, Parsip〈.J., 1989, p. 2.
7. Anonymous.: Communicate to avoid malpractice claims. AVMA Trust Repo ?, 1991.
8. Antelyes, J.: On being compassionate. J. Am. Vet. Med. Assoc., *190*:1534–153t
9. Egan, G.: The Skilled Helper: A Model for Systematic Helping and Interperso tions. Monterey, Calif., Brooks/Cole Publishers, 1975.
10. McQueen, I.: Take an active role in relieving client's grief. Vet. Econ., *30*:64–67,

ʃ

ɔal Communication

ective to encourage grievers either to replace or to rationalize
; yet, most people do exactly that. They offer advice, clichés,
:tualizations because no one has taught them how to do any-
effective or supportive. No one has taught them how best to
grief that naturally and spontaneously occurs in response to

experience has shown that loss itself is not damaging to a per-
:steem and sense of well-being. Rather, it is the way loss is
y grievers themselves and by others as helpers, that really does
e (Lagoni, L., and Butler, C., unpublished data). Unfortunately,
i our collective lack of knowledge and training in the area of grief,
s are usually mishandled. Ignorance and incompetence keep grief
s from proceeding in normal, healthy ways.
ıe vast body of knowledge about loss and grief is transferrable, and
ny techniques that are effective when helping one another with grief
ıchable. This revelation is exciting because it tells us that the more we
about loss and the more skillful we become in responding to it, the
ɔ we can counteract the feelings of powerlessness that occur during
f. It tells us that, by simply gaining knowledge and skill in the areas of
ɔf education, facilitation, and support, we can dispel feelings of awk-
ırdness and helplessness.
We have already provided a basis for understanding loss, grief, and the
asic principles of helping. Together, knowledge and skill are empower-
ıng. They give us confidence and a higher tolerance for emotional pain.
They help people maintain a higher comfort level when discussing, responding to, or even experiencing loss, death, and feelings of grief. Feeling

118

comfortable and confident in the face of grief is the key to handling it. It is therefore important to become familiar, not only with the facts, but also with the numerous communication techniques pertinent to helping others deal with loss and grief.

In Chapter 5 we introduced you to the TEAM model. This model can be thought of as a recipe for helping. In this chapter and the next we provide you with information regarding the ingredients of that recipe. These ingredients are the verbal and nonverbal communication techniques that help you attend to the emotional needs of clients.

Both verbal and nonverbal communication techniques are adaptable to any communication exchange. They are especially useful, however, during times of loss when the grief response pushes anxiety to an all-time high. We believe that, if you can master the art of communication enough to help people during grief, you can easily handle any other client-relations issue that may arise. As you gain experience with using both the verbal and nonverbal language of death and grief, you become more comfortable "doing the unthinkable" and "speaking the unspeakable." You learn that you can allow owners to view their dead pets' bodies or say words like "dying" and "dead" and not feel shattered by your clients' responses to them. Thus, after you are comfortable communicating about death and grief, all other modes of communication seem easier. Let us begin to build your confidence by first learning more about the nonverbal communication techniques useful when helping people deal with normal grief.

NONVERBAL MESSAGES

You may be surprised to learn that most messages sent between people are conveyed nonverbally. In fact, psychologist Albert Mehrabian has said that only 7 percent of our ideas and emotions are communicated verbally.[1] More specifically, body language expert Paul Seaser is quoted as saying, "Communication is 7 percent words, 38 percent tone of inflection, and 55 percent nonverbal visual."[2] That means, 93 percent of one's thoughts and feelings are communicated without words.

Effective communication is much more than an exchange of words. It is also *what* is said, *where* it is said, *how* it is said, *why* it is said, *when* it is said, and to *whom* it is said. Communication is also what is *not* said: The nonverbal part of communication. Nonverbal communication is conveyed through facial expressions, body postures, gestures, and hand movements. It takes place not only when people speak, but also when they write, read, gesture, and listen.

The nonverbal part of communication is important because it helps people bridge the gap between what is said and what is interpreted. In other words, it helps people add meaning to what they are hearing. For example, you add meaning to what another person tells you by listening to their spoken words and by watching the nonverbal cues that accompany them. As a veterinarian, you may say to a client who is feeding his pet excessively, "You're killing your dog with kindness" and, depending on the nonverbal cues accompaning your statement, he may interpret it as praise, criticism, or anything in-between.

Body Language

Nonverbal cues, or body language, are often called the "silent language" and are one of the most common forms of nonverbal communication. Body language is composed of hand movements, facial expressions, eye contact, gestures, and posture. The clothes and colors people choose to wear are also part of communicating through body language. Nonverbal cues and behaviors send clear messages. Examples of some of the messages they send are in Table 6-1.

Table 6-1
The Messages in Body Language

Although body language communicates unspoken thoughts and feelings, common sense must be used when interpreting it. Cultural differences must also be considered when interpreting nonverbal communication. Here are some examples of common messages sent by body language.

Body Language	Message
Gestures	
Nose rubbing	Puzzlement, confusion
Arms folded across chest	Defensiveness, anxiety, cold
Hand to mouth	Surprise, sorrow
Neck rubbing	Pain, stress
Fingers tapping	Bored, nervous, impatient
Posture	
Collapsed	Discouraged, hopeless, tired
Erect	Confident, proud
Clothing	
Exposed neck and throat	Open and receptive
Covered neck and throat	Vulnerability
Colors	
Black	Power, respect (as in mourning)
Blue	Neutrality
Red	Passion

Eye contact, or lack of it, is one of the most telling forms of nonverbal communication. Research has shown that most people blink about 15 times per minute. The average period between blinks is about 2.8 seconds in men and slightly under 4 seconds in women. Each person seems to have an individual rate of blinking, which is maintained as long as the external environment is not changed. The rate may be altered by changes in the surroundings or by the person's mental state. Any cause for excitement usually increases the blink rate considerably.[3] Thus, aside from those used to lubricate and cleanse the eye, all other eye blinks are forms of communication. For example, when someone is lying, the pupils of his or her eyes grow larger; and when someone is uncomfortable, he or she blinks excessively. The absence of blinking connotes intense interest. One blink at a time sends a message of understanding from listener to speaker and says, in effect, "go on."

In the February 18, 1991, issue of *Newsweek* magazine, it was reported that analysis of videotape of Saddam Hussein's speeches during the Persian Gulf war showed that he blinked 113 times per minute during his Cable News Network interview with Peter Arnett.[4] A "normal" blink rate for someone speaking on camera is 30 to 50 blinks per minute, with more than 50 classified as "high." Experts saw Saddam's high blink rate as a clear indicator that his outward display of control was mostly pretense. Other examples of communication through eye contact are shown in Table 6-2 and Figure 6-1.

As you work with clients, begin to notice how their body language and eye contact differ from one situation to another. Start by observing how

Table 6-2
The Meaning of Eye Contact

Eyes are considered one of the most telling aspects of nonverbal communication. The eye movements listed below are common in western society and usually convey the meanings indicated. However, cultural differences must be considered when interpreting communication conveyed through eye contact.

Eye Movement	Message
Looking to the side or avoiding contact	Insecurity, dishonesty, preoccupation, shyness
Looking up	Intellectualizing
Looking down	Dealing with feelings
Looking up, to the side	Looking for approval
Rolling	Dislikes what is being said
Misty	Sadness
Slow blinking	Listening intently
Fast blinking	Anxiety, lying
Glaring	Hatred, anger

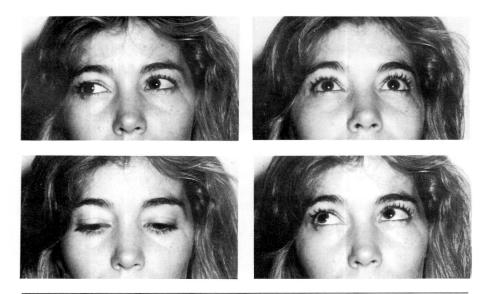

Figure 6-1 These photographs are examples of communication through eye movement. The meaning of each is discussed in Table 6-2.

high-strung, belligerent clients use closed body language and divert their eyes, whereas calm, receptive clients use open body language and direct eye contact. Notice also how your clients' use of open and closed postures evokes the same responses from you. Remember, in a communication feedback loop, you alternate between the positions of sender and receiver; therefore, you should monitor not only your clients' eye contact and body language, but your own as well.

Tears

Because crying is one of the most prominent nonverbal manifestations of grief, it deserves special attention in this discussion. People cry when they are grieving because it is a natural reaction to pain. Crying is an outward expression of an inner feeling. It is a mechanism for releasing emotion. Crying is what many people do when they are hurting. Therefore, tears associated with pet loss "fit the situation" and, in fact, are often an essential part of the grieving process.

Much has been learned about crying over the past few years. For example, William H. Frey, a biochemist considered to be the world's leading authority on human tears, has determined that not all tears are the same.[5] He reported that irritant or reflex tears (stirred by onions or dirt, for example) and emotional tears (stirred by sadness or joy) do not have the same chemical content. Emotional tears contain 20 to 24 percent more protein than do irritant tears. They also contain elevated amounts of hormones and neurotransmitters. The cause of these differences has yet to be discovered; however, Frey theorizes that emotional tears remove substances that are released into our bodies during times of stress. Just as other excretory processes, such as exhaling, perspiring, urinating, and defecating help maintain homeostasis in our bodies by removing waste and harmful substances, so does emotional tearing. Frey also believes that identifying the types and origins of proteins, hormones, neurotransmitters, and other substances specifically elevated in emotional tears will help us understand the biochemical basis of emotion and stress.

Frey's research supports what is intuitively known about crying: people generally feel better after they do it. In his study of a group of 106 male and female subjects, he found that 85 percent of women and 73 percent of men reported that they felt better after crying.[5] One woman said that she "felt clearer, that it was easier to see reality" after crying, and another said, "after a good cry, [she] was more willing to deal with the situation." In another study, researchers found that widows who had acquaintances who made it easy for them to cry and express their intense feelings were healthier than widows who experienced less encouragement from others to weep and to discuss their feelings of grief.[6]

Frey says, "People have the right to be human, to feel, to cry. They need to know there is no need to deprive themselves of the natural, healthy, release of emotional tears." Interestingly, however, one of the biggest obstacles to helping is the helper's fear that he or she may cry. We have overheard many conversations in which veterinarians discourage clients from being present at their pets' euthanasias. Later, when we have asked the veterinarians why they discouraged the owners' presence, many have told us that they were afraid they themselves would cry and "lose control" in a professional situation.

In reality, crying shows compassion and empathy for pets and their owners. We have *never* had a client tell us that they disliked it when a staff member cried with them. In fact, it touches clients deeply when you cry with them. If you cry easily you might say to a client, "It is natural for me to cry during times like this. I cry easily. I can still do my job, though, and be here for you and Pepper."

Because tears are natural reactions, they should not be fought or stifled. They should be expected, prepared for, and nurtured. Both research and clinical experience lend credibility to the idea that you should support your clients' tearful behaviors, not inhibit them.

The Practice Environment

When pet owners bring their companion animals to your practice, they learn a great deal about you from the physical environment that surrounds them. While you are with clients, you can *talk* all day about the significance of the human-animal bond and the support you are prepared to offer them at the deaths of their companion animals, but, if you have neglected to convey these same messages through the nonverbal cues in your practice environment, your communication will be far less believable.

As the TEAM model showed, you want to establish trust and rapport with pet owners from the time you first meet them as clients. You want to structure your practice environment so it acknowledges the human-animal bond and is conducive to lending emotional support. The idea is to provide clients with nonmedical help during the healthy times of their pets' lives so that they will also trust and rely on you when their pets are injured, ill, or dying.

Think for a moment about the stressful situations in which you sometimes find yourself. What makes you feel comfortable when you visit your own doctor, dentist, or tax accountant? Is your sense of comfort based on the furnishings, the color scheme, or on the type of lighting that is used (Figs. 6-2 and 6-3). Is it based on the way the staff is dressed or on the cup of coffee you are offered the moment you arrive? All of these elements are known to affect clients' feelings about and their confidence in a veterinary practice.

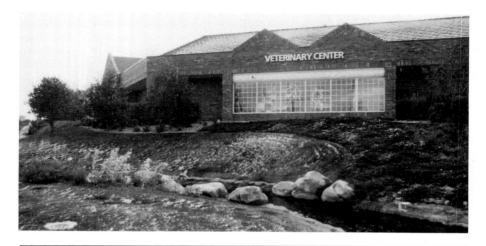

Figure 6-2 The outside of this veterinary practice appears clean, professional, and new. These environmental cues send messages to pet owners about the veterinarians practicing inside.

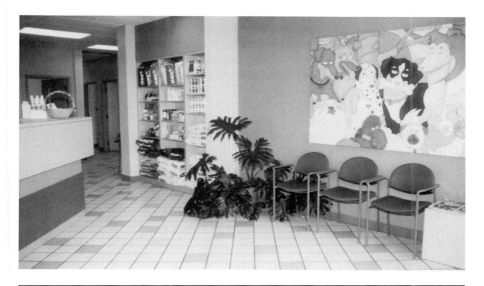

Figure 6-3 The inside of this veterinary practice is warm and inviting. The reception area is clean and large enough to accommodate several owners and their animals.

There are many ways to design your practice to make it more attractive to pet owners. Several of these are described in articles published in veterinary-oriented journals and magazines like *Veterinary Economics* and *DVM*. Most of these articles, however, overlook the specific ways in which you can design your practice so it will accommodate people's pet loss-related crises and grief. Let us look at some of them.

Public Areas

Many of your clients spend idle time in your waiting room and at your reception desk. In terms of pet loss and grief, you can do several things to educate, facilitate, and support clients while they wait. In most veterinary practices, reminders of death and grief are kept out of sight, thus perpetuating the illusion that animals live forever and discouraging pet owners from preparing and planning for their pet's deaths. When the subjects of pet loss and grief are tastefully introduced into the practice environment, however, the environment itself does some client preparation for you.

In the waiting room, framed poems or posters that refer to both the joy and sadness of animal ownership and death and pictures, plaques, or artwork that memorialize special pets can be displayed (Fig. 6-4). Many veterinarians reserve a special place on a wall for these memorials and regularly rotate the items they have on display. Other veterinarians create

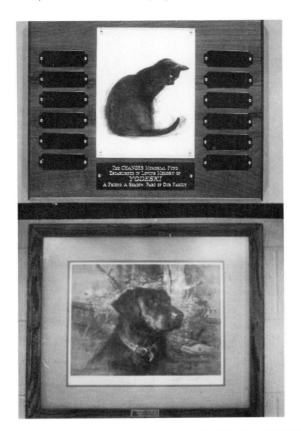

Figure 6-4 Memorials, in the form of plaques or pictures, are created in honor of special animals. They can be prominently displayed in waiting areas or examination rooms.

bulletin boards showing pictures of companion animals (Fig. 6-5). These can be captioned with the animals' names and their birth and death dates. Although these techniques may sound a bit morbid as you read about them here, they tend to be comforting to clients when they are used in practice. Clients who have lost beloved pets want to know that they have not been forgotten. Therefore, your sincere efforts to remember their pets means a lot to them.

The reception desk is a convenient place to display pamphlets about pet loss and grief and to place referral items like pet loss counselors' business cards and information about support groups offered in your area (Fig. 6-6). Because a classic manifestation of grief is confusion and an inability to concentrate, most pet owners appreciate receiving printed material about pet loss when it is offered as *a supplement to and as a reinforcement of* their

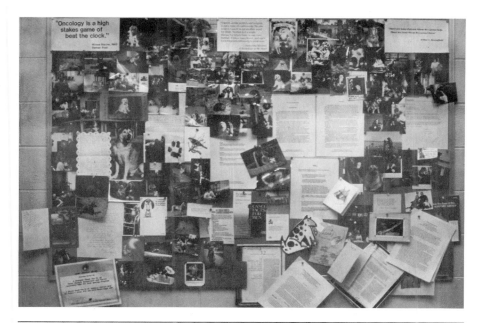

Figure 6-5 A bulletin board is covered with pictures of pets and notes of appreciation from satisfied pet owners. Pets *and* their owners get attention in bond-centered practices.

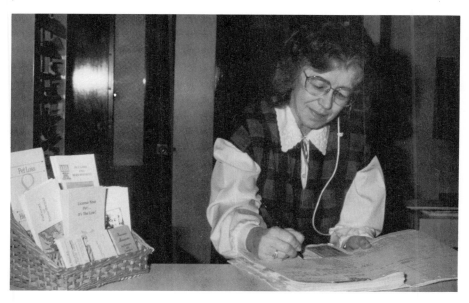

Figure 6-6 Sensitive veterinarians display pet loss–related materials, along with basic pet care information, in reception areas where clients can easily find them.

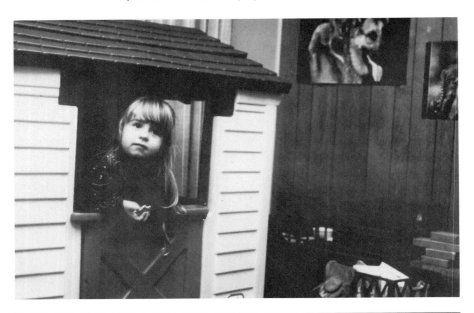

Figure 6-7 Play areas for children range from simple to elaborate. Veterinarians sensitive to the needs of families begin by creating a small play space that is visible and accessible to examination rooms (so that children can play within the sight of their parents). This area is stocked with books and toys for children of different developmental levels. These items can often be purchased at garage sales and second-hand shops or may be donated by loyal clients.

veterinarian's verbal expressions of sympathy and support. Printed materials also serve as a catalyst for more meaningful conversations about pet loss.

The public area of your practice is the place to calm your clients' anxieties. Because research on the human-animal bond indicates that blood pressure and heart rates are lowered by watching fish swim in aquariums,[7] you can equip your waiting room or reception desk with one or more tanks. Other "mascot" animals can also help ease tension. Some veterinarians bring their own dogs or cats to work with them, letting them socialize with clients in the waiting area.

No real evidence supports this notion, but we suspect that the blood pressure and heart rates of your clients who are parents are also lowered when you devote an area of your waiting room to children's play! Parents often feel torn between wanting to give their undivided attention to ill or injured pets and wanting to supervise their young children. A well-designed, well-equipped play area often keeps young children occupied long enough for parents to spend quality time with you and with their companion animals (Fig. 6-7).

Private Areas

You may want to have an area of your practice that offers your clients more privacy than the main waiting room. This room may be an examination room or even your own office. Wherever it is located, the room can be used for consultations, visitations, and even euthanasias; therefore, it should be equipped with comfortable seating, soft lights, and books or pamphlets about pet loss. If possible, the room should also have a video-cassette recorder and television monitor so clients can watch educational videotapes. A telephone and a box of tissues should be standard items. Access to information regarding necropsy, body care, and referrals to professional grief counselors should also be provided. Although you do not want to overwhelm clients with resources concerning grief and the arrangements that need to be made after death, pet owners cannot explore their alternatives and resources without accurate information (Fig. 6-8).

If a room is specifically designated for use during client-present euthanasias, several additional features are helpful. Clean, soft fleeces or blankets for pets to either lie on or be covered with are nice features. Pads that can be placed on examination tables or on the floor also provide patients and clients with extra comfort and make the practice environment seem less sterile (Fig. 6-9). Blinds that cover windows and Do Not Disturb signs on examination room doors further protect the privacy of grieving clients (Table 6-3). Other items and arrangements that make a room more appro-

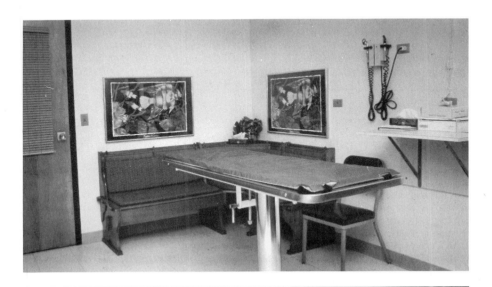

Figure 6-8 This room is designed to soften the typical sterile medical environment and thus provide comfort to pet owners and their pets. A cloth-covered pad is placed on the examination table to cushion the pet during treatment or euthanasia.

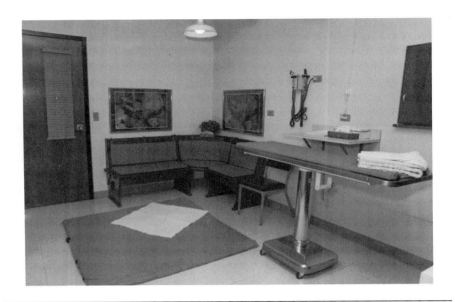

Figure 6-9 This room is designed for client comfort. The large cloth-covered pad on the floor allows pets and pet owners to spend extended time together during visitations, treatments, or euthanasias.

Table 6-3
An Examination Room Designed for Client Comfort

A standard examination room can be modified to provide pet owners with a private, comfortable area when visiting or euthanizing their companion animals. The following items are used in a modified examination room at the Colorado State University Veterinary Teaching Hospital. The costs are estimates. Many items were donated by student and community organizations or by clients in memory of their pets.

Item	Estimated Cost
Warm color of paint (or wallpaper border)	$20
Adjustable mini-blinds for the door windows	$75
"Please Do Not Disturb" signs for the doors	$10
Small pad for exam table, large pad or mat for floor	$120
Washable pad covers (three small, two large)	$70
Comfortable seating (loveseat or wooden corner bench with cushions)	$675
System for lowered lighting	$100
Television monitor, videocassette recorder and educational videos	$500
Display rack stocked with materials (brochures, pet cemeteries, counselor referrals, *etc.*)	$50
Pictures	$90
Bulletin board or scrapbook for pictures and cards	$50
Miscellaneous (clock, mirror, used blankets, towels)	$50
Sample urns, caskets, *etc.* (demonstration models)	no charge
Total	$1810

priate for use during client-present euthanasias are discussed in Chapters 8 and 9.

Certain clients will more readily respond to your nonverbal communication about pet loss and grief than others. These clients will feel more comfortable about asking you for help. They are also likely to feel reassured about their chosen plan of action, be it treatment or euthanasia, because they will be aware of the caring atmosphere that you have created in your practice environment.

NONVERBAL COMMUNICATION TECHNIQUES

Now that you understand the significance of nonverbal communication, it is important to learn how to use several basic nonverbal techniques to communicate your message to clients more effectively. Six nonverbal techniques are described in this chapter. They are demonstration, written material, adapting the environment, attending, active listening, and responding with touch. When used in conjunction with the TEAM model of helping, these techniques make your communications with clients even more effective.

Demonstrations

Demonstrations are very effective forms of nonverbal communication. They can help clients learn the proper way to administer drugs at home or learn the specifics of the euthanasia procedure (Fig. 6-10). Demonstrations can also be used to describe an illness or disease process and to explain surgery plans or test results. They are a way to simplify and to "walk clients through" complicated and overwhelming medical information.

Verbal descriptions generally accompany demonstrations. Sometimes tours of your veterinary facilities can also enhance a demonstration. When used together, verbal descriptions, tours, and demonstrations give clients a step-by-step idea about what is likely to happen to their companion animals while they are under your care.

It is helpful to conduct demonstrations during the Alternatives and Resources part of the TEAM model. When clients have a visual understanding of what certain treatments or euthanasias entail, it is often easier for them to decide whether or not those options are right for them. Videotapes that show the key points of several treatment protocols, surgical procedures, and methods for conducting client-present euthanasias are available. Offering these videotaped demonstrations to your clients to watch, either at your clinic or at their homes, can also aid in their decision-making processes.

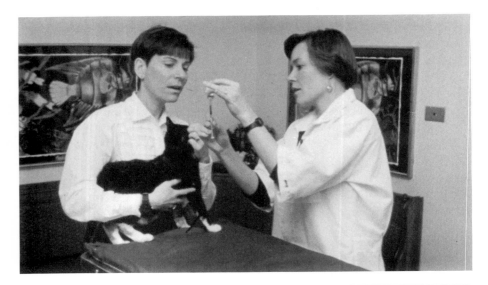

Figure 6-10 Veterinary professionals help owners give pets the care they need by pairing verbal descriptions with demonstrations of simple medical procedures. In this photograph a veterinarian shows an owner how to give her diabetic dog an injection.

Written Information

Providing clients with written information is another form of nonverbal communication. It is also helpful to use during the Alternatives and Resources part of the TEAM model. Much of the medical jargon and information familiar to you is very foreign-sounding and unfamiliar to average pet owners. Therefore, it helps to write things down or to draw pictures for clients (Fig. 6-11). Drawings and written materials also allow pet owners to take information home so they can describe their pets' situations accurately and in full detail to other family members.

When the subject matter is emotional, it is tempting to hand clients a packet of materials and hope that the message will somehow get through. In terms of grief, however, written material should be used primarily to *enhance* potentially emotional discussions *not to replace* them. Printed materials are most effective when the information reinforces points that have previously been verbally discussed.

Written information is especially helpful when working with highly emotional pet owners who are unable to concentrate on the facts of the case. We did, however, witness one occasion when the intent of this technique backfired. A veterinary oncologist spent several hours working with a distraught owner explaining the necessary diagnostic procedures and cancer treatment protocols available to his pet. The veterinarian realized, however, that he was not getting anywhere with his client, who seemed just as confused after the lengthy discussion as he had been when they started. In desperation, the clinician went back to the beginning of their discussion and wrote down the four things he would do for the animal during the next several hours. With the intention of simplifying and clarifying the process for his client, he gave the list to the pet owner and left the room. Before he had gone ten steps down the hall, however, the owner ran out of the examination room, frantically waving the clinician's list. "Dr. Sogard," he called. "Wait a minute! You forgot to take the list of what you're going to do with Bingo today!"

Structuring the Environment

Structuring the environment means paying attention to the elements of your office, examination rooms, and consultation areas that are easily moved and changed. It means arranging chairs, examination tables, and other furnishings so they invite, rather than suppress, emotion. This kind

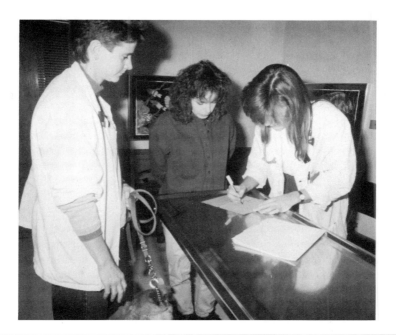

Figure 6-11 The veterinarian can ensure that a client understands exactly what is happening to her pet by writing down the important facts about the animal's condition and the available treatment options. The veterinarian can also clarify information by drawing a picture of the disease process, medical condition, or surgery plan.

of moment-to-moment adaptation of the environment tends to facilitate uninterrupted communication, which, in turn, facilitates the "finishing business" aspect of grief.

Environments are structured in many ways. For example, chairs are moved so conversations can take place face-to-face and away from barriers such as desks or examination tables. The physical use of space is also easily adapted. For example, within examination rooms, euthanasias can be performed on an examination table, on the floor, or on a gurney rolled over near the window so pet and pet owner can be near the outdoors. Euthanasias can also be performed outdoors or even in the veterinarian's private office. The point is to think ahead, plan, and prepare these spaces so they can be easily adapted to accommodate whatever may occur within them.

When anxiety is high, people tend to get "frozen into position." They forget that they can stand up if they are sitting, walk around the room if they are standing, or even leave the room altogether if they need a few minutes to be alone. You can help clients and yourself overcome this rigidity by remembering that you can adapt the physical elements of your environment however and whenever you choose. It is useful to use this communication technique during all phases of helping. In terms of your use of the TEAM model, it is most helpful to use while you are establishing trust and rapport, exploring alternatives and resources, and setting action plans in motion. Here is an example:

> You have just told Nancy Dixon that there is nothing more you can do for her dying cat. As the realization of her cat's impending death sinks in, you see that her eyes begin to fill with tears. In response to this nonverbal cue, you pick up the box of tissues that is close at hand, move your chair closer to hers, and offer her a tissue with which to dry her eyes. Later, as the discussion turns to her cat's body care, you leave the room for a moment and return with an urn filled with the actual cremains of a cat. With her permission, you show the cremains to her as you explain the cremation procedure. When the decision to euthanize the cat is made, you comply with Nancy's wishes to conduct the procedure outdoors and escort her to the site where the death will occur. At this time, the whole procedure begins again as, together, you adapt the outdoor environment, perhaps by spreading out some fleeces or a blanket, to fit such an occasion.

Attending

According to educator and communication expert Robert Bolten, attending is a form of nonverbal communication that uses body language to indicate that careful attention is being paid to the speaker.[8] Attending means giving physical attention to another person. Thus, when on the receiving end of the communication feedback loop, helpers keep their body postures open, attentive, and lean slightly forward (Fig. 6-12). This shows that the helper is available, present in the moment, and unintimidated by what is happening.

Attending behaviors include direct eye contact, nonjudgmental facial expressions, encouraging gestures, open body postures, affirmative head nods, and direct observation of what is occurring. When using this technique, helpers face their clients squarely and speak to them directly at an eye-to-eye level. If the client sits down, the helper sits down too. If young children are present, helpers squat down to their level when they greet them or talk to them directly.

In veterinary medicine, many distractions can get in the way of attending behaviors. They include pager messages, questions from staff members, phone calls from other clients, and the need to write notes in patients' case files. The animals themselves are also distractions. They move around, make noises, and generally divert everyone's attention from the main point of the conversation. Because nonattentiveness often results in additional phone calls to clarify procedures and clients' noncompliance with treatment plans, it is a good idea to remove pets from the room when the goal is to attend to your clients and to have them attend to you.

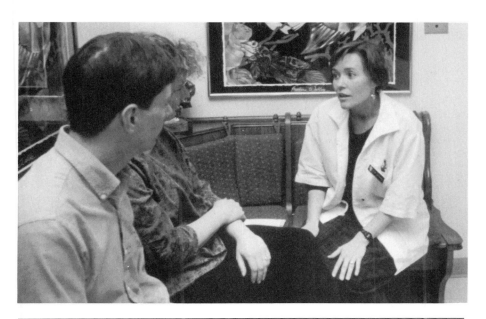

Figure 6-12 A helper is in an attending position when she leans slightly forward and maintains eye contact with the pet owner.

Attending is certainly one of the mainstays of developing trust and rapport. However, because clients want and need to know you are there for them throughout their pets' dying processes, it is an important technique to use during all four phases of the TEAM model.

Active Listening

Listening is a skill. A difference exists between merely hearing someone and actively listening to what they say. The word *listen* is derived from the two Anglo-Saxon words *hlystan,* which means hearing, and *hlosnian,* which means to wait in suspense. Active listening is the combination of hearing what another person says with an attitude of suspenseful waiting. This kind of listening denotes an intense psychological involvement with the person sending the message.[8]

Actively listening to others as they talk and sort through problems is a powerful form of help and support. It may be the most effective way to help and support clients who are distressed. Yet, listening is difficult because we listen much faster than we speak. Although we speak at an average rate of 125 words per minute, we listen at roughly 500 words per minute.[8] Thus, as listeners or message receivers, we have a strong tendency to think ahead of the person who is speaking. In thinking ahead, we often make assumptions about what the other person is likely to say and either become eager to contribute our own thoughts to the conversation or become bored, letting our minds wander off onto other tangents of thought. In eagerness, we often interrupt or steer conversations off track. In boredom, we often lose track of conversations altogether. When we are not listening carefully to what other people are saying, we are most often using their speaking time to collect our own thoughts and to decide what, in response, we want to say (Fig. 6-13).

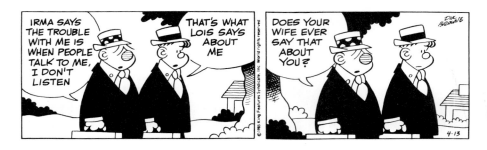

Figure 6-13 Reprinted with special permission of King Features Syndicate.

The quality of listening is affected by various other factors, including:

- physical status (fatigue, illness, hunger, intoxication),
- emotional state (feelings like being upset, excited, anxious, preoccupied),
- distractions (noise, daydreams, other activities),
- gender.

The gender issue is particularly interesting. Research has shown that both men and women are more likely to interrupt and to disagree with female speakers than with male speakers.[9] In one study, researchers[10] found that, in conversations between male-female pairs, regardless of their individual attitudes toward sexual equality, men interrupted more, accounting for 68 percent of the interruptions.

Another study shows that ideas and topics introduced by men are almost always picked up for discussion, whereas the same is true for only one third of topics introduced by women.[11] Fishman[12] found that in male-female conversations, the topics raised by men were much more often developed than were those raised by women, largely because of women's greater "interaction work" (answering questions, providing active conversational support). She concluded that conversations were under male control but were mainly produced by female work. West and Zimmerman[13] found that when women tried to develop topics in their turns at talk, men often gave minimal responses, which, along with more frequent male interruptions, became mechanisms by which men controlled the topic in mixed-sex conversations.

Most people think of women as the more talkative sex, but men actually talk more than women.[14] The longest speaking times recorded are men talking with other men[15] and are defined as displays of power.[16] These statistics have particular significance in veterinary medicine because clients are primarily women, staffs are primarily women, and a high percentage of veterinary students and practitioners are women.

Gender issues aside, however, we are all accustomed to listening to the factual, rather than the feeling, content of conversations. And, even when feelings are heard, we are accustomed to diminishing any negative emotions by changing the subject or ignoring what has been said. Listening for the affect or for the emotional content in conversations is very difficult. Yet, this is what the communication technique called "active listening" is about. Active listening means that you listen for messages that seem emotionally charged or important and respond to them without judgment or bias. Active listening conveys genuine concern and nonjudgmental acceptance. It is a technique that lets clients know that what they have to say is important.

Active listening incorporates attending behaviors such as eye contact and open body posture, but goes further in that it actually encourages the other person to talk. Two verbal communication techniques that encourage speakers to continue are called paraphrasing and asking questions. These are discussed in the next chapter. Two predominantly nonverbal communication techniques important to the process of active listening are necessary silences and minimal encouragers. Let us first take a closer look at these factors.

Necessary Silences

Silence is a necessary part of active listening. Yet, remaining silent while others vent their feelings takes practice. It is difficult to sit in a room with someone who is sobbing or reviewing painful events. But when deep emotion is present, silence is often precisely what is needed. Emotional conversations, within the context of helping relationships, move very slowly. Both senders and receivers often need a few minutes to process what has been said before they respond.

When anxiety is high, it is tempting to engage in "nervous babble" to fill in the silent, empty spaces. Silences become much more comfortable for everyone when they are acknowledged and used as an effective communication technique. You can acknowledge and use your clients' silences by limiting your comments to phrases like:

"Take your time. I'm right here for you."

"I can imagine how hard it is for you to talk about this. I won't be uncomfortable if you cry."

"Your tears are okay. I would cry, too, if I were facing this situation."

"All of this is overwhelming."

"You've been very quiet for awhile now. Would you like to continue talking or would you like some time alone?"

Minimal Encouragers

Minimal encouragers are simple responses that encourage people to talk more. When using minimal encouragers, it is not the content of what is said that enhances the conversation, but rather the strategic placement of brief comments, made in an appropriate tone of voice, that elicit more storytelling. Minimal encouragers are generally nonjudgmental in nature. They do not change the subject or directional flow of emotional conversations. Instead, they keep conversations going and, in most instances, deepen their emotional content.

As a helper, the purpose of using minimal encouragers is to let people know you are an active participant in the communication taking place between you. It also lets them know you are interested in gaining more information from them. Examples of nonverbal minimal encouragers include head nods, eye blinks, hand motions, and supportive touches.

These are even more effective when paired with such phrases as:

"Go on."

"Tell me more about that."

"Uh huh."

"Hmmm."

"I see."

"Wow."

"Really?"

"And?"

"For instance?"

Most inexperienced helpers talk too much; therefore, the importance of learning to listen cannot be overemphasized. Like talking, however, listening can be overdone. Nothing is more frustrating than relating a story to someone who does not add a comment or two along the way. In fact, extremely quiet listeners sometimes make the speaker feel even more anxious.

It is valuable to find a balance between using silence and minimal encouragers when helping clients deal with their emotional responses. In fact, active listening is one of the most important communication techniques to use throughout all four phases of the TEAM model.

Responding with Touch

During emotional times, a light touch on a person's arm or shoulder can be very comforting. Touch shows care and concern and often takes the place of reassuring words. During pet loss, touch lets pet owners know they are not alone with their feelings of grief (Fig. 6-14).

Touch seems to have a calming affect on many people. It often helps them slow their thoughts and to steady themselves emotionally. Some evidence also suggests that touch affects the body physiologically, slowing heart rate and lowering blood pressure.[17] Thus, touch can be used to soothe a grieving client or to bring someone who is rambling back to the point. Here is an example of how touch works. When helping, you can raise your hand in front of you, with your palm open and facing the client, to indicate that she needs to slow down. Then, by firmly placing your hand

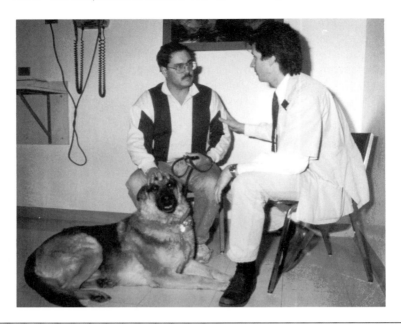

Figure 6-14 When pet owners appear distressed, veterinarians can comfort them with a light touch on the arm or shoulder. Most pet owners appreciate this sensitive gesture.

on her arm and keeping it there, you can indicate that she needs to stop talking and listen to you.

For the most part, touch is used quite naturally in the interchanges that take place between veterinarians and clients. With practice, you can learn to read your clients' body language and, therefore, know who is (and who is not) receptive to touch. When using touch with clients, neutral or "safe" areas to touch are the shoulders and arms. Areas of the body that are not viewed as neutral or safe include the neck, hands, torso, lower back, and legs. In general, people, particularly children, dislike being patted on their backs or heads. This behavior connotes a sense of superiority on the helper's part and can be viewed as condescending.

If you are not sure how the people might respond to touch, just ask. Say, "We have been through a lot together over the past few days. Could I give you a hug before you leave?" They will tell you if they are comfortable with your request. Be sure to use touch in ethical ways, especially with clients of the opposite sex, because comfort can be misinterpreted as a sexual advance. As a veterinarian, if touching or hugging clients makes you squirm, a substitute technique is to touch their animals with great sensitivity and care. Pet owners often decide whether or not they can trust you based on the way you touch and handle their animals.

Although touch can be used at anytime, within the context of a helping relationship, it is probably most effective when it is used to build trust and rapport with clients. Specifically, when working through the TEAM model, it is effective to use touch to help clients focus, to provide them with structure, and to signal the end of communication interactions.

CONCLUSION

Although nonverbal behavior appears to be random, research tells us that it has an identifiable structure and can be predicted.[18] For example, we expect that when people are happy, they smile, and when they are sad, they cry. We also expect that when people are cold, they shiver, and when they are frightened, they run away. All of us share these preconceived notions about how people will behave in certain situations. Because we share these ideas, it is possible for us to agree on what nonverbal behaviors say, what they do not say, when they should occur, when they should not occur, and why.

Because we share this knowledge, we also expect that people's nonverbal communication will be accompanied by words that match their facial expressions, gestures, tone of voice, and body language. It is very confusing when words say one thing and behaviors say something else. Therefore, nonverbal and verbal communication must be congruent. The term congruent means an agreement of fit. In the communication field, it means that nonverbal and verbal messages are compatible and appropriate to one another and that the message given verbally matches the one that is broadcast by the body. Let us go on to Chapter 7 and see how verbal communication techniques can be paired with nonverbal factors to convey a message of help to clients.

REFERENCES

1. Mehrabian, A.: Communication without words. Psychology Today, p. 53. September 1968.
2. Seaser, P.: Body language: Actions speak louder than words. Fort Collins, Colo., The Coloradoan, p. 8, April 22, 1989.
3. Moses, R.A.: The eyelids. *In* Moses R.A., and Hart, W.M., eds.: Adler's Physiology of the Eye: Clinical Application, 8th ed. St. Louis, C.V. Mosby Company, 1987, pp. 1–14.
4. Don't blink. Newsweek. February 18, 1991.
5. Frey, W.H., and Lanseth, M.: Crying: The Mystery of Tears. Minneapolis, Winston Press, 1985.

6. Maddison, D., and Walker, W.L.: Factors affecting the outcome of conjugal bereavement. Br. J. Psychiat., *113*:1057–1067, 1967.
7. Katcher, A.H., Friedman, E., Beck, A.M., and Lynch, J.: Looking, talking, and blood pressure: The psychological consequences of interaction with the living environment. *In* Katcher, A.H., and Beck, A.M., eds.: New Perspectives on Our Lives with Companion Animals. Philadelphia, University of Pennsylvania Press, 1983, pp. 351–359.
8. Bolten, R.: People Skills: How to Assert Yourself, Listen to Others, and Resolve Conflicts. New York, Simon and Schuster, 1979.
9. Kennedy, C.W.: Patterns of verbal interruption among women and men in groups. Paper given at 3rd Annual Conference on Communication, Language, and Gender, Lawrence, Kansas, 1980. Annotated bibliography by Thorne, B., Kramarae, C., Henley, N., eds.: *In* Language, Gender and Society. Rowley, Mass., Newbury House Publishers, 1983.
10. Octigan, M., and Niederman, S.: Male dominance in conversations. Frontiers, *4*:50–54, 1979.
11. Killian, P.: Isn't anyone listening? Network: A Magazine for Colorado Women, *2*:36, 1986.
12. Fishman, P.M.: Interaction: The work women do. Social Problems, *25*:397–406, 1978. Revision *in* Thorne, B., Kramarae, C., and Henley, N., eds.: Language, Gender and Society, Rowley, Mass., Newbury House Publishers, 1983, pp. 89–101.
13. West, C., and Zimmerman, D.H.: Small insults: A study of interruptions in cross-sex conversations between unacquainted persons. *In* Thorne, B., Kramarae, C., and Henley, N., eds.: Language, Gender and Society. Rowley, Mass., Newbury House Publishers, 1983, pp. 102–117.
14. Doherty, E.G.: Therapeutic community meetings: A study of communication patterns, sex, status, and staff attendance. Small Group Behavior, *5*:244–256, 1974.
15. Ayres, J.: Relationship stages and sex as factors in topic dwell time. Western Journal of Speech Communication, *44*:253–260, 1980.
16. Sattel, J.W.: Men, inexpressiveness, and power. *In* Thorne, B., Kramarae, C., and Henley, N., eds.: Language, Gender and Society. Rowley, Mass., Newbury House Publishers, 1983, pp. 118–124.
17. Lynch, J.J., Thomas, S.A., Paskewitz, D.A., Katcher, A.H., and Weir, L.D.: Human contact and cardiac arrhythmia in a coronary care unit. Psychosom. Med., *39*:188–192, 1977.
18. Bandler, R., and Grinder, J.: The Structure of Magic I: A Book about Language and Therapy. Palo Alto, Calif., Science and Behavior Books, 1975.

7

Verbal Communication

Many people feel that we are born knowing how to communicate and that the ability to talk with one another is what separates us from the lower forms of life. Yet, communication experts say that effective communication techniques are actually learned[1] and can be improved with practice. As with any skill, innate abilities certainly help, but ongoing practice is essential to achieve mastery. Consider the example of a concert pianist who is born with natural talent but who must work diligently to perfect her skills. How many pianists do you know who reach the highest levels of their profession without practice? Not many. The same is true for effective communicators, especially when it comes to developing skills in the use of verbal communication techniques.

With verbal communication, what you say is not as important as how you say it. The context in which your words are spoken has the greatest impact on the message you are trying to convey.

VERBAL MESSAGES

The effectiveness of verbal communication is influenced by many variables. These variables include word choice, grammar, voice tone, volume, and pitch. Effectiveness is also affected by the emphasis and inflection placed on certain words and the pacing of overall speech. We know from research that voice tone and the pacing of words have the most influence on the meaning of spoken words.[2] Voice tone and pacing make significant contributions to what is actually communicated. For example, if, as a helper, you use appropriate words to describe a situation, but speak very quickly, you may be seen as rushed, nervous, insensitive, or unsure of yourself. If you speak the same words too slowly, however, you may be viewed as dull, boring, or even condescending. It is particularly important for you to monitor your voice tone when working with clients who are under stress, because words that are spoken softly and at a slightly slower pace than normal are viewed as more comforting.

The words you choose are also important. According to researchers Campbell and Helper,[3] when health care professionals use medical jargon in the presence of clients, their credibility is enhanced and clients' confidence in them is increased. They also note, however, that jargon can alienate clients. Therefore, if technical terms must be used, they should also be explained in plain language. The word *lymphosarcoma*, for example, means nothing to the average pet owner. The word *cancer*, however, does. As a helper, therefore, you gain common ground with your clients when you share an understanding of the meaning of words. Then, true communication begins.

CLICHÉS

It is very difficult to both initiate and sustain any kind of emotional communication. Because emotions are so threatening, many helpers look for ways to distract clients from pain by keeping them busy or cheering them up. Others change the subject altogether when conversations become emotional. Attempts to shut down emotional conversations can also take many other forms. These include giving pep talks, offering advice, and scolding people for "wallowing in their feelings." None of these methods, however, is effective when helping people who are feeling sad, scared, or vulnerable.

Communication interchanges during grief become awkard for two main reasons. The first is that if you *have not* experienced a major loss yourself, it is often difficult to relate to the deep level of pain that grievers experience. When you cannot relate, you tend to help "from your head" instead of "from your heart," offering what you believe to be words of comfort.

The second is that if you *have* experienced major loss in your life, you may not want to re-experience the deep level of pain that you felt at the time of your loss. Because another's loss can trigger your own unresolved feelings of grief, you may avoid grievers or try to move them from a feeling level to a less intense, intellectual level of conversation. Again, you offer what you believe to be words of comfort as a way to deal with others' and your own losses.

Intellectualized responses are commonly referred to as clichés. Clichés are trite sayings that represent attempts to find answers to problems that

BOX 7-1

Clichés of Grief

"If there is anything I can do just call me."

"I know just how you feel."

"Time will heal."

"He had a long life. Think of all your good memories."

"You have other pets," or "There'll be other dogs."

"God needed another dog in heaven."

"Try to stay busy."

"Out of sight, out of mind."

"Life goes on. . ."

"She is holding up so well."

"Support groups are for weaklings."

"You must be strong for your children."

"Children are flexible, they'll bounce back. . ."

"Big boys don't cry."

"If you look around you can always find someone who is worse off than your-self."

"It is better to have loved and lost, than never to have loved at all."

"Count your blessings."

"Only the good die young."

"God never gives us more than we can handle."

"God needs him more than you do."

"What you don't know, won't hurt you."

"No sense dwelling on the past."

"No sense crying over spilt milk."

This list was partially drawn and adapted to pet loss from Erin Linn's 1986 book *I Know Just How You Feel: Avoiding the Clichés of Grief.*

have no answers. Clichés attempt to provide simple, intellectualized solutions to emotionally significant and overwhelming problems. Trite sayings fall short of expressing your true feelings and can sound offensive and insensitive to grievers. If you speak from your heart with honesty, clichés are unnecessary.

Clichés come in many forms. According to Erin Linn, author of *I Know Just How You Feel: Avoiding the Clichés of Grief*,[4] five of the basic ones are discounting, hurry-up, guilt for grief, replacement, and God's will or punishment clichés (Box 7-1). Some of you have probably used these phrases during times of loss. We have used them ourselves. It is not our purpose to embarrass you or to admonish you for making this common mistake. Rather, our purpose is to enlighten you about how grievers hear the "words of comfort" that we offer them. Examples of the five kinds of clichés and their pertinence to veterinary medicine follow.

A Discounting Cliché: "If there is anything I can do, just call me."

This statement sounds caring, but can be perceived as a brush-off. It probably does more to soothe your sense of powerlessness as a helper than to provide real help to your clients. Most bereaved persons are confused and depressed after a loss and cannot muster the energy or initiative to ask for help from others. As one pet owner told us:

> Even though my veterinarian told me to call if I needed anything, I
> couldn't because I was afraid that I was the only person who had
> ever grieved that deeply for a pet. I really wish he would have called
> me and asked how I was doing. That would have taken a lot of
> pressure off me.

Also, asking for help is risky because those who occasionally reach out to others with specific requests sometimes find people unwilling to help, for one reason or another, although they offered previously.

Several reasons explain why inexperienced helpers commonly place the burden of reaching out for help on clients' shoulders. For example, they do not want to bother them, catch them at a bad time, or remind them of the trauma of loss. This line of reasoning tends to isolate clients and gives them the message that others are not interested in simply listening to their feelings about loss.

A better approach to helping is to say:

> "I will call you (tonight, tomorrow, next week), and, if there
> is anything that you need me to do for you, you can let me
> know then."

Do not say you will call, however, unless you truly intend to call. Also, do not be content with leaving messages and waiting for clients to get back to you. Leave messages that you called, but then get back to them yourself as soon as possible.

If you are especially close to a client who is grieving, it is helpful to call them every day or so. After a week or so, it is usually alright to taper off your calls, but only if you tell the pet owner that this is your intention. Calls can be kept short (10 minutes or so) and can be used to help your client focus his or her attention on the many tasks involved in adjusting to loss. Whenever possible, call during a gap in the client's routine that was once filled by the pet (for example, the time set aside for walking the dog after work). Grievers benefit from having some structure imposed on their lives, and phone calls can provide such structure if they are ones on which they can depend and to which they can look forward. In short, when offering your help to grieving clients, state your intentions clearly and concretely, and then make sure you follow through.

Another Discounting Cliché: "I know just how you feel."

When you say "I know just how you feel," you are assuming that you know how your clients feel because you remember how you felt or how you would feel in a similar situation. No one can truly know, however, how another person feels. Your clients' grief responses are the result of thousands of experiences and intervening variables unique to their own lives. Saying that you know how clients feel discounts their losses and compares them with a loss you either knew of or experienced.

If "I know just how you feel" is followed by "My cat died, too, and I'm still not over him," the comment can shift the focus of the conversation from the client to you, the helper. If, as a helper, you allow this shift in focus to occur, the interchange does more to meet your personal needs than those of your client. Better statements to use are:

"I can only imagine how you must be feeling."

"What has this been like for you?"

or

"I have been through a similar experience. Would you feel comfortable talking to me about yours? What happened?"

A Hurry-up Cliché: "Time will heal."

This cliché implies that clients are powerless over the manifestations of grief and that the best they can do is passively wait for time to lessen their pain. Ineffective helpers usually make this statement because they want their clients to pull themselves together and not to dwell on their losses. In other words, they want them to hide their pain while they are in public and to do their grieving in private. What they really want is for the client to get "back to normal" so they can also "get back to normal" and once again be comfortable in their presence.

Grief is difficult and complex. It ebbs and flows and varies in intensity. When grief is present, time moves very slowly, and each day can seem like an eternity. Therefore, the idea of time as an ally is not a comforting thought for one who is in the midst of grief. It is tempting to try to get clients to look ahead and to focus on a time in the future when they will feel better. Such approaches, however, discount the feelings they are currently having. A better comment to make would be:

"You must feel as if this pain will never end. I just want you to know that I feel sad about Jake's death, too."

This lets clients know that you understand their situations and are with them in the present moment. Knowing they are not alone with their pain is often great comfort in itself.

A You Should Feel Guilty for Grieving Cliché: "He Had a Long Life. Think of All of Your Memories."

The first statement implies that one who lived a long life does not need to be mourned. It also implies that the loss should have been anticipated and that the client should feel guilty about grieving an "expected" loss. The second statement implies that the client should be satisfied with memories of their loved ones and should feel grateful for whatever time they had together. Memories are a poor substitute for the real thing, however, and are often bittersweet. Additionally, some clients' memories include the myriad of unpleasant situations that can surround a loss and may be anything but comforting to them.

Instead, say:

> "You were together for so many years. Tell me about some of
> your special times together."

This encourages clients to talk about their experiences and to review the special parts of the relationships they had with the pets who died. After talking about and reviewing memories, clients may come to some positive conclusions about their situations on their own. This approach is far preferable to having others tell them how they should feel.

A Replacement Cliché: "You have other pets" or "There'll be other dogs."

The first statement implies that pet owners share bonds with their pets as a group and that one individual will not be missed. The second statement implies that one companion animal can take the place of another. Regrettably, these same kinds of statements are also made to parents who experience the deaths of children. Insensitive statements like, "You're young, you can have more children" or "At least you have other kids to love right now" send the message that some (especially young) loved ones are replaceable and that their deaths occur without significant impact on our lives. In regard to pet loss, it is more helpful to say:

> "Captain will always have a special place in your heart."

Or,

> "I know you miss Captain a lot. No one will ever take his
> place."

A God's Will or Punishment Cliché: "God needed another dog in heaven."

When clients are grieving, they often draw on spiritual beliefs to help them through hard times. Therefore, suggesting that a pet's death was God's idea may not provide comfort. In fact, when you use this cliché, a source of spiritual support is also presented as the direct source of pain. This connection may create confusion toward God and cause clients to feel even more isolated.

When clients are grieving they also feel anger. You may think it is helpful to try to diffuse that anger by bringing meaning to their losses or by assigning responsibility to someone or something greater than yourself. Blaming losses on God, however, may not lead to desired results. Suggestions that God played a role in a pet's death may be particularly confusing for children who do not have the cognitive abilities to understand death, much less the "will of God." Comments about God should only be made if religious beliefs are first introduced by the clients themselves.

To conclude this section on clichés, we relate one of the most touching, comforting interactions we have seen between a pet owner and a veterinarian. This example involved a senior student who had worked all night to save a dog who was in the critical care unit. After the dog died, the student knew that she did not have to go out to the lobby to face the clients, but she had talked with them several times and wanted to acknowledge their loss. As she approached them, she began to cry. So did the pet owners. When she got close enough to them, she put her arms around their shoulders, pulled them both close to her in a hug, and said, "I don't know what to say to you. I know how much you loved Corky. I grew very fond of him, too, over the last two days." The interchange was short, but sincere. During the course of it, she gave them concrete, descriptive details of Corky's condition while in the critical care unit. She also described the details leading up to his death and reassured them that he had died in the presence of people who cared about him. Later, the clients wrote a letter to the hospital director, telling him how much it meant to them that the student had come to talk to them, had cried, and had told them about how much others had cared for Corky too. It was confirmation for them that Corky had again done what he did best—worm his way into other people's hearts. How different this exchange would have been if the student had approached them with composure and said no more than, "I know just how you feel."

VERBAL COMMUNICATION TECHNIQUES

We have told you about the dangers of relying on clichés and about what is not helpful to say to clients. Now we will discuss some ideas of what to say to clients to make your helping more effective. The following collection of verbal communication techniques form the basis of any helping relationship. The six basic techniques described here are called acknowledging, normalizing, giving permission, asking questions, self-disclosure, and paraphrasing. Two advanced techniques are also discussed. They are gentle confrontation and immediacy.

Acknowledging

Acknowledging is defined as recognizing the existence or truth of something. In matters of loss and grief, verbal affirmation is the primary form of acknowledgment. For example, acknowledging pet loss means using realistic words like "dead" and "died" instead of euphemisms like "passed away" or "put to sleep." Concrete terms help pet owners accept the reality of their pets' deaths and begin the process of grieving. It also means saying aloud, "I know Pepper's death is a great loss for you," and "I can see how painful Pepper's death is for you." The acknowledgment of pet loss also takes place when pet owners receive condolence cards, follow-up telephone calls, and encouragement to openly express their emotions. As a helper, you can continue to acknowledge your clients' grief when, on subsequent office visits, you ask, "How have you been doing since Pepper died?" Numerous research studies show that survivors of human loss want to talk about their dead loved ones.[5] The same seems to be true for pet owners. Talking about their pets reassures them that their companion animals have not been forgotten.

When using the TEAM model, acknowledging helps build trust and rapport. As a communication technique, it is also helpful to use when clients are in the process of evaluating their problems and exploring their alternatives and resources. Acknowledgment encourages people to continue to focus on the task at hand, be it decision-making or saying goodbye. Acknowledging your clients' dilemmas, struggles, efforts, and progress lets them know that you respect and understand them. It also reassures clients that you will support their plan of action when it has begun.

Normalizing

The goal of normalizing is to lend credibility to others' thoughts, feelings, behaviors, and experiences. As we have said previously, pet loss is often a trivialized and socially negated loss. Therefore, even some pet owners are surprised by their intense feelings of grief when their companion animals die. Manifestations of grief can seem quite odd and disturbing when they are not clearly understood. It is helpful to inform clients that it is normal for a wide range of emotions to accompany loss. Normalizing grief can take place before, during, or after death. It is most helpful when supported by written or videotaped materials.

One simple way to normalize grief for clients is to provide them with what we refer to as "five minutes of grief education." By "five minutes of grief education," we mean a brief spiel that you can use regularly to explain to clients the normal manifestations and progression of grief. Creating this spiel requires you to keep a mental notebook containing basic information about the grief associated with pet loss. It also requires you to decide, on a case-by-case basis, what words and information are appropriate to use to briefly get this information across to your clients. Just as you have a spiel that you use to explain colitis, lymphoma, or feline infectious peritonitis, you can develop a standard spiel to use when educating your clients about grief.

Your five minutes of grief education should include basic information that would help normalize the grief experience for your clients. It should include, for example, information about the time frame and intensity of grief, the predictable manifestations of grief, how the grief process varies from one griever to another, and the reliable coping skills and resources available to support grievers. Depending on the animal's medical status, grief education should also give clients some ideas about planning ahead for their pets' deaths, saying goodbye, and memorializing their companion animals. In addition, you should be sure to let your clients know whether or how you plan to support them. For an example of what you might say during five minutes of grief education, see Box 7-2.

When normalizing grief, a veterinarian might say:

> "You have every right to cry and to feel lonely without Titan.
> You two were together for 12 years. You were best friends.
> It's normal to miss him."

Or,

> "It's very draining to say goodbye to your best friend. I'm not
> surprised to hear that you feel exhausted."

It is very helpful to normalize your clients' thoughts, feelings, behaviors, and experiences throughout the entire helping relationship. As a technique used in conjunction with the TEAM model, normalizing is probably most effective when establishing trust and rapport, referring clients to outside resources, and assisting them with their action plans.

Giving Permission

Giving permission means encouraging clients to voice their needs and wishes without fear of judgment. Professionals are perceived by many clients as authority figures. Therefore, clients who are intimidated by authority may hesitate to ask for what they want or to make certain requests that are important to them. For example, if they are intimidated by you, they may not ask for a soft surface on which to lay their animals, to clip some of their animals' fur, to be able to feed their pet one last time, or to be present at their pet's euthanasia. Sadly, intimidated clients may put their own pretenses and fear of embarrassment before their own wishes and regret it later.

When veterinarians offer their clients options and choices about ending

BOX 7-2

Five Minutes of Grief Education

It is appropriate to educate your clients about grief before, during, and after their pets' deaths. The basic content of your educational spiel should be adapted according to each loss situation. Information about euthanasia procedures or helping children with grief, for example, can be included when appropriate.

Obviously, information about grief is not delivered in the form of long, dry monologues. It is more common for it to be delivered within the context of a conversation, with clients responding, crying, or asking questions along the way.

Grief education is most effective when it is supplemented with written materials. The following is an example of 5 minutes of postdeath grief education. Note that the topics covered include typical grief manifestations, a time frame for grief, the individual characteristics of grief, ideas about memorializing, and referral information.

> Bill, we all experience grief when we lose an important relationship, whether our loss is a human family member or a pet, like your dog Jeanie. How feelings of grief are expressed varies from one person to the next. Somehow, though, we all find our own personally meaningful ways to get through important losses.
>
> When grieving, it is not uncommon to cry a lot—or to feel like crying a lot. You may feel sadness, depression, anger, guilt, and even some relief in response to your loss. You might find yourself uninterested in your usual activities for a while as you try to adjust to a new life without your special companion. You may also have a hard time concentrating on even the most basic tasks and your eating and sleeping routines may be disrupted. Some people find that grieving makes them feel extremely tired and they become irritable and even angry about their losses.
>
> Even as time goes by, it may be hard to accept that Jeanie is really dead. You may find that you think about her frequently and miss her deeply. You may even think you hear, see, or smell her. These sensations, these emotions, are common during times of loss. All of them are normal.
>
> Grief can be very unpredictable. One minute you may feel fine and the next minute you may feel awful. That's why there is no specific time frame for grieving. It may take days, weeks, or months to come to terms with Jeanie's death. It may take a year or longer to adapt. You'll have your first holiday season without her (your first birthday, hunting trip, competition, vacation). Those can be tough times to get through. The important thing is to find your own pace with it.
>
> Expect that others may want you to feel better before you are able, Bill. You will probably find that everyone in your family grieves in their own way. That is to be expected. You all had a different relationship with Jeanie. Your grief will be different, too.

You might find it helpful to think about some ways to memorialize Jeanie. Some people make a scrapbook of pictures or special objects. Others have a funeral, plant a tree or bush in their pet's honor, or make a donation to an animal-oriented organization in remembrance of their animal. Whatever is most meaningful to you will be the best memorial for Jeanie.

When my dog died I talked to others about how much I missed him and that seemed to help me get through the rough times. You might want some additional support along the way, too. There is a pet loss support group in town and several grief counselors who understand the special bonds people have with pets. I'd like to give you some information about them [business cards and brochures]. There are also good books available in our library about pet loss [bibliographies].

My staff and I would like to support you, too. We know Jeanie was a family member and her death has had a significant impact on your life. We want you to know that we will be thinking about you during this difficult time. How should we leave it between us? Would you like to contact us if you'd like to talk further or would you prefer that one of us call you in the next week or so to see how you are doing?

Predeath education should focus on preparation, decision-making, and predictions about how grief is likely to manifest. *Education during grief* should take advantage of "teachable moments." For example, if a client says, "I don't know why I'm acting like this. After all, Dusty is just a dog," you might say, "Yes, Dusty is a dog, but he is also your best friend. If your best human friend were dying, you'd be very upset. This situation is no different than that. It's very normal to be feeling and behaving this way." *Postdeath education* should normalize and validate grief and give grievers permission to openly express their feelings. Postdeath education is still effective when it is offered a few days after a death because clients are often in shock immediately after a loss has occurred. They also may not have consciously experienced many of the manifestations of grief.

treatments, saying goodbye, or being present at euthanasias, they sidestep intimidation and give clients permission to say and do whatever is necessary concerning the ends of their pets' lives. Examples of giving clients permission to voice their desires include:

> "It's important to me that we care for Bandit in a way that is right for you. Do you have any specific requests?"

Or,

> "I know you have a unique relationship with Bandit. If there is anything you would like to say or do for Bandit before he dies, please don't hesitate to tell me."

If, for some reason, you are unable or unwilling to permit a client to carry out a specific request, try to refer them to another resource who may be better able to help them.

Like acknowledging and normalizing, the technique of giving permission should be used throughout all four phases of the TEAM model.

Asking Questions

Asking questions goes hand-in-hand with the nonverbal skill of active listening. Through active listening, you ascertain the problem. Through asking questions, you gain valuable information about the circumstances surrounding the problem. The client's answers to your questions tell you more about the client, the situation, and the dynamics specific to this particular human-animal relationship. Questions can also help you surmise the obstacles to decision-making and what, if anything, clients want to do about their problems.

Although questions are very helpful communication techniques, they are sometimes difficult to verbalize because asking them may offend your sense of politeness or make you feel you are being intrusive. In our society, we value privacy and want to respect it. Most beginning helpers report that they hesitate to ask tough questions because they do not want to offend clients or cause them any discomfort. In reality, however, most helpers avoid asking questions because they want to protect themselves from hearing their clients' answers. For both helpers and clients, answers to emotionally charged questions may elicit emotions such as sadness or anger. They may also bring to light client requests or needs that helpers do not want to handle.

Failure to ask clients questions can lead to problems, however, because assumptions about your clients' needs hold many consequences. Problems can be avoided by specifically asking clients about what you are observing or perceiving. Asking questions about what your intuition is telling you can create short-term anxiety but can greatly reduce stress in the long-term. Examples of some questions that are particularly difficult to ask are:

"Do you have any thoughts on how far you want to go before stopping treatment?"

"Shall I start the euthanasia procedure now?"

"Have you made any plans to care for Jake's body? Would you like me to tell you about your options?"

"Mrs. Jones, you've called with a question every day for the last week. Is there something else you're wondering about, something that is difficult to talk about?"

"I understand your daughter died of the same disease. What has this been like for you?"

"How would you like to take care of your bill?"

Questions take several forms. The most helpful questions are open-ended rather than closed-ended. A closed-ended question can be answered with a simple "yes," "no," "fine," or any other one- or two-word answer. Open-ended questions, on the other hand, demand and elicit additional information. Open-ended questions create opportunities for clients to tell you about what they are experiencing, thus helping you explore and discover the intricacies of their problems.

Open-ended questions begin with "how" or "what" rather than with "why." "How" and "what" questions elicit thoughtful explanations. "Why" questions often elicit an answer of "I don't know." "Why" questions also tend to put clients on the spot and to make them feel that you are asking them to explain themselves to you. Be cautious about using open-ended questions, however, when you are working with a limited time frame. One well-placed, open-ended question can launch a lengthy client monologue. A list of sample open-ended questions is given in Box 7-3.

Because listening is vital to establishing rapport with clients and to understanding their problems, the technique of asking questions, particularly those that are more difficult to ask, is probably used most effectively during the middle two phases of the TEAM model. The more questions you ask, the more information you will have regarding your role in a TEAM-based helping relationship.

Paraphrasing

Paraphrasing is *not* parroting back exactly what has been said by another person. Parroting is annoying and, in most cases, serves no useful purpose. In a helping relationship, paraphrasing is defined as the restatement of a client's communication, in slightly different words, to test the helper's understanding of the comment. When a helper paraphrases a client's comments, it reassures the client that the message got through. It also provides the client with the opportunity to clarify his or her meaning if the helper's understanding is inaccurate. Paraphrasing gives clients the feeling of being genuinely heard and understood.

Paraphrasing is one of the communication techniques most frequently used by helpers. Different levels of accuracy and difficulty exist in paraphrasing. The first level involves the simple restatement of facts. Most people use this level of paraphrase in everyday conversations without realizing that it is a communication technique. An example of paraphrasing with the simple restatement of facts is:

Client: "My dog is a yellow lab and is 3 years old."
Helper: "Oh, you have a 3-year-old lab."

BOX 7-3

Typical Open-Ended Questions

The following questions will encourage clients to talk more openly with you.

- "What has been happening?"
- "How would you describe your relationship with Patrick?"
- "What was your goal in coming here?"
- "What is your personal experience with this disease?"
- "What is your response to all of this?"
- "What are you thinking or feeling?"
- "How do you feel about the treatment we have provided?"
- "What is your biggest concern at this point?"
- "Could you tell me more about how you came to your decision?"
- "What kinds of things will be important to you in regard to Ben's euthanasia?"
- "What are your expectations of me? of my staff?"
- "What is the most positive part for you in all that has happened?"
- "Who have you considered talking to about this?"
- "What kind of support do you have from others in your life?"
- "How can I best support you through this?"
- "We have a good sense about what Ollie needs. What do you need?"
- "What can we do to make this situation easier for you?"
- "What else would you like to discuss?"
- "How should we proceed from here?"
- "What could we have done differently?"
- "How have you been doing since Pepper died?"

The second level of paraphrase involves paraphrasing the feelings heard to determine whether the client's feelings are properly understood. Examples of paraphrasing feelings are:

> **Client:** "I'm thrilled about the success of the treatments. I never expected Muffin to respond so well!"
> **Helper:** "You sound really excited about Muffin's progress."

> **Client:** "I don't know which treatment option to chose. This is all so overwhelming."
> **Helper:** "You sound confused."

The third level involves paraphrasing the emotional content of a conversation. This form of paraphrase is particularly helpful when people are experiencing emotional crises. Persons who are under stress may attempt to cover-up their feelings or have difficulty identifying them altogether. By paraphrasing words and feelings, helpers can focus conversations on the emotions that accompany the facts. Examples of paraphrasing the emotional content of conversations are:

> **Client:** "I've had it! I can't seem to get anyone to understand what I am going through. You would think my family would be sensitive to me right now. They know how much Boots means to me. I know I am probably expecting too much, but I'm really mad about their lack of interest in this situation."
>
> **Helper:** "Now, when you need your family the most, you feel they aren't there for you. It sounds like you're hurt and angry."
>
> **Client:** "I don't know what to do. Nobody understands how hard this is."
>
> **Helper:** "It sounds like you haven't found many people who understand how important Boots is to you."
>
> **Client:** "I don't know what I will do if Boots dies while I am at work. I'll never forgive myself."
>
> **Helper:** "You're worried that she'll die without you and then you'll feel guilty."
>
> **Client:** "Boots stood by me when everyone else abandoned me. She has been so good to me."
>
> **Helper:** "No one else has loved you like Boots."

Easy ways to begin paraphrase statements are, "It seems like . . . ," "It sounds like . . . . ," or "If I hear you correctly, you feel . . . ." One simple way to paraphrase is to repeat the last few words of what a person says. This type of paraphrase indicates that you are following the conversation and signals your client to continue talking. Let us use an earlier example to demonstrate this approach:

> **Client:** "I've had it! I can't seem to get anyone to understand what I am going through. You would think my family would be sensitive to me right now. They know how much Boots means to me. I know I am probably expecting too much, but I'm really mad about their lack of interest in this situation."
>
> **Helper:** (Simply picking up the end of the sentence) ". . . and you're mad about their disinterest."

A final form of paraphrase is the summary. When summarizing conversations, what people say is condensed and then related back. Again, this technique ensures that the messages sent were heard correctly. For example, helpers might summarize all of the client statements used as previous examples by saying:

> **Helper:** "I want to make sure that I haven't missed anything. Here is what I've heard you say so far. You're feeling isolated from your family and angry at them because of their disinterest. You're fearful that Boots will die while you are at work and that would be devastating for you. Most importantly, Boots is your best friend and has been there for you during hard times. All of this sounds like it is very difficult for you."

After this, the client has the opportunity to either affirm or correct the helper's understanding of the situation.

When paraphrasing people's words and emotions, it is also important to, in a sense, paraphrase their voice tone and pacing as well. For example, if your client is loudly ranting and raving about how angry he is, you should respond in a voice that matches his in volume and energy. If you paraphrase anger using a quiet voice that is void of emotion, you are likely to elicit more anger and even sarcasm from your client. Therefore, when you are using paraphrase to establish trust and rapport, it is important to match your client's voice tone, volume, and pacing. As rapport develops, however, you can lower your voice and slow your pace. This approach will slow your client's side of the conversation as well and will create an atmosphere more conducive to helping.

For the most part, your medical training has taught you to solve problems. When you are learning how to be a helper, it is often tempting to sidestep paraphrasing and jump directly into problem-solving. Once you have made medical recommendations, however, feelings must be addressed. If they are not, clients may be afraid to share their deeper concerns.

Paraphrasing will probably sound mechanical to you at first, and this is to be expected. Just as you struggled to learn how to tie sutures, you will probably struggle a bit while you learn to use this basic communication skill. Many students and practitioners say they do not initially see the value in paraphrasing. They feel it is too simplistic and awkward to use. They are also worried that the technique might be discovered by clients. Yet, as they practice using the various forms of paraphrase, they begin to notice its positive effects on communication.

Paraphrasing is used by helpers throughout the four phases of the TEAM model. Its use is almost always appropriate. In fact, we refer to paraphrasing as a "punt mechanism." By this, we mean that when you feel you are "in over your head" and have no idea about what to say next, you can always paraphrase. Then, even if your clients realize that you cannot really "help" them with their problems, at least they feel heard and understood.

Self-Disclosure

Self-disclosure is defined as sharing personal experiences when they may be appropriate and useful to clients. When helping others with grief, self-disclosing about your own experiences helps clients feel less isolated. It also normalizes grief for clients because they learn that someone they respect and admire has also felt the effects of loss.

When you use self-disclosure, you allow yourself to be human with clients. In other words, for a moment, you drop the role of expert and expose your true self to another person. Self-disclosure occurs on both verbal and nonverbal levels. Self-disclosing statements are heartfelt and related to what is taking place. Although crying is obviously not a communication technique, tears are a prime example of self-disclosure on a nonverbal level. Verbal examples include such statements as:

> "As I stand here watching you cry I feel so much compassion for you and your family. Shortstop's death has touched us all very deeply."

> "I'll never forget what you and I have been through while trying to save this little guy."

> "Your family's struggle with the decision to help Bud die brings home to me how difficult it will be for our family to deal with the death of our old horse. These decisions are never easy."

> "I've lost two wonderful cats to the same kind of cancer. This euthanasia was really hard for me today."

> "When I am in this position with my dog, I hope I can handle it as beautifully and as openly as you have today."

It is very important to keep statements of self-disclosure brief. Don't shift the focus away from grieving clients to yourself. If you disclose something about yourself and your clients question you further, you can talk briefly about the situation, but then return to the situation at hand. This can be done by saying something like:

> "I'll be happy to tell you about my experience at another time. Let's go back to you. This is your special time with Buddy."

When it is used correctly, self-disclosure is effective during any part of the TEAM model. Because it tends to be easier for most of us to talk about ourselves than to listen to others, however, we recommend that you use it sparingly and primarily for the purposes of establishing rapport, normalizing grief, and reassuring clients regarding their chosen plan of action.

ADVANCED VERBAL COMMUNICATION TECHNIQUES

Sometimes clients become "immobilized" by their reactions to loss. In these situations, it is almost impossible for them to absorb information, to make decisions, or to grieve normally. When your case-management goals include helping clients to again become "mobilized," it is helpful to know about two advanced communication techniques that can assist you in moving cases ahead.

Gentle Confrontation

Confrontation represents an advanced form of caring. When it is used, however, it must be for the good of the client and be presented in a gentle manner. Gentle confrontation can be used to point out discrepancies or inconsistencies in what has been said or done. It can also be used to set limits on clients' behaviors or expectations and to help them adjust or "reframe" their ways of thinking. Confrontation can also be used to narrow the content of a conversation. It should not be used, however, to talk clients out of their ways of thinking.

As a communication technique, gentle confrontation takes many forms. It may be a question, indicating that what the client has said is confusing to you. It may also be a statement in which the client's belief system or interpretation of events is challenged. Here are some examples of gentle confrontation:

> **Client:** "My family doesn't care at all what happens to me or my animals."
> **Helper:** "I wonder if you really believe that? You've shared lots of special stories with me about how kind and caring your husband and children are. Do you think they would neglect you or your animals intentionally?"

Or you might say:

> **Helper:** "I hear a lot of anger in your voice and yet you say you're not angry."

> **Client:** "I could have done more to save her. I wasn't there for her when she needed me."
> **Helper:** "I try not to talk people out of their feelings, but I'm going to have to disagree with you on this one, Mary. It sounds to

me like you are being hard on yourself unnecessarily. I've seen you do this before over the last several months."

Or you might say:

> **Helper:** "What I have to tell you will be difficult for you to hear, Mary. I do think you could have done things differently and I'd like to help you learn from this situation so you won't repeat your mistakes in the future."

Clients who are dealing with loss and grief often lose sight of personal and professional boundaries. In the midst of their fear and panic, they may push the limits of the helping relationship that you have established with them. Clients in need, particularly those in desperate need, are often demanding and obnoxious. They may behave in ways that, in any other situation, they would not. As a result, gentle confrontation is a necessary part of providing grief support because it helps you set limits. With it, you can sensitively, but firmly, help clients understand the established policies of your practice. For example, you can say something like:

> **Helper:** "It's obvious to me that you are disappointed that you can't visit Nugget in the critical care unit. I know this is disturbing to you. However, I feel I have been very clear with you, from the start, regarding our policies. As I've said, we do not allow owners to visit their pets in the critical care unit because it potentially compromises the medical care given to other patients."

Sometimes, confrontation falls on deaf ears and clients either maintain or increase their demands. In these cases, the confrontation may escalate as well. For example, in answer to a client's continued badgering about critical care unit visitation rights, still using a quiet voice, you might say something like:

> **Helper:** "There are many decisions you do have control over regarding Nugget's care, such as which diagnostic tests to run, what kinds of drugs to give, which course of treatment to follow, and when to stop treatment. You do not, however, have control over our critical care unit's visitation policy. I know this is creating a great deal of stress for you and I'm sorry about that. However, If you are unable to live with our rules, I will assist you in transferring Nugget to another veterinarian."

Gentle confrontation may also be used to narrow the content of the client's conversation. Some clients ramble on about topics unrelated to animal care, making it difficult for you to cover pertinent topics with them. Clients sometimes steer conversations off track because they do not want to make difficult decisions or hear what you have to say. Gentle confrontation allows you to redirect conversations that have gotten off track. You can say, for example, something like:

> **Helper:** "I'd like to hear more about your daughter's graduation when we have more time, but we need to make some decisions about Fluffy's treatment before I move on to my next patient."

Or,

> **Helper:** "I get the sense that there is a lot you could tell me about the dog show, but I must tell you that I am most interested in discussing Fluffy's treatment."

When used effectively, we have seen gentle confrontation actually improve poor relationships between veterinary professionals and pet owners. Your willingness to be honest and forthright may actually increase your clients' respect for you because the structure imposed by setting limits and boundaries is often appreciated by clients who are feeling "out of control."

Immediacy

Immediacy is a higher level response than either gentle confrontation or self-disclosure because, as a communication technique, it combines both these features. The purpose of immediacy is to comment on the unspoken feelings or thoughts that exist within an interpersonal relationship. The use of immediacy requires you to talk openly with your clients about the experiences that you are sharing in the present moment. For example, when using immediacy, you might say:

> "Sharon, I feel like something just changed between us. Did my last comment offend or hurt you in some way?"

Unspoken thoughts and feelings may exist within helping relationships because clients want to avoid confrontations with you, protect their own feelings, or because their intense emotions keep them from identifying and speaking about what they are experiencing.

You can use immediacy in the form of a statement or a question. Here are some examples:

> "I think there is more to your story than what you are telling me because, when I just said the word cancer, you nearly collapsed out of your chair."

> "Am I correct in feeling that I upset you a moment ago when I brought up the subject of money?"

> "I feel like you and I have discussed this treatment option at length and yet you still seem confused."

"I get the feeling that you're angry with me for some reason
but I'm not sure why. Have I done something to offend you?"

Most people are accustomed to participating in indirect communication
that is geared toward protecting others' feelings. What they are unfamiliar
with is straightforward communication. Therefore, using immediacy to
directly comment on clients' thoughts, emotions, and behaviors may be
intimidating for some. Immediacy should be used within the context of a
well-established helping relationship. If it is used too soon or too harshly,
clients may feel exposed or judged and may react defensively.

CONCLUSION

Becoming an effective communicator requires practice. It takes commitment to confront sensitive issues rather than walk away from them. It also
takes dedication to ongoing skill-building and training. To that end, numerous, currently available educational programs focus on communication
skill-building. University continuing-education courses, crisis-training programs, and various weekend workshops abound. Many are offered outside the field of veterinary medicine in the realm of human services. As a
veterinarian, you can attend or send all or part of your staff for training.

When you possess the ability to communicate effectively, you maintain
confidence in your ability to move through the interpersonal crises that
arise. Whether conflicts involve clients or staff, your skills can allow you to
remain calm and assured that, no matter what happens, you will know
how to handle it. You can feel good about the work you do and about
yourself. When you are committed to ongoing, open communication with
your clients and staff, you also enjoy a more successful practice and personal life.

We close this chapter with a suggestion to you that you start practicing
the communication skills presented in this book. Use the teaching hospital
or clinic in which you work as a living laboratory for honing your skills.
Remember, as the great educator and family therapist Virginia Satir said
about communication:

> "You can read about swimming, you can watch others swim, but
> you don't really know what it's all about until you take the plunge
> yourself."[1] (p. 101)

The following case study illustrates how difficult clients are often grieving clients and how communication techniques (asking questions and normalizing grief) can often turn tense, negative veterinarian-client encounters into positive relationships.

A Case Study

Lee Gutierrez, Senior Veterinary Student

Anxieties about death aren't always directly associated with a euthanasia or traumatic death of an animal. There are occasions when just the potential of the loss of the pet, no matter how remote, may cause a person to become anxious and uneasy. The signs of apprehension may vary, but the end result is an uncomfortable, sometimes difficult, client. The concept of addressing the client's fright is just as timorous to the practitioner as is the fear of loss of a pet to the owner. However, if these fears can be confronted, the client may then be capable of coping with the situation in a clearer and more stable frame of mind.

I would like to share with you a situation where confronting the client's fear of loss of a friend not only helped the professional relationship with the client, but helped the client herself to cope with the decisions being made and the prognosis for her pet.

Mindy Brown presented with Jacque, a 4-year-old standard poodle with a history of acute seizure activity and postural deficits on the right side. Jacque was diagnosed with a 2×3 cm mass on the caudolateral aspect of the right temporal lobe of the brain. Computed tomographic enhancement was used to describe a discrete lesion. The most evident differential diagnosis for the case was meninglioma. It had several of the characteristic signs of such a neoplasia.

The next step was to determine what treatment regimen to follow in order to treat this tumor. As Mindy was initially reluctant to spend money, all the options were offered to her, including the National Cancer Institute protocol for meninglioma treatment which would be free of charge. However, suddenly money was not the issue and the life and well-being of her buddy was all that mattered. She chose surgery and follow-up radiation.

In the meantime, Mindy was very concerned to find out all that she could about the procedures being performed and the disease process that was in progress. Her manner of going about her "investigation" was to call the student on the case—me—constantly to ask questions of the surgery, radiation treatment, and the process of the disease. To oblige her, I told her as much as I felt she would understand, and some I knew she would have to look up, in an attempt to make her feel at ease with the situation. Surgery, however, revealed no discrete mass, but a relatively normal gross appearance to the brain tissue. Samples of the brain were taken and submitted for histopathology. The result of the biopsy was granulomatous meningioencephalitis, a disease process that would significantly diminish the animal's life span. Thus, the prognosis diminished even though the follow-up treatment was essentially the same.

It was at this point that the owner became difficult to deal with. She wasn't blatantly rude, but seemed to be much more insistent. Her anxieties could be felt over the phone. Per normal, the case was transferred to other students as the weeks went by. Mindy, however, continued to call me after being frustrated with the other students and the other students being frustrated with her. I had a strong idea from her concern with the diminished life span of the dog that Mindy was concerned about the dog dying, but I didn't know how to bring it up without being offensively blunt. I'm sure that I was as afraid of asking her about how she felt about Jacque dying as she was about thinking about it. It was at this point that I consulted with one of Colorado State's grief counselors.

Carolyn suggested that I simply and politely ask, "I'm going to take a chance with you, Mindy. I feel that you are frustrated and very anxious about what is happening to Jacque. Are you afraid that Jacque is going to die?" I did as was suggested and was immediately confronted with tears from the owner. We then discussed that feeling these emotions was very normal and very acceptable. She seemed finally able to pinpoint what had been bothering her, as if she herself didn't understand what was making her feel that way. We talked a bit more and cried a bit more. It was at this point that Mindy was more able to cope with what was happening to Jacque. The panic-stricken phone calls ceased and the demanding questions seemed to go by the way side.

The point made is that even though discussing death is oftentimes very difficult for both the clinician and the client, if you can take the initiative and break through your own anxieties, then the situation will be much more at ease and everyone will benefit. The clinician has developed a loyal, trusting client and the client feels much more at ease and able to cope.

REFERENCES

1. Satir, V.: The New People Making. Mountain View, Calif., Science and Behavior Books, 1988.
2. Fudin, C.E.: Basic skills for successful client relations. *In* Cohen, S.P., and Fudin, C.E., eds.: Problems in Veterinary Medicine: Animal Illness and Human Emotion, Vol. 3. Philadelphia, J. B. Lippincott, 1991, pp. 7–20.
3. Campbell, J.H., and Helper, H.W.: Persuasion and interpersonal relationships. *In* Campbell, J.H., and Helper, H.W., eds.: Dimensions in Communication: Readings, 2nd ed. Belmont, Calif., Wadsworth Publishing Company, 1970, pp. 132–137.
4. Linn, E.: I Know Just How You Feel: Avoiding the Clichés of Grief. Incline Village, Nev., The Publisher's Mark, 1986.
5. Maddison, D., and Walker, W.L.: Factors affecting the outcome of conjugal bereavement. Br. J. Psychiat., *113*:1057–1067, 1967.

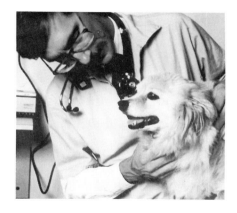

III

Veterinarians as
Helpers during Loss
and Grief

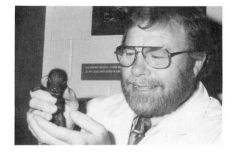

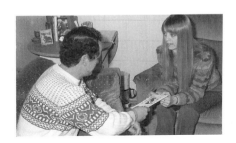

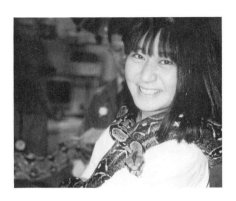

8

Helping during Small-Animal Euthanasia

In the first two sections of this textbook, you learned how to recognize significant human-animal relationships, acknowledge normal grief responses, establish a bond-centered practice, and develop helping relationships with your clients. In this section, you will learn how to apply the principles of a bond-centered practice and the communication techniques discussed previously to the procedures surrounding both small- and large-animal euthanasias.

No other medical procedure has as great an impact on you, your staff, and the quality of your veterinarian-client relationships as does euthanasia. When euthanasia is performed well, it can soothe and reassure all involved that the decision to end an animal's life was correct. However, when euthanasia is done poorly (that is, thoughtlessly or without compassion and sensitivity), it can deepen, complicate, and prolong grief for everyone.

As Andrew Edney says:

> Euthanasia management is the most sensitive time for the client-veterinarian relationship. Handled well, it is a great service to an owner who can be appreciative enough to remain a client and continue to keep pet animals. Poor technique and an insensitive attitude will do more to damage practice relationships than practically anything else.[1] (p. 217)

What constitutes poor technique in euthanasia management? Even more importantly, what do euthanasias that are conducted with compassion and sensitivity involve? This chapter attempts to answer those questions in terms of small-animal euthanasia. Chapter 9 covers the subject in terms of large-animal euthanasia. Strategies for following-up with pet owners after their companion animals' deaths and for managing your own loss-related stress are discussed in Chapters 10 and 11, respectively.

A HISTORICAL VIEW OF EUTHANASIA

It seems that euthanasia has always been an accepted part of veterinary medicine. In our research, we were unable to find any historical references or rationales specific to the time at which euthanasia was formally incorporated into the veterinary medical field, perhaps because veterinarians are not the only professionals who perform euthanasias. Research scientists, humane society workers, animal control officers, wildlife conservation officers, animal health technicians, and zookeepers also facilitate animal deaths (Fig. 8-1). In fact, many more companion animals are euthanized in our country's animal shelters than in veterinary clinics.[2] Because euthanasia is performed for different reasons and under different circumstances by

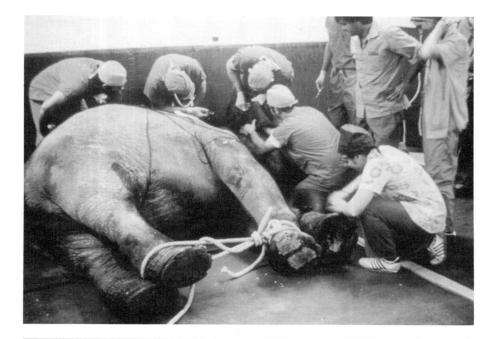

Figure 8-1 When zoo animals become ill, veterinarians work hard to save their lives. When nothing more can be done medically to save these animals, veterinarians must also help them die.

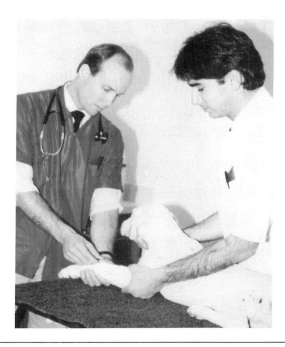

Figure 8-2 Some euthanasias occur behind closed doors, out of sight of owners, with only veterinary staff members present.

each of these groups, the moral, ethical, and emotional issues are somewhat different for each. The recommended medical procedures also vary.

Until now, most of the progress made in the area of euthanasia has been toward identifying the proper drugs and methods that can be used to induce painless and humane animal deaths.[3] Equal attention has not been paid to establishing similar humane protocols for human participation in the event. In fact, researchers and educators have only recently begun to study the moral, ethical, and emotional ramifications of witnessing and conducting euthanasia.[4,5]

In veterinary medicine, human participation (in the form of client presence at euthanasia) has traditionally been discouraged. Thus, the process has been conducted as a somewhat routine, albeit uncomfortable, medical procedure. Typically, euthanasias have been conducted in "sterile" environments with only the members of the veterinary staff present (Fig. 8-2). Contemporary veterinary medicine, however, is beginning to see euthanasia in a new light. Because of a new perspective on euthanasia, the procedure is evolving into more than a dreaded clinical task. More frequently, euthanasia is coming to be viewed, by veterinary professionals and companion animal owners alike, as both a privilege and a gift, one that can be lovingly bestowed on dying animals.

Modern veterinarians recognize client-present euthanasia as a powerful practice-builder and a potent grief-intervention tool. After veterinarians experience the profound effects of conducting euthanasias with both their patients' and their clients' needs in mind, most understand why well-planned euthanasias can be effective in building positive relationships between themselves and the pet owners they serve. Thus, many of the euthanasias performed by today's compassionate, bond-centered practitioners are conducted like ceremonies (Fig. 8-3), in which the process itself is treated with the respect and reverence that it deserves.

At some point in your veterinary career, you have probably been told that the term "euthanasia" is derived from two Greek words—*eu* meaning "good" and *thanatos* meaning "death." These words qualify euthanasia as a "good death."[6] Words such as humane, painless, and loving are also associated with euthanasia. Yet, putting these positive attributes aside, euthanasia remains, in reality, the purposeful act of terminating a life. Therefore, the euthanasias of companion animals often affect the individuals involved in intensely emotional ways.

During the last decade, progressive veterinarians, animal health technicians, and grief counselors from across the country have worked together

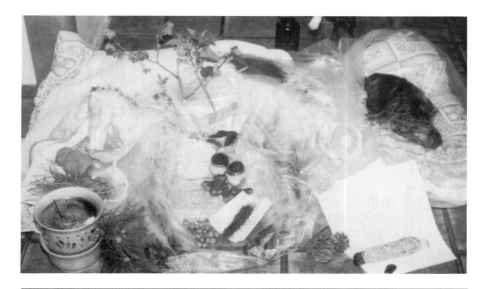

Figure 8-3 This picture illustrates how one pet owner used symbolic items to create a goodbye ceremony after her dog's death. Included in the picture are the dog's favorite toys, treats, a poem written by the owner, and some familiar items from the owner's backyard.

to create and to perfect euthanasia protocols that have both the patients' and the clients' comfort and well-being in mind. These teams of professionals have taken many variables into consideration, including the attitudes of those involved in the euthanasia process, the physical surroundings and emotional ambience of the euthanasia site, and the combination of drugs and methods used to induce peaceful and painless death. How best to prepare clients for their companion animals' deaths and how best to help them plan the circumstances surrounding the euthanasia procedure have also been studied. Protocols representing the most recent work in this important area of veterinary medicine are described in this chapter.

A NEW PARADIGM

In the old model of euthanasia, the standard operating procedure was to discuss the process as little as possible, to involve clients as little as possible, and to complete the act as quickly as possible. Euthanasia was often mentioned only indirectly or euphemistically, and clients were encouraged to simply "drop their animals off" at veterinary clinics so that they would not be burdened by the details of their pets' deaths. It was believed that this impersonal, clinical approach to euthanasia helped to protect both clients and veterinarians from addressing emotions, thus making the process as painless as possible for all involved.

This paradigm probably worked for some, but for others it created different kinds of emotional pain. For many clients and veterinarians alike, it created feelings of guilt, shame, depression, and unresolved grief. The old model of euthanasia was particularly difficult for veterinarians because it placed the bulk of the emotional burden on their shoulders. Usually, with owner's permission, veterinarians were the ones to decide *when, why, how,* and *where* animals should die. In addition, veterinarians usually refrained from formally acknowledging their patients' deaths and from contacting their clients afterward. Thus, the old model forced everyone to grieve in isolation and, in general, did not allow either veterinarians or clients to "finish" their experiences. Many of the veterinarians with whom we have spoken have expressed resentment about this overwhelming responsibility, and many clients have expressed the same emotions about their perceived lack of control over the process.

The standard operating procedure of the new euthanasia model is the exact opposite of that used in the old model. With the new model, it is more common for veterinarians and clients to discuss euthanasia together, directly, and at length. It is also common to allow as much time for the procedure as is needed and possible, to involve clients in the process as much as possible, and to acknowledge animals' deaths and to talk openly about them afterward. The new paradigm is much more congruent with the findings of research in the areas of healthy grief resolution and effective

BOX 8-1

Choices for Pet Owners

This is a sample list that can be used to facilitate the euthanasia planning process. Ideally, it should be given to pet owners several days or weeks before their pet's deaths. The following information can be used to prepare a client handout.

After you realize that the time for your pet's euthanasia is near, it is helpful to do as much planning and preparing ahead of time as possible. The purpose of this list is to make you aware of the many choices that you have about your pet's death. Please discuss any decisions about which you are uncertain with your veterinarian.

When preparing for your pet's euthanasia, it is helpful to:

- Ask your veterinarian to describe the methods and details of the euthanasia procedure.
- Decide whether or not to be present during your pet's euthanasia.
- Decide who else (if anyone) you would like to have present during the euthanasia. (If you wish to be alone during the procedure, you may still want to ask a friend or family member to accompany you to the appointment so you will have support before and afterwards.)
- Plan the logistical details of your pet's euthanasia
  When should it take place?
  Where should it take place?
  How will you care for your pet's body?
  What will you transport/bury your pet's body in if you take it with you?
- Consider a post-mortem examination. Postmortems can potentially answer the questions you may have regarding your pet's illness or injury.
- Think about how you want to say goodbye or memorialize your pet.

practice management.[7,8] Therefore, the new model is both sensitive and pragmatic.

The key word when conducting euthanasias within the new paradigm is *choice*. As much as your clients may love their companion animals, they are probably underinformed consumers of veterinary services. They may not always realize, therefore, that they have choices. For them to make wise and timely decisions when faced with their pets' deaths, they must be provided with information and choices (Box 8-1). In the new paradigm, clients are given choices about as many details as possible. The emotional burdens are shared, and, as a team, veterinarians and clients decide about when, why, how, and where companion animals should die. This paradigm fits well into a bond-centered practice.

When people make conscious choices, they feel empowered.[9] Thus, they are more likely to feel they are making decisions that are right for them. Even in loss-related crises, clients feel that they have an element of control when they are presented with options and choices to consider. As Mark Trueblood states:

> There is no set way to handle euthanasia or the death of a pet. The subject is too complex to be handled in a cookbook fashion. But a primary part of this job is being able to communicate to clients what their pet needs and when. I think the key to advising the client about the pet's condition and what choices he or she has is to be sensitive and caring, because every situation is different.[10] (p. 34)

Obviously, we use the new paradigm when making recommendations about how you can conduct euthanasias in your bond-centered practice. It is important for you, however, to remember that not all clients will want or require this kind of time or attention when euthanizing their companion animals. Based on our experiences, each client will make different choices. Some will choose total involvement and will orchestrate a fairly complex euthanasia process. Others will choose minimal involvement, opting for only a goodbye hug as they leave the examination room. All of your clients will, however, appreciate being given the option to be as actively involved as *they* choose to be in the euthanasia planning process and in the actual procedure.

THE FIRST CHOICE: DECIDING WHY TO EUTHANIZE

Animals are euthanized for various reasons. These reasons can be broadly grouped into four categories:

1. To terminate the suffering of animals who have been severely injured or who are dying from disease or illness.

2. To address behavior problems that may or may not be resolvable and that, if aggressive in nature, could present a danger to people.

3. To deal with deteriorating quality-of-life issues, in which animals may not be in severe pain, but whose existence has been compromised by loss of function due to disease or age.

4. For "convenience," in which euthanasias usually involve healthy animals for whom owners no longer want to take responsibility.

These categories are somewhat arbitrary and may overlap. For example, an animal may be ill or injured and may require extensive nursing care to recover. This animal may also suffer during the recovery process, may not be guaranteed a cure, and may require resources above and beyond those which the owner is capable of providing. If you were asked to categorize the euthanasia outcome of this situation, you might place it in category one, three, or four, depending on your personal moral and ethical beliefs. Further discussion of some of the ethical and moral dilemmas involved in euthanasias and animal deaths is presented in Chapter 14.

In this chapter, we discuss the practical methods you can use to help your clients before and during the small-animal euthanasias that you feel are justifiable. Many of these methods refer to helping clients prepare and plan for their pets' deaths. This preparatory process may occur over a period of weeks or months in cases of long-term, chronic illnesses. On the other hand, the process might be collapsed into a matter of minutes in cases of acute illnesses, injuries, or traumas. We want to focus on the ways in which euthanasias can be conducted so that your patients', clients', and staff members' needs (including your own) are all given sensitive consideration. As Patsy Mich states:

> Knowing what to expect at the time of euthanasia minimizes the client's anxiety, as well as my anxiety, so that together we can help the animal die in the very best way possible, respecting the dignity of all concerned. It is imperative that the client can live with his or her decision, that my staff is comfortable with the way the situation is handled, and that I can live with having performed this euthanasia.[11] (p. 4)

THE SECOND CHOICE: DECIDING WHEN TO EUTHANIZE

Clinical experience has shown that most pet owners instinctively know when their companion animals' battles to recover from disease or injury are over. Experience has also shown that, when veterinarians have been honest and straightforward with clients regarding their pets' conditions, veterinarians and clients tend to come to the same conclusions about euthanasia concurrently. Nonetheless, introducing the subject of euthanasia is often uncomfortable for veterinarians and companion animal owners alike. However, veterinarians must inform clients when they feel the appropriate time to consider euthanasia has arrived. After clients have decided to proceed with euthanasia, veterinarians must also take time to prepare them for what lies ahead. Research has shown that longer preparation time diminishes the intensity of grief reactions[12] and that anticipatory grief acts as a mitigating influence on postdeath grief.[12,13] Client-present euthanasias, therefore, begin with thorough preparation. Preparation minimizes the regrets, the "what ifs," and the "if onlys" that inevitably follow companion animal death.

Introducing the Subject

Many of us have experienced a parent, spouse, friend, or family member saying, "If anything ever happens to me, I want you to . . . ." Because it is frightening to think of our loved ones' deaths, we may have responded with, "Don't be silly; nothing is going to happen to you." Yet, by denying the inevitability of death and avoiding a discussion of what our loved ones' wishes are, we may make it more difficult for everyone if death-related decisions must be made in the midst of a medical crisis.

As with any discussion of death, veterinarians often have difficulty knowing when to begin talking to clients about euthanizing their companion animals. Although all clients intellectually understand that their pets will inevitably die, some may feel awkward discussing euthanasia during the same office visit in which they are being encouraged to try a new treatment option. Practicing veterinarians differ greatly in their opinions regarding the best time to introduce the subject of euthanasia. Some believe that the subject should not be mentioned until animals are near death. Others believe that it should be discussed when animals are diagnosed with terminal conditions, even if those conditions do not pose immediate threats to the animals' lives. We know a handful of veterinarians who engage clients in general discussions about euthanasia, along with discussions about other client services, during the first meeting, regardless of the nature of the office visit.

Although no right or wrong answer exists to address this dilemma, it is generally true that the more preparation time that is made available for death and euthanasia decisions, the more comfortable you, your staff, and your clients can be with the process. Companion animal death is much more of a crisis if clients have not had the time or opportunity to decide what their wishes are and if you have not been made aware of your clients' wishes.

How you refer to euthanasia, and the detail in which you discuss it, depends on each individual situation. Some case examples follow:

> Mr. and Mrs. Smith and their two children, ages 7 and 9, bring their new yellow Labrador puppy in for its first examination and vaccinations. After establishing rapport, you make the point that you take a life-span approach to animal care. This means that you and your staff will be there to support them and their family dog from the time of his first puppy examination throughout his adult health care maintenance and geriatric care. You also reassure them that, when the time comes to think about saying goodbye to their canine family member, you and your staff will assist them in making that process as meaningful as possible. As with any new client,

you take the Smiths on a tour of your clinic, showing them the euthanasia room along with the rest of your medical facility.

Your long-time client Mr. Jones brings in his 7-year-old spaniel, Buddy, who has been showing exercise intolerance while hunting. You discover a heart problem which, although manageable for now, will shorten the dog's life-span. You tell Mr. Jones that Buddy is responding well to treatment, but that the course of his condition is somewhat unpredictable. Gently, you tell Mr. Jones that Buddy may live for several months or even several years but that he is probably going to lose Buddy sooner than he had planned. You invite Mr. Jones to sit down with you and ask him if he would like a cup of tea or coffee. As you structure a more informal conversation with Mr. Jones, you ask him to tell you more about his bond with Buddy. After listening for awhile, you tell your client that you will provide Buddy with the best in veterinary care but that the time will come when, together, you and he will have to make some difficult decisions about Buddy's quality of life, as well as about his death. You present Mr. Jones with the option of learning more about your methods of conducting euthanasia now or later, when the time for decision-making is closer.

Ms. Black brings in her 17-year-old cat, Lulu, who you discover is in renal failure. Lulu's condition is not stable, and she is likely to worsen within several days. Ms. Black is a new client who has just moved to the area, so you do not have a professional history with her. As you gently stroke her cat, you tell Ms. Black that Lulu is not likely to live more than several days and that she is going to have to say goodbye to her soon. You also tell Ms. Black that, when you can do nothing more for Lulu medically, you will be there to support her emotionally and to help her decide about the circumstances of Lulu's death. As Ms. Black begins to cry, you calmly and quietly tell her that you feel it would be reassuring for her to have some information about how euthanasias are conducted in your clinic. You invite her to sit down with you, place Lulu on her lap, and ask if she would like a cup of coffee or something else to drink. Then, you hand her a tissue and, with her permission, gently proceed to describe the euthanasia process in detail, comforting her and answering her questions along the way. In conclusion, you ask if she would like to borrow a videotape that depicts the euthanasia process as you've described it, so she can more easily share this information with her family.

Making the Decision

No doubt, both clients and veterinarians struggle with the timing of euthanasia. Yet, as veterinary professionals wait and watch the companion animals whom they have grown to love and respect deteriorate, they are obligated to discuss with owners what signals to look for as death draws near. In doing so, they ease client anxieties and also accurately educate them about what lies ahead. You can facilitate your clients' decision-making processes in many ways. In fact, decision-making is an area in which use of the TEAM model and use of both verbal and nonverbal skills are appropriate. It is also an area in which maintaining a conscious awareness of the four helping roles (educator, facilitator, source of support, and resource and referral guide) that you hold with clients proves to be invaluable. Some classic examples of what you can say and do to assist clients with euthanasia-related decision-making follow:

- When clients ask, "What would you do if this was your pet?"

Clients who ask this question are looking for reassurance. Basically, they want to know whether you will support them, regardless of the decision they make. As an authority figure and a trusted professional, your approval is important to them. Rather than stating your definite personal opinion, it is probably more effective to answer with something that resembles one of the following statements. Remember to pair your words with nonverbal communication techniques.

"If Georgie were my pet, I would be as confused and as upset as you are."

"If Georgie were my pet, I would want someone to tell me that, from this point on, I couldn't make a wrong decision. I would also want someone to tell me that they would support me if I wanted to continue treatment and that they would also support me if I felt the time had come to stop. And that is what I'm telling you. I will stand behind your decision."

"Georgie isn't my pet and what I might do if she were and what you should do now are probably two different things. You are the expert on Georgie. I know how hard you've tried to save her and I know that this is one of the most difficult decisions you will ever face. However, I can't make this decision for you. I can only support you through it."

- When clients ask, "How will I know when it's time?"

Clients who ask this question are asking for guidance and structure. Anticipating death and knowing that it is near can be intimidating, overwhelming, and anxiety-provoking. Therefore, having solid, concrete information about what to watch for and what to do may make it seem more manageable. For this reason, it is not enough for you to simply answer your clients' question with, "You'll just know." If specific medical signs such as seizures, disorientation, or tenderness in the abdomen can be detected by owners, be sure to tell them. It is even a good idea to write a list of any medical symptoms that clients may encounter. Such a list can serve as an easy reminder. Beyond reviewing the medical aspects of the case, here are some suggested statements that may help clients to clarify their fears regarding their pets' final days. As always, pair these words with nonverbal communication.

> "Dorothy, one concept that may help you decide when it is time to euthanize Blue is the idea of a 'bottom line.' By this I mean a guideline by which we can measure his level of deterioration and quality of life. Now, bottom lines are different for everyone. For some, the bottom line is their pet's lack of interest in drinking, eating, or in going for walks. For others, it is the agony of watching their pet struggle to breathe or to get comfortable in bed. For many clients, the bottom line is their pet's incontinence, the inability to walk or to get up from the floor, or the inability to respond to them as before. Any of these characteristics can aid your final decision. Do you have an idea of what the bottom line might be for you and Blue?"

> "Over the next several days, you will want to try to distinguish between pain and suffering for Blue. Pain can be medicated, but suffering is much harder to remedy. If Blue is experiencing significant discomfort (a term that refers to both pain and suffering), his eyes will probably tell you. His pupils may be dilated, and his eyes may appear glossy. Also, he may not pay attention to detail, sound, or movement in the room, and he won't lift his head when you talk to him.[14] If Blue is in pain, he may cry out if you touch or try to move him. If Blue is suffering, he may be lethargic or sulky. He'll have what we call 'the ain't doing rights' and will seem sick and unhappy, as if he had the flu. When Blue seems to have more bad days than good days or even more bad hours than good hours, you'll know that, in some way, he is suffering. Fortunately, in veterinary medicine, we have the privilege of humanely ending Blue's suffering. Then, together, we can give him a peaceful death."

"I believe that you will know when it is time because Blue will tell you. You and Blue have always been able to communicate. That hasn't changed. Even now, if you get down on the floor, lay beside him, and look into his eyes, he will tell you when he is ready to go. Together, you can make the decision about when it is time to help him die."

- When clients ask, "How can I go through with this? How can I bring myself to schedule an appointment?!"

Clients who ask these questions are dealing with panic and anxiety. At this time, they need a balanced blend of freedom and structure, firmness and understanding. You can help clients to handle anxiety in many ways. One of the best ways is to assist them in thinking through the consequences of their actions (or inactions.) The following suggested statements need to be made with a soothing tone of voice and without a hint of impatience or scolding. Nonverbal communication techniques go a long way toward mitigating panic and anxiety.

"I understand that it's hard to make an appointment to euthanize Butch. It seems so final. However, I want you to know that you can change your mind and cancel if you find you can't go through with it. Let's schedule an appointment and see what that brings us."

"I know it's difficult to actually make an appointment for euthanasia. However, I want you to think about the consequences of not making an appointment. With Butch's condition, he may die at any time. Also, his death may be a fairly painful one for him and a disturbing one for you to witness. Alternatively, he may die alone, without you with him, or you may come home one day and find his body. The other fact to consider is that, if you schedule an appointment, I can assure you that Butch's death will go the way we have planned. However, if you wait until it is an emergency, I may not be the veterinarian on duty, and his death may be less than a comforting experience for you. I'd like to make an appointment during a time that I know I will be available to you. Then, if you change your mind, we'll go from there."

"I understand that by scheduling an appointment for euthanasia, you feel you are the one taking Butch's life. Sometimes I feel that way, too. However, it's important for both of us to remember that disease is taking his life and that all we are doing is sparing him a painful death. Our task now, as difficult as it is, is to shift our thoughts from providing him with quality of life to providing him with a quality death. Shall we schedule an appointment during a quiet time of day so we'll be able to help one another through this?"

Sometimes clients become "stuck" in the decision-making process and simply cannot move forward toward euthanasia. During these times, you may find yourself facing moral and ethical dilemmas if you truly feel euthanasia is in the animal's best interest. Several techniques that you can use when you feel that you must be more persuasive with clients are discussed in Chapter 13.

THE THIRD CHOICE: CLIENT PRESENCE

When we first began the Changes Program at CSU, most of the veterinarians either discouraged or did not allow clients to be present at euthanasias. When we asked the veterinarians why they adhered to this general policy, one of their common responses was, "Clients never ask me if they can be present, so I take that to mean that they don't want to be there." When we talked to clients after their pets had been euthanized, however, we heard a very different perspective. Examples of their common reactions to the issue of client presence were:

"I didn't even know I had a choice. I would have liked to have been there for Toby the way she was always there for me."

"I wanted to ask if I could be there, but I was afraid to bring up the subject. My veterinarian seemed so sure that I shouldn't."

"I thought my veterinarian would think it was sick or morbid that I wanted to be with Ginger when she died. But now I don't know what death was like for Ginger. I find myself wondering, 'was it peaceful or did she suffer?'"

"I wanted to be there, but I didn't think I could handle it. Other people have told me that it's gruesome to watch. But now, even though I know she's dead, I keep thinking maybe she really isn't. It feels like it was all just a dream."

"My veterinarian told me I shouldn't be and I figured she knew best, but now I feel guilty for not being there. It also makes me feel suspicious of her. What did she do to Max that she didn't want me to see?"

What accounts for the discrepancy in perceptions between clients and veterinarians over this issue? From the perspective of companion animal owners, veterinarians are authority figures. Even when veterinarians show great compassion, it is still intimidating for some owners to ask to be at their animals' deaths. Thus, if veterinarians do not directly offer companion animal owners the choice to be present, owners may assume they do not have this option.

Why Clients Want and Need to Be Present

Eddie Garcia has this to say about client-present euthanasia:

> For years, I encouraged clients not to be present during euthanasia because I assumed they did not want to see their animal put down. I now know the opposite is true. Recently, I contacted several of my good clients whose pets I had to euthanize in past years, and asked them if they would have preferred to be present. I was surprised when every one of them said more or less the same thing. 'I never mentioned this to you, but I wish I could have been there. I want to be there if we have to do this again.'
>
> Most clients think their veterinarians do not want them to be present when their pets are euthanized, and so choose not to ask to witness the event. I strongly believe that the client should be given the option, and so I ask them, 'Do you want to be present?" Some will ask, 'What do you think I should do?" I tell them, 'It's perfectly alright for you to be there if you want to be.'
>
> All things considered, I believe it is appropriate and beneficial to give clients the opportunity to be with their pets when euthanasia is performed. It is very important to allow a client to have a few private moments with the pet beforehand, whether or not they wish to be present at death. Most tell me how much they appreciated these last minutes to say goodbye to their pet.[15] (p. 11)

During medical treatment, it is not uncommon for veterinarians, staff members, and clients to become a team and to develop relationships based on mutual respect and trust. When treatment efforts fail and it is time to consider euthanasia, it is normal for all involved to want and need to say goodbye to the animals whom they have cared for and loved. Saying goodbye means finishing business and drawing closure to relationships. Client-present euthanasias provide opportunities to accomplish these tasks because they allow pet owners to say goodbye to their companion animals, not only before or after death, but at the moment death occurs. By being present, owners also know that the last thing their animals heard and felt were their soothing words and their loving touches. Owners and veterinary team members also have opportunities to comfort one another and to openly express personal feelings of grief. This factor is important because these two variables, support and emotional catharsis, are known to have positive effects on people's overall grief outcomes.[7,16]

Clients have several other reasons for wanting to be present when their companion animals die. A review of these reasons follows.

Preventing Long-Term Denial

One of the normal reactions to death is denial. At first, death or loss does not seem real. All of us have remarked "I just can't believe it" after experiencing not only personal losses, but on hearing about such national tragedies as the assassinations of the Kennedys, the explosion of the Challenger, or the declaration of war in the Persian Gulf. Denying that death has occurred or will occur is a normal coping mechanism. When functioning as a *healthy* coping mechanism, denial allows people to accept and adjust to loss in their own way and at their own pace. If not provided with some sort of concrete evidence that death, tragedy, or loss has actually occurred, however, people may remain in denial indefinitely. This is not healthy. Witnessing a peaceful death or viewing loved ones' bodies after death provides grievers with a sense of finality and allows their grieving processes to begin or to continue.[17,18]

Much of what is known about the importance of viewing dead bodies comes from research and clinical experience with parents of stillborn babies. At one time, infants who were stillborn were taken from parents immediately with no allowance for further contact. Now, the opposite is true. When babies are stillborn, hospital caregivers provide parents with as much contact as possible, thus making the baby and the event real to them and providing them with a focus for their grief. Today, parents are most often encouraged to see, hold, touch, and talk to their babies who have died. They are also offered mementos like a lock of hair, a footprint, the hospital bracelet, and the birth and death certificates. They are also encouraged to give the stillborn baby a name and to hold an appropriate memorial service.[19] As painful and gut-wrenching as this sounds, most who experience it agree that the searing pain is somehow comforting, healing, and far preferable to the alternative of not seeing or holding their babies.[20]

Like parents of stillborns, pet owners who are not provided with the option of viewing their dead pets' bodies may have difficulty accepting the reality of their loss. Consider this example:

> A private practitioner approached us at a state veterinary conference where we were presenting a lecture on pet loss and euthanasia. She stated that the reason she attended our lecture was to find out what she could do about a troublesome client whose dog had recently been euthanized at the owner's

request. The client was not present at the death (nor was she asked if she wanted to be) and she did not view her dog's body after his death. Several days later, the client rushed into the veterinarian's clinic and accused her of not euthanizing her dog. She was sure she had just seen it riding in a car that had passed her on the street. No amount of reassurance from the veterinarian could convince her otherwise.

As discussed in Chapter 2, it is normal for pet owners to have visual, auditory, and olfactory "hallucinations" or reactions after their pets die. For example, they may think that they hear their pets moving about in their houses or yards, hear them barking or meowing to go outside, or smell their "wet dog" or other distinctive odors. These hallucinations are normal manifestations of grief; however, these normal manifestations can escalate to levels of irrational intensity if owners are denied the choices that support and facilitate the healthy progression of grief. If the client in the case described above had been with her dog when he died, had seen his body afterwards, or had been educated about normal symptoms of grief by her veterinarian, her symptoms probably would not have led to her unfortunate and inaccurate conclusion.

Preventing Guilt about Abandonment

In Chapter 1, we mentioned that many owners feel that their pets support them through difficult times in their lives. We also discussed the fact that many owners feel that their pets have always been there for them when they needed them. Owners who feel this way, and who are denied the choice to be present at their pets' euthanasias, often feel that they abandoned their companion animals just when their animals needed them the most. The guilt associated with feelings of abandonment can last for years. Consider this case brought to our attention by one of our clients:

> When my cat Mittens was put down, I couldn't find the courage to be there. My husband advised me to just drop her off at the vet's and let him take care of it. When I did that, the vet didn't even take the time to talk with me. A staff person took my cat and disappeared with her into the back room. I never saw her again and I never heard one word from the vet. If I had known then what I know now, I would never have let Mittens die like that. I'm sure she was frightened and felt I abandoned her. I'll never forgive myself for that.

Knowing What Death Was Like

Many people have never witnessed death. Because our society shelters us from death, what we imagine death to be is often worse than the reality.

Almost every pet owner we have talked with who has witnessed their pet's well-planned euthanasia has remarked, "I had no idea it would be so peaceful. It's such a relief to know she didn't suffer."

Owners often invest a great deal emotionally and financially in caring for their pets throughout their lives. It is comforting for them to know that, at the end, they also gave their pets good deaths—ones that they saw for themselves were painless and compassionately administered.

Common Concerns of Veterinarians about Client-Present Euthanasia

You remember from Chapter 2 that most of us are relatively uninformed about what grief is like and about the ways in which we can help grieving persons. One of the common myths about grief is that we can spare people pain by protecting them from a painful experience. Without question, it is emotionally painful for owners to watch their dearly loved companion animals die; however, clinical experience with owners has shown that *not* being present when companion animals die potentially increases feelings of pain and distress. It also has shown that being present can facilitate resolution of the loss and the grieving process. The words of Cecelia Soares bear this out:

> As difficult as it may seem to veterinarians who are involved, it has been my experience that clients who are present at the euthanasia of their pet are less likely to have problematic grief reactions, including nightmares and unpleasant waking fantasies. Being present also defuses myths about the euthanasia process, although clients need information prior to the procedure to prepare them for the effects of the death process.[21] (p. 3)

The veterinarians with whom we have spoken seem to have five basic concerns about client-present euthanasias. Brief descriptions of these concerns follow.

There May Be Negative Effects on Animals

Veterinarians worry that if owners become emotionally upset while present at euthanasia, they may negatively affect the behavior and increase the anxiety levels of their animals. Subsequently, animals who become frightened may become more difficult to handle, thus making the euthanasia procedure more difficult to complete.

Something May Go Wrong with the Procedure

Veterinarians are concerned that, if animals become more difficult to handle, something is more likely to "go wrong" during the euthanasia procedure. Specifically, veterinarians are concerned that animals may struggle or cry out. Veterinarians may also feel that, in the midst of a difficulty, they might miss the venipuncture or make a mistake in front of their client.

Clients May Not Cope Well

Many veterinarians question the efficacy of their clients' coping skills. They reason that, if clients cry and exhibit emotional distress when simply discussing their pets' deaths, the actual witnessing of their companion animals' deaths may be more than they could handle. Veterinarians fear clients may faint, get sick, or even become hysterical if present during euthanasia.

Veterinarians also worry about the effects of client-present euthanasias on their clients' perceptions of them and their practices. They fear that clients will only remember images of their pets' deaths and that those images will overshadow and negate all other good memories. One common fear is that clients will forever associate their veterinarians with sad experiences and their pets' deaths. Thus, clients will avoid their painful memories by switching veterinarians.

It Will Take Too Much Time

The fourth concern of veterinarians is that client-present euthanasias will take too much of their time and be too emotionally draining for them and the members of their staffs. They fear that these experiences will be so demanding that they will not be able to continue with their normal case loads.

I Might Cry

The final concern that veterinarians have is that, if they allow clients to be present at euthanasias and actually witness their clients' open expressions of grief, their own feelings of grief will be triggered. Many veterinarians feel that crying in front of clients is unprofessional and inappropriate. These veterinarians also express concern that, if they are upset, they will not know what to say or do to help their grieving clients.

Although all of these concerns are legitimate, the experiences of veterinarians who conduct client-present euthanasias suggest that, when euthanasias are well-planned and facilitated, the opposite of what these fears and worries predict actually happens. When both patients and clients are adequately prepared for euthanasia, these difficulties *rarely* occur. If they do occur, clients have been prepared to face them.

Veterinarians can do several things to ensure that their fears will not be realized. For example, to guard against patients struggling if they are very rambunctious, they can lightly sedate animals as soon as they arrive at the euthanasia site or, alternatively, ask owners to give their animals a mild medication before coming to the clinic. The use of a catheter also minimizes the possibility that "something will go wrong."

Many people, including veterinarians, do cry during euthanasias, but it is important to remember that open displays of emotion are normal responses to loss and grief. People who display intense emotion usually just need permission to express their feelings and to be reassured that they are normal and "OK." This principle also applies to veterinary professionals. One of the most frequent comments we hear from clients is, "It meant so much to me that the doctor cried, too. I could tell how much my pet meant to her."

Client-present euthanasias take more time; however, when client-present euthanasias are well-planned and sensitively conducted, no other part of veterinary medical care engenders more loyalty to your practice. When clients are given choices, have their emotional needs anticipated and met, and witness their pets dying while surrounded by people who love and care about them, they are forever grateful. During lunch one day, two veterinarians practicing in the Denver area told us that nothing seems to matter to clients more than how they conduct euthanasia. We could not agree more. These veterinarians feel their advocacy of client-present euthanasia has had a definite positive effect on building their clientele (Box 8-2).

Most veterinarians have been trained to offer treatment choices to clients, from the "Cadillac version" to the bare minimum. For the same reasons, clients should be offered similar choices when their animals die, ranging from being present for euthanasia to viewing the body after death. These choices should be offered in a neutral manner, with information presented regarding advantages and disadvantages. It is not fair to your clients to say "Well, you can be there if you *really* want to be, *but*. . . ." We have encountered clients who changed veterinarians after learning that other practitioners would indeed offer them choices about their presence at euthanasia.

Although client presence has value, encouraging client presence must be done with care. You should never aggressively talk a client into being present at a euthanasia. Some clients very clearly decide to leave their animals in their veterinarian's hands to be euthanized. This option is as acceptable as any other, and clients should not be deterred from this decision when their choice is an informed one.

Some owners want to be present or feel that they "should" be present at euthanasia but doubt their abilities to do so. They may have been told by friends or family members that they "shouldn't put themselves through

BOX 8-2

Letter from a Client after Her Pet's Euthanasia

June 17, 1991

Dr. Rod Straw
Laurel Lagoni, M.S.
Angela, Senior student
CSU Veterinary Teaching Hospital
Fort Collins, CO 80523

Dear Friends,

   I want to thank you all for the fine care you gave Titian. More importantly, I want to tell you how grateful I am for the sensitivity and compassion you offered to us at the time of euthanasia. Your gentle understanding and careful explanations helped me to deal with a difficult decision. Your willingness to provide options for me and Titian turned what I feared would be a very difficult clinical and disturbing experience into one that brought both peace and acceptance.

   I learned a great deal that day about loss. I know now that even out of great grief and pain, something wonderful can happen. I am changed because of the experience and better able to reconcile this loss and others to come. It seems Titian gave me one last gift—a better understanding of myself. I am so glad I was there for her as well. Despite the emptiness in our family, I know that because of your warmth and support, I left having gained more than I lost.

   If ever a day passes when you doubt or despair about a job well done, remember me and Titian and know that you made a valuable difference in our lives. Your deep respect for life and animals brings great comfort to those you serve.

Many thanks,

Karen Shaw
and family

that.'' They also may fear that death is too frightening to witness based on beliefs they have held since childhood. These kinds of misconceptions about euthanasia are damaging to the field of veterinary medicine. They imply that the methods used are less than humane. It is important to pet owners to know that their animals' deaths are facilitated with sensitivity and compassion. Thus, in these cases, it is the veterinarian's responsibility to describe the euthanasia experience so that owners can make educated and informed choices.

Explaining the Procedure

To decide whether or not to be present, clients usually need information about what the actual euthanasia procedure entails. The veterinarian's role during this time is to provide detailed information about the process of euthanasia and to exhibit nonjudgmental support during the decision-making process. For instance, attending veterinarians at the CSU Veterinary Teaching Hospital consistently provide owners with information similar to the following. Altogether, these explanations take about 10 minutes. It should be emphasized that this information is not delivered in a dry, continuous monologue because, during the veterinarian's explanations, it is not uncommon for owners to cry or to interrupt with questions.

> "Mary, we know that Pepper is very important to you and to your family. Therefore, we are committed to making this experience as meaningful and as positive for you as possible. To decide whether or not you want to be with Pepper when he dies, you need accurate information about euthanasia. Would you like me to explain the procedure to you now?" With the owner's permission, the veterinarian continues.
>
> "The first thing we may do in preparation for Pepper's euthanasia is to take him back to our treatment area, shave a small area of fur, and place an intravenous catheter in a vein, most likely in one of his rear legs. The use of a catheter simply means that we can administer the euthanasia solution more smoothly. It also means that we can accomplish what we need to accomplish without interfering with your desire to pet or to hold Pepper's head and front paws.
>
> "After this, Pepper will be brought back to you, and you will be given time to spend with him, if you so desire. Then, when all of us agree that it is time to proceed, we will begin the euthanasia process. The method we prefer to use involves three injections (Fig. 8-4). The first is merely a saline solution flush. This insures that the catheter is working. The second is a barbiturate, usually thiopental, which places Pepper into a soothing state of relaxation. The third injection is the euthanasia solution, usually pentobarbital sodium. This injection will actually stop Pepper's heart, brain activity, and other bodily functions, and ultimately cause his death. Many people are surprised by how quickly death takes place as it occurs within a matter of seconds.
>
> "You should also know that, although humane death by euthanasia is painless and peaceful, Pepper may urinate, defecate, twitch, or even sigh a bit. He will not be aware of any of this, however, and he will not feel any kind of pain. In addi-

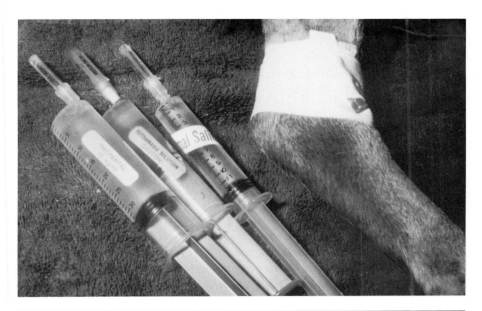

Figure 8-4 Three injections (saline solution, thiopental, and pentobarbital sodium) are given during the euthanasia procedure. A catheter is placed in the animal's rear leg to facilitate the smooth injection of drugs. This also allows the owner to stay by the animal's head and front paws during the procedure.

tion, Pepper's eyes may not close. Do you have any questions about any of this?" If the owner expresses understanding, the veterinarian concludes with, "Mary, after Pepper has died, you can stay with his body for as long as possible."

This explanation is greatly enhanced when the conversation is conducted in a private, quiet setting with both owners and veterinarians sitting or standing at the same eye level. It is also enhanced when veterinarians show their sense of compassion by offering tissues or gentle touches to owners who cry or openly express their feelings.

If clients are interested, veterinarians can provide them with a tour of possible euthanasia sites. For example, your clinic may have a special room or an inviting outdoor area that clients would appreciate seeing. In addition, the American Animal Hospital Association offers a videotape portraying a version of client-present euthanasia similar to the one described in our example. It is called "The Loss of Your Pet." Clients can view this tape while they are at the clinic, or they can check it out for viewing at home. The clients we know who have toured clinics or viewed videotapes tell us that they have found these visual representations to be extremely helpful. Knowing what to expect helped to calm their anxieties about being present at their companion animals' euthanasias.

THE FOURTH CHOICE: EUTHANASIA LOGISTICS

The fourth group of choices clients face when preparing for euthanasia is planning and agreeing on the logistic details of the procedure. For example, appropriate times and settings for the procedure must be determined. Owners must also decide who else, if anyone, they want to accompany them to the euthanasia. With proper preparation, for example, children often choose to be present when their companion animals die. See Chapter 12 for more information on children and pet loss.

As more and more clients choose to be present when their pets are euthanized, careful planning is required by you and your staff. A euthanasia that occurs smoothly and with compassion and sensitivity does not just happen passively (Box 8-3). It requires members of the clinic staff working together as a team. Examples of how things can go wrong without prior thought or planning are illustrated in the following case examples. The names we use are fictitious, but all these examples actually happened:

> At the ABC Pet Clinic, client-present euthanasias are done in one of the boarding wards. The receptionist showed Julie Munson to the room where she was left sitting on the bare, concrete floor with her dying dog while waiting for the veterinarian to perform the euthanasia. After several minutes, the veterinarian entered the room, and without first speaking to Julie, attempted to remove an upset and aggressive cat from one of the cages in the same room. Muttering that he needed to return this cat to an impatient owner, the veterinarian lost his temper and began poking the cat through the door of the cage with a broom handle. Not only did Julie have to wait for her dog to be euthanized, she also had to contend with commotion and insensitivity as she attempted to say her last goodbyes to her dog.

> Tom Martin took his cat to the XYZ Clinic to be euthanized because the cat was old and ill. As the veterinarian attempted to inject the drug into a leg vein, the cat became frightened and began to struggle. In the ensuing struggle, the cat's leg was broken as the veterinary staff attempted to restrain it. Rather than giving his cat a painless, humane death, Tom Martin now feels that he betrayed his cat by choosing euthanasia.

BOX 8-3

Insensitivity toward Clients

After 38 years of practice, it wasn't until I retired that I became aware of an insensitivity toward clients that had not occurred to me while in the situation. It was brought to my attention by a friend who had taken her cat to be put to sleep after an extended illness. She asked, "Why didn't they prepare me for what was to happen?"

What she hadn't understood was why they clipped the hair from the leg, why they 'held the cat down,' as she perceived it. And why had no one told her that there might be muscular twitching after it was dead, that the eyes would remain open, and that it would not be cold for sometime afterward? She had been very reluctant to bury a warm cat with open eyes.

These are things veterinarians understand, of course, and in my practice days I answered client's questions as they arose. But it never occurred to me to explain to each client all the details if they were to watch the euthanasia or bury the pet at home. Perhaps others who have been equally negligent might take note.

Helen E. Rider, DVM
Beaverton, Oregon

From: Letter to the editor, J. Am. Vet. Med. Assoc., 195:852, 1989.

At their veterinarian's suggestion, John and Mary Carr scheduled an appointment to euthanize their dog during the lunch hour. As the veterinarian had told them, this was usually her slowest time of day and the time during which she would best be able to help them. When the Carrs arrived for their appointment, they were shown to an examination room. They were then told that the doctor was running late and would be back from lunch very soon. When the veterinarian did arrive soon afterwards, she was carrying a bag and a beverage from a fast-food restaurant. She greeted them with happiness in her voice and a bounce in her step and said, "I hope you don't mind if I finish my lunch while I do this. I have another appointment scheduled right after this one." Needless to say, the Carrs were deeply offended by the veterinarian's flippant attitude and never went back to her.

None of these emotionally painful and ethically questionable situations should have occurred. They are examples of thoughtlessness and poor technique. They represent how *not* to conduct client-present euthanasias. The proper ways in which to prepare for client-present euthanasias are described further in the following sections.

Appointment Times

Ideally, euthanasia appointments are scheduled for the least busy parts of the day, such as early morning, during a lunch hour, the last appointment in the afternoon, or even after hours. Think of yourself as well as your client when you schedule appointments, however. Client-present euthanasias take a certain amount of energy and, if you usually collapse with fatigue after 4:00 P.M., you will feel more like attending to clients during an earlier part of the day. Clients who bring their animals to the clinic for a euthanasia appointment should be given first priority over everything else except medical emergencies. They should also be immediately escorted to wherever the euthanasia will occur.

Location

Clients should never be left to sit in a busy waiting area. Instead, they should be taken to the previously agreed on euthanasia site. In a bond-centered practice, it is most likely that this site would be an examination room, especially equipped with some or all of the features described in Chapter 6. If you and your staff have prior knowledge regarding what your client will want and need during the procedure, the site can be prepared

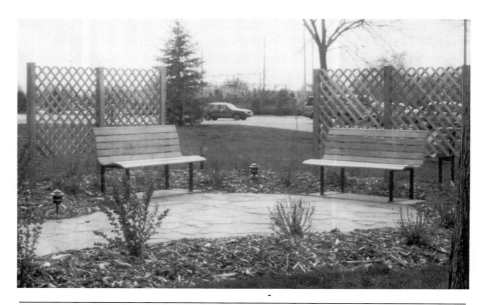

Figure 8-5 Many clients whose animals have always loved the outdoors (or hated the veterinarian's office) are comforted when they can help their animals die in nonclinical, natural settings.

BOX 8-4

A Ceremonial Home Euthanasia

This is an excerpt from a letter written by a veterinarian practicing in Colorado Springs, Colorado. It is a good example of what veterinarians need to be prepared to address during home euthanasias. It also shows that emotional ceremonies can be healing for all who are involved.

I had an *experience* last Thursday night with an in-home euthanasia that was incredibly moving. I'll briefly detail it: Dijin was a 15½ year old Malamute who clinically was demonstrating hind limb ataxia progressing into paralysis. He was bright and alert although he had moments of loss of clarity. . . . The owners decided, with a great deal of courage, mixed with sadness and mingled with fear, that the quality of Dijin's life had reduced sufficiently for them to desire that he be put to sleep in the home. They desired a ceremony, which consisted of placing Dijin in his favorite spot in front of the fireplace, and us all eating dinner surrounding him, offering him bites off our plates. Then, when we had finished, we lighted candles and . . . all joined hands. . . . His "mom" read a statement. She had written a farewell living eulogy for Dijin and all of us were weeping. I tried to set a catheter (Butterfly) in Dijin's leg, but he was resisting. So, I gave him a tranquilizer of xylazine (1.5 mg/#) and Ketamine (1 mg/#) into a lumbar muscle. After he settled down, I was able to place the catheter. I then spoke of Dijin's strong spirit being too powerful for his physical body and related a personal story of my own Malamute's death, under circumstances out of my control. I praised Dijin's mom for her courage to do the right thing for Dijin even in the face of her own painful loss of his presence. . . . I stayed for another hour after his physical death as we cried and wept and spoke of Dijin and spoke of our own special memories. They kept his body and hand-carried it themselves to the Humane Society for cremation and to save the ashes, intending to use the ashes to fertilize the soil in their garden. . . . I hope this account moves you as much as experiencing it affected me. The only loss in this work is the physical presence of Dijin. In all other respects, all of the people involved grew with their love and their grieving.

ahead of time. For example, if you know your client would prefer that the euthanasia take place outside, you can place tissues, handout materials, and some type of covering for the ground outdoors beforehand (Fig. 8-5).

Some veterinarians find that many of their clients prefer euthanasias to be conducted at their homes. Thus, they are offering home euthanasia as a special service. Because you are performing this service on someone else's "turf," we strongly recommend that home euthanasias be conducted by a team of at least two veterinary professionals. We also recommend that they be done after regular office hours. Typically, following these guidelines requires you to expend more of your time and manpower, so we also

BOX 8-5

Checklist for Euthanasia Materials

Clients sometimes wish to have their pets euthanized outdoors or in their own homes. If you are going to be traveling away from your clinic to conduct euthanasias, take an abundance of supplies. It is always better to be overprepared than underprepared.

Use the following checklist to ensure that you will be adequately prepared for all euthanasias taking place in locations other than your clinic exam rooms.

- Clippers and blades—be sure that the plugs on your equipment will work with any kind of electrical outlet (grounded or not grounded). Carry an adapter to ensure success in any situation.
- Scissors and tape.
- Alcohol and 4 × 4s—you may also need a surgical scrub to prepare the skin for an intravenous catheter.
- Intravenous catheters and caps—take various sizes and types of catheters. Some catheters work better than others depending on the age and condition to the animal being euthanized.
- Syringes and needles—overestimate the number that you may need.
- Heparinized saline flushes—overestimate the amounts that you need.
- Tranquilizers—for example, acetylpromazine 0.11 to 0.25 mg per pound, intravenously.
- Euthanasia solutions—for example, thiopental sodium, 8 mg per pound by slow intravenous infusion before sodium pentobarbitol, 40 mg per pound by intravenous infusion.
- Fleeces, rugs, or blankets—lay pets on soft surfaces and partially cover them if there are injuries or surgical incisions. Bring something to transport the body in if you take it with you after death.
- Facial tissues, printed materials, business cards—anything relevant to grief education or to making referrals.

Adapted from *The Understanding Client Pet Loss* workbook in the American Animal Hospital Association's Educational Videotape Series on Pet Loss and Bereavement, p. 16.

suggest that you charge accordingly. We have found pet owners to be very understanding about the extra effort required and willing to pay more if the service is provided at a reasonable charge. The two most important things to remember about conducting home euthanasias are to be prepared to address strong emotions and to take multiple quantities of anything and everything you might possibly need for the procedure so you will not be caught without a needed item. An excerpt from a description of an emotional, ceremonial home euthanasia and a sample materials list are provided in Boxes 8-4 and 8-5, respectively.

Procedural Details

Regardless of where the euthanasia occurs, procedural matters should be addressed before the day of euthanasia if possible. Consent forms (Fig. 8-6) should be signed, and arrangements for payment should be made. If yours is a trusted client, a bill can even be sent after the event. However, *do not* include a bill with a condolence card or letter. Before the appointment, you should also suggest to owners that they bring a friend or a less-involved

---

EUTHANASIA/POST-MORTEM/
CREMATION RELEASE
Veterinary Teaching Hospital
300 West Drake Road
Ft. Collins, Colorado 80523   WEIGHT:_____
(303) 221-4535

We understand that the death of an animal can be an emotionally difficult time. With that in mind, your compliance in filling out this form is much appreciated. Be advised that you have the right to be present at this animal's euthanasia, if you so desire. Grief counseling (Changes program) is also available to you at your request. _____

Animal's Name_____
                                                                BRAND   TATTOO
I certify that I am the owner, or authorized agent of the owner, of the above named animal. I release the above named animal to Colorado State University's Veterinary Teaching Hospital for:

                                                                                                                          FEES

1. Euthanatize (stop life of) my animal and.. YES   NO

    a) Return the body to owner/agent for burial... YES   NO

    b) Veterinary Teaching Hospital will dispose of the body............................. YES   NO

    c) Cremate the body... YES   NO_____

        cremains returned to owner... YES   NO

        cremains returned to owner in an urn.. YES   NO_____

        cremains shipped to owner.. YES   NO
        (must be shipped if outside of Ft. Collins)

        cremains disposed of by the Veterinary Teaching Hospital............. YES   NO

        cremains returned to Dr._____

2. Perform a post-mortem examination (autopsy).. YES   NO

Has this animal bitten, seriously scratched, or exposed anyone to rabies within the past ten days?........ YES   NO

If insured, has the insurance company release for euthanasia been obtained?.. YES   NO

To the best of my knowledge, the information I have provided on this form is true. I understand that my wishes will be carried out immediately upon signing this agreement. Fees for these services have been explained to me.

Owner/Agent signature_____Date_____

Owner/Agent verbal/telephone release obtained by_____Date_____

Witness' signature_____Date_____

Euthanasia performed with _____Time_____Date_____
                                    (Drug used and amount)

Clinician's signature_____

Figure 8-6 The euthanasia consent form used by the Colorado State University Veterinary Teaching Hospital.

family member with them for support and also to assist them with the drive home.

Saying Goodbye and Memorializing

Clients should be encouraged to think about the ways in which they want to say goodbye to their pets before death. Many owners want to spend special time with their pets, engage in favorite activities, take pictures, or make videotapes of their companion animals. When they are prepared for death, the last days owners spend with their pets, when they know that their time together is short, can be very special and can become some of their most treasured memories.

Some pet owners also want to make plans to memorialize their pets. Memorializing helps to bring meaning to loss and helps to draw closure to relationships.[19] There are countless ways to memorialize companion animals. Several of these are explained in Chapter 10.

Body Care

Whenever possible, decisions about body care should also be made before euthanasia. Owners should be offered all of the options available to them, and each should be explained with honesty and sensitivity (Box 8-6). The cost of each option should also be disclosed. It is helpful to use visual aids during this explanation. For example, if veterinarians make caskets or urns available for owners to purchase, samples can be shown to them (Fig. 8-7).

Body care options can be explained by either veterinarians or technicians. Again, it is important to emphasize that this information is not delivered in the form of a dry, continuous monologue, given that owners often respond to it by crying or by asking several questions. When offering body care options for small animals, veterinarians and staff at the Colorado State University Veterinary Teaching Hospital say something like:

> "Mary, we can offer you three options for taking care of Pepper's body after he dies. The first option is that you can take him with you and bury him in a pet cemetery or in another appropriate place. If that is your choice, we encourage you to bring something in which you will feel okay about transporting his body. This might be a blanket or a box. We also have caskets available if you would like one.
>
> "Second, we can cremate Pepper's body and either dispose of the cremains for you or return them to you, if you so desire. If you want them returned to you, you may want to choose an urn or another kind of container. Some people like

BOX 8-6

Options for Body Care

Various body care options available for companion animals are explained below. Because costs vary dramatically across the country, estimates are not included in this figure. However, this information should always be provided to clients during their decision-making process. Understanding the methods and costs involved with each of these options allows clients to make informed choices. The following information can be used to prepare a client handout.

An animal's body is cared for depending on the owner's wishes and circumstances:

Burial

Home: A pet owner who lives in a rural area or in a community that allows home burials for animals should be advised that an animal's remains should be placed in a thick liner bag inside a container that can be sealed. The body should then be buried at least 3 feet in the ground, away from any water sources. These precautions diminish the likelihood that other animals will dig at a pet's grave.

Cemetery: When home burials are impossible, pet cemeteries provide the pet owner with a final resting place for a pet. Many pet cemeteries offer options ranging from simple burial to complete funerals. They also provide caskets. Almost all pet cemeteries will send a representative to pick up an animal's body. A pet owner may choose to make arrangements for a pet directly with the cemetary or work through a veterinarian.

Communal: Some pet owners elect to care for their pets' bodies without ceremony. Therefore, they choose communal burial. This means that their animals are buried along with others, usually on the grounds of a pet cemetery, humane organization, or city landfill. Wherever the burial site, it is important that pet owners who choose this option are told the truth about it.

Cremation

Individual: Individual cremation is increasingly popular among pet owners. With many people renting homes or planning future moves, cremation provides a way for them to keep their pets' cremains with them. Owners have two choices with this body care option. That is, to have a pet's cremains returned to them or not returned. If returned, many owners preselect an urn or other special container in which to permanently place their pet's cremains. Alternatively, other pet owners choose to ceremonially bury or scatter their pet's cremains during a memorial ritual. If a companion animal was a family pet, cremains are often divided among various family members, allowing each to maintain a bond with the pet. Many crematories allow owners to be present while pets are being cremated, thus showing respect for an owner's wishes.

Communal: When it is not important to an owner to have a pet cremated individually, several pets can be cremated en masse. The cremains are then distributed by the crematory. Most crematories bury or scatter the cremains, either on the grounds of their business or in natural settings.

Box continued on following page

Rendering

When large animals die, it is very difficult to bury them and very expensive to cremate them. Because of these difficulties, most people send their horses, llamas, mules, cows, and so forth to rendering plants. These businesses use animals' bodies for animal foods, fertilizers, and even kitty litter. Rendering is a way to reuse or recycle animals' bodies after they are dead.

to keep their companion animals' cremains and some like to spread them in an appropriate location. Because so many people today move quite often, many owners choose cremation so they can take their companion animals' cremains with them. Some clients find it useful to see what cremains look like. It helps make their decision real. Are you interested in seeing some cremains?" If clients answer yes, show them an urn containing some cremains. Be sure to explain whose cremains they are.

"Your third option, Mary, is to have us take care of his body for you. Although I wish I had a more aesthetically pleasing option to offer you, my only option is _____." (Veterinarians should fill in the blank with whatever is accurate, usually mass incineration, mass burial, or delivery to a rendering company.)

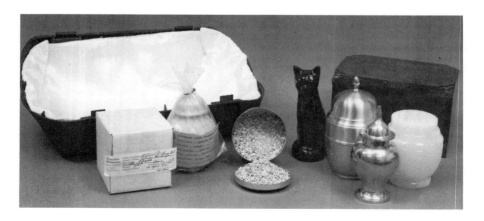

Figure 8-7 Veterinary professionals can use brochures, pictures, and sample items (for example, caskets, urns, cremains) when helping pet owners make decisions about body care. If you do not have access to a pet crematory, check with the human mortuary or crematory in your area. Many are also willing to cremate pets but may not advertise the service.

Because most mass burials occur in landfills, owners should be given this information. If it is accurate, owners can be told that an area of the landfill is set aside for animal burial. Clinical experience has shown that, for some owners, after their companion animals are dead, their bodies no longer have meaning for them. Typically, these owners have no objections to mass burial in a landfill. In fact, when given the option of mass burial at the city landfill, one client quipped, "That's perfect for my dog. His favorite thing to do was to get into the garbage!"

Because the thought of burying their companion animals at the landfill might be abhorrent for other owners, however, veterinarians have an ethical responsibility to offer this information to anyone who considers this option. Clinical experience has shown that the omission of pertinent details often serves to complicate owners' grief. For example, an elderly woman who decided to have her veterinarian dispose of her dog's body was simply told that her dog would be buried in a mass grave. A month after her dog's death, she contacted her veterinarian and told him she wanted to know where the mass grave was located so she could visit her dog. At that time, the veterinarian reluctantly told the woman that the mass grave was located at the landfill. The woman found this information extremely upsetting and told the veterinarian that, had she known this during her decision-making process, she would have certainly chosen another body care option. Based on this miscommunication, the woman chose to take her business to a different veterinarian when she adopted another dog 6 months later.

Necropsy

At times, it may be desirable to perform necropsies on animals who have died. For example, you may have a patient who dies unexpectedly, without obvious cause, or a client who wants a definitive diagnosis regarding their companion animal's disease. Necropsy is important because it can potentially provide everyone involved with some answers about why an animal died. This information is also often desired out of concern for other companion animals living in the household. When necropsy is warranted, the option must be tactfully introduced and explained to clients. Several points are relevant to tactful discussions of necropsy.

Most pet owners are unfamiliar with the term necropsy and have more understanding of the term autopsy. Researchers suggest that "postmortem examination" is an even more acceptable term for lay people than is autopsy.[22] Whatever word you choose to use, you are more likely to receive your clients' cooperation if they have a thorough understanding of the benefits of the procedure.

For example, owners may be told that postmortem examinations provide the last opportunity to potentially learn all of the facts about their animal's illness and cause of death. They may also be told that it is some-times easier to accept death, or the decision to euthanize, when everyone knows that death was inevitable. Do not rely on this last rationale too heavily, however, because it can lead to further complications if the results of the postmortem do not agree with your diagnosis or if an answer is not found. For some pet owners, another benefit of necropsy is that knowl-edge of the cause of death is often necessary for settling insurance or legal matters.

Some owners are comforted when they are reminded that both human and veterinary medicine can benefit from necropsies, especially if nearby universities are researching problems that pertain to a patient's case. This aspect of necropsy may be especially appealing to breeders who want to attempt to eliminate certain predispositions for established heritable dis-eases from their blood lines. When considering necropsy for research pur-poses, however, owners must be informed that certain precautions may be required so that the research value of the tissue is not inadvertently de-stroyed. For example, some euthanasia solutions and some methods of tissue preservation, such as freezing, may alter some necropsy results. Thus, the procedures you may need to follow might not allow them to have the kind of goodbye they desire with their pets. If your clients like the idea of contributing to research, be sure to consult your pathologist so that a realistic post-mortem plan can be established before the euthanasia.

The last option you need to explain to pet owners is the concept of cosmetic necropsy. In cosmetic necropsies, only selected tissues are re-moved. Cosmetic necropsies are usually recommended when an owner wants to attempt to obtain a diagnosis, but also wants a pet's body re-turned for burial. It is extremely important to let owners know, however, that cosmetic necropsy will potentially hinder the pathologist's ability to evaluate pertinent tissues and may ultimately preclude a definitive diagno-sis. In a cosmetic necropsy, tissue that is removed is often replaced with crumpled newspapers or paper towels, and the incision is then sewn to-gether. Animals are also cleaned of blood and body fluids. It is important to check the suturing to insure that bodies don't "leak" after they are returned to owners.

Whether necropsies are complete or cosmetic, they should never be done without owners' knowledge or permission, and owners should never feel that they were bullied or "talked into" agreeing to the procedure. After they have agreed, owners should be informed of the results *as soon as possible*. Quite often, preliminary results can be obtained within a few days. Final results, however, can take much longer and owners should be made aware of this fact.

To explain the concept of a postmortem examination, David Getzy, CSU pathologist, suggests you say something like:

"The postmortem examination involves looking at the external and internal organs of the animal and includes opening of the body and body cavities and dissection of the tissues." (Getzy, D., Personal communication)

Getzy feels that this explanation is vague enough not to bring up morbid visions but sufficient to let owners know that a postmortem examination is an invasive and implicitly destructive procedure.

BOX 8-7

Checklist for Euthanasia Procedures

Several steps facilitate client-present euthanasias. The categories used here are somewhat arbitrary but can be used by veterinarians to assist clients with the process.

Before the procedure, it is helpful to:

- Inform clients that the time to consider euthanasia has arrived.
- Educate clients about the methods you use to facilitate the process.
- Prepare clients for what may happen during the procedure (possible side-effects, their own grief manifestations).
- Offer clients a choice about being present.
- Help clients plan the logistic details of euthanasia (where, when, body care, body container, bringing a friend for support).
- Offer reading materials, videotapes, tours.
- Ask clients to sign consent forms and pay their bills ahead of time.

During the procedure, it is helpful to:

- Ask another veterinary professional to team the case with you.
- Prepare the euthanasia site.
- Place a catheter.
- Offer clients time alone with their pets.
- Pronounce the animal dead.
- Allow clients to clip fur, remove collars, or carry through with any activity that may be symbolic and meaningful to them.

After the procedure, it is helpful to:

- Notify other clients who are waiting for appointments if unexpected delays arise.
- Position and prepare the body for viewing, storage, or transport.
- Escort clients out a side or rear door.
- Update client files and records.
- Send condolence cards or letters.
- Make follow-up telephone calls.
- Make referrals to support groups or grief counselors, if appropriate.
- Plan and carry out debriefing or stress management strategies.

One of the best ways we have found to facilitate the various decisions and logistic plans that take place before euthanasia is to ask clients to think about how they will feel when they look back on their pets' deaths. What do they need to do *now* so they will feel at peace with themselves *later*? What details will be important to them? What set of circumstances will be reassuring to them? We have found that one detail out of order is enough to negate the entire, otherwise positive, process for some clients. Because so many details must be considered when helping clients plan a euthanasia, we have found it helpful to use a checklist. A sample list is included in Box 8-7.

FACILITATING CLIENT-PRESENT EUTHANASIAS

As with home euthanasias, it is highly recommended that *all* client-present euthanasias be conducted by a team of at least two veterinary professionals. This allows those assisting the veterinarian to also focus on owner needs and allows the veterinarian to concentrate on the medical aspects of the euthanasia procedure.

It is also highly recommended that, if an owner has elected to be present, the use of a catheter be carefully evaluated. Catheters are not always necessary, and they do not always improve the medical procedures involved with euthanasia. They are, however, often an enhancement to the emotional side of euthanasia because they provide extra insurance that animals will die peacefully, without adverse side-effects. As previously explained, if the veterinarian decides to use a catheter, it should be placed in the rear leg of a small animal. If veterinarians are concerned about the added cost of using catheters for euthanasias, nonsterile, previously used catheters can be placed.

After the intravenous catheter has been placed and the animal has been returned to the euthanasia site, owners should be given the opportunity to spend a short time alone with their companion animals, if they so desire. If owners are left alone to say their last goodbyes, the veterinarian should specifically state when he or she will return. For example, the veterinarian may say, "I will be back in about 10 minutes." If clients want more time and you can afford to give it to them, do so.

Alternatively, veterinarians may ask owners to somehow signal a member of the veterinary staff when they are ready to proceed. If owners are asked to signal, the task must be made as simple as possible. It is very probable that, during this time of intense grief, owners will be able to do no more than to crack open a door or wave a hand in a staff member's direction. Therefore, at least one member of the veterinary team must remain close by so he or she can watch for the client's summons.

If, after about 10 minutes, owners are still saying good-bye, the veterinarian can approach them and gently say, "It is time for us to proceed. May we begin?" Most owners will indicate their answer by either nodding or shaking their heads. If their answer is "no," it is appropriate for the veterinarian to give them 5 or 10 minutes more. Any permission, however, must be made in a calm, quiet voice with no overtones of impatience. Owners have often reported that they felt rushed through the euthanasia process by their veterinarians and feel this negated the other positive aspects of their experiences.

When owners are ready to proceed, it is normal for veterinary team members to feel somewhat awkward as they enter the environment in which the euthanasia is to be performed. Many wonder what they should say or do to comfort their grieving clients. Sometimes, no words are necessary. A touch on an owner's arm or a hug around their shoulders communicates support and understanding quite well.

Before veterinarians begin the lethal injections, they should again tell the owners that they are ready to begin. Whenever possible, syringes should be kept out of sight (for example, in the pocket of a laboratory coat or a smock) and handled very discreetly, because some people become very alarmed at the sight of syringes and needles. Anxiety is usually high at this point, and sometimes owners have momentary episodes of panic. If this happens, it is advisable for veterinarians to halt the procedure and to attend to the client before continuing. Veterinarians can say something like, "This is always the most anxious and difficult moment, Mary, but we have all decided this is best for Pepper. Let's all take a deep breath and say goodbye one more time." Alternatively, veterinarians may take advantage of this moment to self-disclose about one of their own experiences with euthanasia. A statement like, "I was with my own dog when she was euthanized last year and I had a moment of doubt, too. But, looking back on it now, I know I did the right thing for her. This is the hardest part, Mary, and, for Pepper's sake, I'm going to continue now." It goes without saying that, if clients become adamant about stopping the procedure, it should be stopped, if it is still medically possible to do so. In our years of experience, however, we have never encountered this situation.

After the procedure has begun, the drugs should be injected quickly, with little or no delay between them. As they are injected, each should be named so that owners are kept abreast of how the procedure is progressing. For example, veterinarians might say, "Mary, I am injecting the first solution, the saline flush, to make sure the catheter we have inserted is working properly." After that has been done, the next might be announced by saying, "Now I am giving Pepper a barbiturate that will make him sleepy and help him drift off and relax." When it is time for the last injection, the veterinarian might say, "Now I am injecting the final drug." Aside from these statements, it is best for veterinarians to remain silent.

Most owners want to focus on saying goodbye to their animals and find comments, questions, and chatter distracting to their concentration.

While you are performing the euthanasia, the person assisting you should be standing or sitting quietly near the owner. Owners should be allowed to focus on their pets and to say goodbye, but assistants should be instructed to stay close by and to lend both emotional and physical support should the client need it.

This method of facilitating euthanasia usually goes so quickly and smoothly that most owners do not realize when their pets have actually died. It is very important, for the veterinarian to use a stethoscope to listen for a final heartbeat. When the veterinarian can do so with certainty, the animal should also be pronounced dead. Veterinarians should do this with a clear, simple statement such as "Mary, Pepper is dead." At this time, owners may gasp, cry, sob, or sigh with relief. They may make remarks about how quickly death came and about how peaceful the experience was. This is a good time for veterinarians to reassure owners about the decision to euthanize their animals. It is also a good time for veterinarians to express their own feelings of affection and respect for the animal. For example, the veterinarian might say, "I'm going to miss Pepper, too. His tail always wagged when he saw me come into the waiting room." These statements may prompt owners to begin a review of their pets' lives. They may share special or funny stories. Many owners appreciate the opportunity to talk a bit about their pets and to reminisce about the life that has just come to an end.

When we team euthanasias with veterinarians, we all strive to create a "wake" atmosphere in the room. At wakes, it is acceptable to say not only positive, but also negative things about the deceased. This balance helps to prevent grievers from overidealizing the person who has died. A more balanced perspective is desirable because idealization of the deceased is closely related to chronic grief.[23]

After an animal has died, one of us in the room will usually, at some point, say something like, "I'll bet this guy got into his share of trouble" or "I can only imagine the tricks this old girl used to play on you." Almost every pet owner we have known has picked up the conversation at this point and related wonderful stories about the good and the "bad" sides of life with their companion animal. For example, one pet owner said, "I know I really loved this dog because he chewed up my $3,000 leather couch and I didn't kill him on the spot!" Another said, "This cat brought home little presents, like snakes and mice, and left them all over the house. Sometimes I wouldn't find them for days."

Most of these stories make everyone laugh; however, as owners realize they will never again witness their pets' high-jinks, in the midst of our laughter, their tears begin again. Our "wakes" often go through several of these crying-laughing-crying cycles before everyone feels ready to bring them to an end. It is important to remember that, under these circumstances, we do not encourage the use of humor as a way to "break the tension" in the room or to "cheer people up" after loss. Rather, we use it to make the euthanasia experience real and human and to help pet owners recall all dimensions of their pets' personalities.

FOLLOW-UP AFTER DEATH

After euthanasia, some people want to leave the veterinary facility or site quickly, whereas others need more time alone with their pets. Because many owners have invested so much in the physical care of their companion animals, even after death, their pets' bodies remain important to them. If the euthanasia has been conducted in an examination room, and, if it is needed for the next client's visit, veterinarians can tell owners that they will be back in 10 minutes or in whatever time frame seems reasonable. Alternatively, veterinarians can ask their next clients if they would mind waiting a few extra minutes past their designated appointment times to allow another owner to finish saying goodbye to an animal who has died. Almost everyone is gracious under these circumstances.

Sometimes, family members who have not been present at the euthanasia may want to view an animal's body before it is buried or cremated. As we said earlier, grief experts agree that seeing dead bodies helps people to accept the fact that death has occurred.[18,19] If a pet's body is going to be viewed immediately after death, clients need to be prepared for what they will see and for what will be acceptable for them to do. Here is an example of how we prepare clients to view their pets' bodies at CSU:

"Henry, when you see Pepper, his body will still be warm, but it may be slightly soiled due to the natural release of his bowel and bladder. Pepper's eyes will not be closed and his tongue may protrude slightly from his mouth. Pepper is covered with a fleece from the head down but you may remove it if you want to see his entire body. As you remember, there are stitches on Pepper's abdomen where he last had surgery.

"It's alright for you to touch Pepper, to pet him, and even hold him if you so desire. There is also a brush and a scissors in the room if you want to groom him or clip some of his fur to take with you. I will be happy to go with you when you see him. Would you like me to do that or would you prefer to go into the room alone?"

If the client asks you to accompany him, lead the way and make the first move toward touching, petting, and talking to the animal. This is a prime time to act as a role model for your client so he will have a better idea of

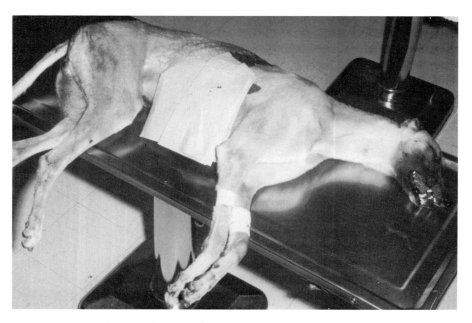

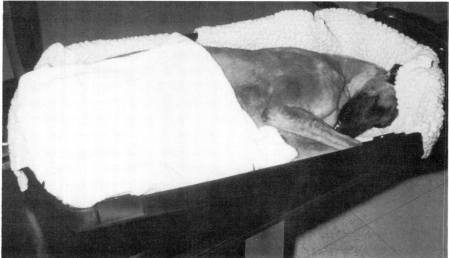

Figure 8-8 Veterinary professionals should position pets' bodies in sleep-like positions if owners plan to view their animals' bodies or pick them up for burial. These photographs represent an insensitive (*top*) and a sensitive (*bottom*) way to present companion animals' bodies.

BOX 8-8

What Clients Like and Dislike

The items listed below represent the comments we have heard most frequently from clients.

What clients like: You can offer small kindnesses to clients before, during, and after pet loss. These small gestures are often what clients remember the most.

- Offering to give pets a treat or a last drink of water.
- Demonstrating your own affection for pets (for example, by petting animals and saying your own goodbyes).
- Offering to let clients clip some fur, keep their pets' collars, and so forth as mementos. In some situations, clients appreciate final Polaroid snapshots of their pets. Pawprints can also be preserved for clients by using either paper and ink or a quick-setting clay.
- Ensuring that you do not use the same examination room that was used for euthanizing a pet the next time your client visits your clinic.
- Using the name of a pet who died and reminiscing about the pet during subsequent interactions with clients.

What clients don't like: There are many small insensitivities you can avoid before, during, and after euthanasia. Unfortunately, these small mistakes are often enough to negate the overall positive effects of client-present euthanasia because they are the images and experiences that clients remember the most.

- Being kept waiting either in the waiting room or at the euthanasia site.
- Being given no warning or explanation prior to visiting their pet, viewing their pet's body, or witnessing a procedure (for example, visiting their pet in the critical care unit, seeing the stitches and shaved areas of their pet's body after surgery, watching as their pet's bladder is expressed before moving the body).
- Handling a pet's body roughly or awkwardly (for example, grabbing the legs and muzzle in order to move the body, letting the head dangle unsupported while carrying the body, dropping part of body).
- Using a cardboard box or a garbage bag to return a pet's body.
- Feeling they were rushed through the euthanasia procedure.
- Hearing others tell them that they should immediately adopt a new pet.

what to do. After you have spent some time talking with and listening to your client, ask again if he would like some time alone. If the answer is yes, leave the room and tell them how soon you plan to return.

When a client wishes to view a pet, the animal's body should be in a position that is pleasing to see. By this, we mean that it should be curled slightly, with the head and limbs tucked into a "sleep-like" position. Positioning the body is especially important if it is to be placed into a casket or other container for burial or transport at a later time. Positioning is vitally important if you are planning to keep the animal's body in a cooler until other family members can view it or pick it up. If an animal (particularly a large dog) is allowed to stiffen, placing it in a casket or even on the back seat of a car is nearly impossible. It is a good idea to keep a box, plastic casket, or other container at your clinic for viewing and storage purposes (Fig. 8-8).

If the owner is not taking the pet's body with them, a staff member should stay with the animal's body at the euthanasia site. Almost every owner we have assisted during euthanasia takes one last look back at their pet before they actually leave. When they see a friendly, familiar face next to their pet, they feel reassured that their companion animal will not be forgotten or treated with disrespect after they leave.

If owners have attended the euthanasia alone, be certain that they feel able to drive themselves home before they leave your clinic. Some owners appreciate time to drink a glass of water or to make a telephone call to a friend or family member as a way to calm themselves before leaving. When owners are ready to leave, they should be escorted through a side or back door, if possible, so that they do not have to exit through the busy waiting area. It can be embarrassing and awkward for clients who have been crying to walk through a crowded waiting area filled with people whom they don't know. It can also be emotionally difficult to see other pet owners with healthy companion animals when theirs has just died.

If clients do not take their pets' bodies with them, you can reassure them while you accompany them to their cars that their wishes for body care will be carried out. If owners do take their pets' bodies with them, take extra care to treat the body with respect and dignity (Box 8-8).

A 10-year-old Siberian Husky underwent exploratory surgery. During surgery, the dog was found to have cancer all through the abdomen. The veterinarian contacted his clients with his findings and, together, they decided to euthanize the dog on the table. The owners expressed their desire to have their dog's body back for burial, and the veterinarian agreed.

Thinking that his clients would probably not want to endure the pain of seeing their pet dead, the veterinarian placed the dog in a large plastic bag and sealed it tightly with a twist tie. When the clients arrived 2 hours later to pick up the body, they knew immediately that their dog was too big to fit into the bag the veterinarian had used. They removed the tie and looked inside. From their perspective, their magnificant dog had been stuffed into a garbage bag and was now contorted into a grotesque posture. With tears in their eyes, the

clients took their dog and left without even thanking the veterinarian.

As they drove away, the veterinarian felt sad, confused,
and a bit angry with his clients. He had done his best for
their dog and handled the body in the way he thought they
would want. He did not understand their reactions.

BOX 8-9

Role Responsibilities for Veterinary Team Members

Euthanasias go more smoothly when each team member clearly understands the
specific tasks they are to perform. The following represents one suggested plan for
the division of duties among veterinarians, technicians, and receptionists. Keep in
mind that clients are often less intimidated by receptionists and technicians, so
they may be more likely to ask them, rather than you, questions about pet loss
and euthanasia. Also, many clients make their first inquires about euthanasia by
telephone, so receptionists must be trained to provide information about the
procedure with both accuracy and compassion.

Receptionists may:

- Accurately and compassionately explain euthanasia when clients
  inquire about it by telephone.
- Schedule euthanasias and facilitate decisions regarding the logistic
  choices involved with euthanasia.
- Meet clients at the door upon their arrival for a scheduled euthanasia, and escort them to the chosen euthanasia site.
- Reschedule other clients, if necessary, due to an unexpected death
  or euthanasia.
- Ensure that the veterinary team is not interrupted during a euthanasia.

Technicians may:

- Explain the euthanasia procedure and field questions.
- Prepare the euthanasia site.
- Place a catheter.
- Attend to clients' needs before, during, and after the procedure.
- Facilitate clients' decisions regarding body care and follow through
  on their wishes afterward.
- Update client files.

Veterinarians may:

- Explain the euthanasia procedure and field questions.
- Structure and guide the euthanasia procedure.
- Sensitively perform the actual euthanasia procedure.
- Escort clients away from the euthanasia site.
- Send condolence cards and letters or make follow-up telephone
  calls.

The preceding case study illustrates how a lack of communication over even a few simple details can damage veterinarian-client relationships. To avoid such problems try to have something other than cardboard boxes or plastic garbage bags on hand to return or transport bodies in. Several items are better alternatives. Blankets, sheets, and even old rugs, for example, can be bought very inexpensively at yard sales or thrift stores. You can also cover cardboard boxes with wrapping or contact paper or ask local carpenters to build plain pine boxes of various sizes for you to have on hand. If you and your client have time to plan for euthanasia, ask them to bring something from home to wrap or transport the body in. Then, you can be certain that whatever is used will be appropriate in your client's eyes. It goes without saying that, if an owner is taking a pet's body home, be sure that the animal's body is not carried out to the owner's car through your busy waiting room.

Obviously, the client-present euthanasia procedures discussed in this chapter represent the ideal. With practice, forethought, and organization, however, it is possible to implement them. For example, when your veterinary staff is well-trained, your technicians, receptionists, and even kennel help can be responsible for making sure that many of the preparatory and after death tasks are accomplished (Box 8-9).

Some circumstances call for modifications in client-present euthanasia procedures. For example, sometimes the veins of very old or ill cats cannot be catheterized. In these cases, it is important to explain to clients why you cannot use a catheter and to tell them that it may take you several attempts before you find an acceptable vein. You may also have cases in which clients have special needs or bring you animals that are nontraditional pets. Some suggestions for helping these clients are discussed in the chapters that follow.

CONCLUSION

When done well, euthanasia is a procedure of which you can be proud. If the trend toward legalizing human euthanasia continues, it is also a procedure about which you will, no doubt, be asked to teach other health professionals in the future.

Due largely to the AIDS epidemic and an aging population, the number of terminally ill patients in the United States is growing rapidly.[24] About 1.3 million Americans die annually in hospitals and hundreds of thousands more die in nursing homes.[25] In 1975, only 41 percent of respondents in a Gallup Poll said that they believed that someone in great pain, with "no hope of improvement" had the moral right to commit suicide. By 1990, that figure had risen to 66 percent.[25] These figures suggest that society, human medical professionals, and patients themselves are beginning to seriously struggle with the issue of human euthanasia.

Other events support this change in beliefs. During recent years, Timothy Quill published an essay in the *New England Journal of Medicine*[26] describing his involvement in a terminally ill patient's suicide. The *American Journal of Forensic Psychiatry* devoted an entire issue to publication and analysis of Jack Kevorkian's article entitled "A Fail-Safe Model for Justifiable Medically-Assisted Suicide,"[27] and Kevorkian himself assisted several people with their deaths by facilitating their use of his so-called "suicide machine." Also, Derek Humphry's book, written for the lay public and entitled *Final Exit: The Practicalities of Self-Deliverance and Assisted Suicide for the Dying*,[28] made its first appearance on the New York Times best-seller list in the number one spot, and Washington state's "Aid in Dying" initiative commanded a 60 percent majority in one opinion poll and was only narrowly defeated in the actual ballot. Plans to introduce assisted-suicide initiatives in California and New Hampshire are currently under way.[29]

As these examples show, more and more people are asking what they can and should do now to try to ensure a dignified, humane death. As stated in a 1991 *Newsweek* article:

> The option that more and more patients, and their families, demand is to leapfrog dying if death is all that awaits. While many people choose death, no one chooses dying.[25]

In response to Kevorkian's aforementioned proposal in the *American Journal of Forensic Psychiatry*, Kenneth Karols said:

> There are situations when rational persons should agree that the most appropriate activity of the physician would be to help end a life of hopeless suffering with painless dignity. Veterinarians do this routinely for animals. Should the physician of humans do less?[30]

Veterinarians need to share what they know about euthanasia with their colleagues in human medicine. Client-present euthanasia is a vital medical procedure as worthy of a medical professionals' time and attention as is surgery. Veterinary medicines' growing acceptance of and knowledge base about ceremonial, client-present euthanasia may one day pave the way for human medicine to begin to see that, along with the withdrawal of treatment and doctor-assisted suicide, planned, family-present euthanasia may also be of great value for people.

REFERENCES

1. Edney, A.T.: Client grief and the art of euthanasia. *In* the Proceedings of the North American Veterinary Conference, Orlando, Florida, January 11–16, 1992, pp. 217–221.
2. Arkow, P.: Animal control laws and enforcement. J. Am. Vet. Med. Assoc., *198*:1164–1172, 1991.

3. Andrews, E.J., Bennett, B.T., Clark, J.D., Houpt, K.A., Pascoe, P.J., Robinson, G.W., and Boyce, J.R.: 1993 Report of the AVMA Panel on Euthanasia. J. Am. Vet. Med. Assoc., 202:229–249, 1993.
4. Hart, L.A., Hart, B.L., and Mader, B.: Humane euthanasia and companion animal death: Caring for the animal, the client, and the veterinarian. J. Am. Vet. Med. Assoc., 197:1292–1299, 1990.
5. Hopkins, A.F.: Pet death: Effects on the client and the veterinarian. In Anderson, R.K., Hart, B.L., and Hart, L.A., eds.: The Pet Connection. University of Minnesota, Minneapolis, CENSHARE, 1984, pp. 276–282.
6. Fogle B.: Attachment–Euthanasia—Grieving. In Fogle, B., ed.: Interrelations Between People and Pets. Springfield, Ill., Charles C. Thomas, 1981, pp. 331–343.
7. Rando, T.A.: Grief, Dying, and Death: Clinical Interventions for Caregivers. Champaign, Ill., Research Press Company, 1984.
8. Lagoni, L., Hetts, S., and Withrow, S.J.: The veterinarian's role in pet loss: Grief education, support, and facilitation. In Withrow, S.J., and MacEwen, E.G. eds.: Clinical Veterinary Oncology. Philadelphia, J. B. Lippincott, 1989, pp. 436–445.
9. Gershon, D., and Straub, G.: Empowerment: The art of creating your life as you want it. New York, Dell Publishing, 1989.
10. Norris, E.: Communicating with clients about death and euthanasia. Vet. Pract. Management, 2:32–39, 1984–1985.
11. Mich, P.: Bond-centered practice plan. Assignment for VM 796Q, Pet Loss and Client Grief, Fort Collins, Colo., Veterinary Teaching Hospital, Colorado State University, 1990.
12. Ball, J.F.: Widow's grief: The impact of age and mode of death. Omega, 7:307–333, 1977.
13. Parkes, C.M.: Unexpected and untimely bereavement: A statistical study of young Boston widows and widowers. In Schoenberg, B, Gerber, I., Wiener, A., Kutscher, D., Peretz, D. and Cam, A., eds.: Bereavement and Its Psychological Aspects. New York, Columbia University Press, 1975, pp. 119–138.
14. Cohen, S.P.: Suffering and euthanasia. In Cohen, S.P., and Fudin, C.E., eds.: Problems in Veterinary Medicine: Animal Illness and Human Emotion, Vol. 3. Philadelphia, J.B. Lippincott, 1991, pp. 101–109.
15. Garcia, E.: Pet loss considered from the veterinary perspective. The Latham Letter, Alameda, Calif. The Latham Foundation, 1986–1987, pp. 10–13.
16. Maddison, D., and Walker, W.L.: Factors affecting the outcome of conjugal bereavement. Br. J. Psychiat., 113:1057–1067, 1967.
17. Fulton, R.: Death and the funeral in contemporary society. In Wass, H., ed.: Dying: Facing the Facts. New York, Hemisphere Publishing Corporation/McGraw-Hill Book Company, 1979.
18. Glick, I.O., Weiss, R.S., and Parkes, C.M.: The First Year of Bereavement. New York, Wiley, 1974.
19. Rando, T.A.: Grieving: How to Go on Living When Someone You Love Dies. Lexington, Mass., Lexington Books, 1988.
20. Worden, J.W.: Grief Counseling and Grief Therapy: A Handbook for the Mental Health Practitioner, New York, Springer Publishing Company, 1982.
21. Soares, C.J.: Grief counseling for euthanasia. The Latham Letter, Alameda, Calif., The Latham Foundation, 1986–1987, pp. 1–4.
22. Morgan, J.H., and Goering, R.: Caring for parents who have lost an infant. J. Relig. Health, 17:290–298, 1978.
23. Stroebe, W., and Stroebe, M.S.: Bereavement and Health: The Psychological and Physical Consequences of Partner Loss. Cambridge, England, Cambridge University Press, 1987.
24. The Associated Press: Physicians state rising need for doctor-assisted suicide. The Coloradoan, December 6, 1992, p. A3.
25. Ames, K., Wilson, L., Sawhill, R., Glick, D., and King, P.: Last Rights. Newsweek, 118:41, 1991.

26. Quill, T.: Death and dignity: A case of individualized decision-making. N. Engl. J. Med., *324*:691–694, 1991.
27. Kevorkian, J.: A fail-safe model for justifiable medically-assisted suicide. Am. J. Forens. Psychiatry, *113*:7–41, 1992.
28. Anonymous.: The ultimate runaway best seller. Newsweek, *118*:57, 1991.
29. Nowak, R.: Final ethics: Dutch discover euthanasia abuse. J. NIH. Res., *4*:31–32, 1992.
30. Karols, K.: Commentaries on Dr. Kevorkian's article. Am. J. Forens. Psychiatry, *13*:45–46, 1992.

9

Helping during Large-Animal Euthanasia

Sometimes the animals that you are called on to treat or euthanize are not household pets. They may be horses and llamas that are considered to be pets or cows and sheep that are valuable to owners, not as companions, but as sources of income. Some large animals are utilitarian animals that are needed to complete daily tasks and special projects or used for riding and showing. Many large animals have both companionship and economic value. The dual nature of these relationships often complicates or intensifies the emotions associated with caring for, and ultimately losing, large animals.

In this chapter, we explore the issues surrounding large companion animal death and euthanasia. We use the term "large animals" to refer to horses, donkeys, mules, llamas, alpacas, cattle, goats, pigs, and sheep. Throughout the chapter, we use the horse as the primary example because horses are the most common large-animal companions, and information about them is, for the most part, generalizable to other large animals. We want to emphasize that the methods described in this chapter are meant to be applied to the euthanasias of companion animals. We do not address the methods used to euthanize animals whose primary function is utilitarian.

Some of the information in this chapter is repeated from Chapter 8. We have done this for two reasons: First, with some adaptation, many of the issues and recommended strategies are identical. For example, the methods used to prepare the owners of small and large animals to be present at euthanasias are, in many ways, similar. Second, many veterinary schools now divide students' learning experiences into small-animal and large-animal tracks. In many cases, the lectures and clinical rotations in which students participate do not overlap. Students in large-animal tracks may not be assigned a chapter dealing with small-animal euthanasia and vice versa. Thus, we thought it best to present the chapters concerning euthanasia in a somewhat independent fashion.

Most of our expertise in the Changes Program with client-present euthanasias comes from working with small animals. We are now beginning to consistently intervene in large-animal cases. Chapter 8 provides a more complete overview of the euthanasia process and covers some topics, such as decision-making, necropsy, and viewing bodies, that are not covered in Chapter 9. In terms of learning the most you can about client-present euthanasia, it is most effective to read both chapters.

As with Chapter 8, this chapter does not concern itself so much with the medical aspects of euthanasia. Rather, its focus is on how to make the emotional side of the experience more positive as you work with highly attached large-animal owners who want to be involved, in some way, with their companion animals' euthanasias. How do you assess which clients are highly attached to their animals? The Keys to Attachment listed in Chapter 1 give you a place to start. They apply to owners of large, as well as small, animals. Keep these points in mind as you observe, listen, and question clients about the bonds that they have with their animals and about their needs and wishes concerning euthanasia.

Throughout this chapter, the philosophic principles of establishing bond-centered practices and of developing helping relationships are applied. When appropriate, suggested communication techniques are also provided. As you know from reading Chapter 5, an important tenet of building helping relationships is knowing your clientele. Therefore, the best way to begin learning about the ways in which to meet the needs of large-animal owners during client-present euthanasias is by gaining a better understanding of the large-animal owners themselves.

UNDERSTANDING OWNERS OF LARGE ANIMALS

Some predictable differences may exist in the levels of attachment and the emotions displayed or felt by female, male, and adolescent owners. We must, however, caution you about making assumptions about owners' attachments to their animals or about what owners want in terms of treatment or euthanasia. Your actions should never be based on the age, gender, outward appearance, or financial status of owners. For example, the toughest-looking cowboys and ranch hands, who appear to have ridden right off the range to your clinic, are often highly attached to their horses and deeply moved by their deaths.

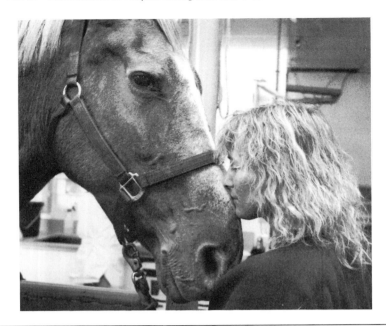

Figure 9-1 It's hard to say goodbye to a friend. PHOTO COURTESY OF GEORGE KOCHA-NIEC, JR., *THE ROCKY MOUNTAIN NEWS.*

Overall, the levels of attachment shown by large-animal owners seem to be increasing. While writing this text, we conducted an informal poll of large-animal veterinarians and asked them about the attachment behaviors they observe while working with horse and llama owners. The veterinarians with whom we talked unanimously agreed that the large-animal owners whom they encounter today appear to be more attached to their animals than were the owners with whom they worked 10 years previously. These veterinarians also said that their current clients seem more likely to show their attachments through expressions of grief, such as crying, wishing to say goodbye, or clipping some mane or tail hair (Fig. 9-1).

It is highly probable, however, that owners' attachment levels have not really changed over the years. Instead, an increase in their outward expressions of feelings might be attributed to society's increased awareness of the significance of the human-animal bond and to an increasing tolerance for emotional reactions to loss. In veterinary medicine, many professionals are more perceptive about what their clients are feeling and, thus, are more comfortable indicating to them that expressions of grief are acceptable.

In the following section, three categories of large-animal owners are discussed. They are horse owners, llama owners, and food animal owners.

Horse Owners

When owners and animals spend time together on a daily basis, special bonds clearly develop between them. Consider these descriptions of the human-horse bond told to us by Susan Williams and Carol Story, two CSU clients:

> The bond between horse and human is one that is hard to put into words. The relationship is magically born, rather than deliberately created. A true horse person knows the magnitude of this bond.
>
> As a professional horsewoman, I have talked to many, many people over the years about their feelings toward their horses. Amazingly, nearly every really serious, hard-core horse lover describes the same sort of behavioral pattern. Starting at a very early age, from her earliest memories, she loved horses, wanted a horse, played "horse," dreamed about horses, constantly talked about horses, and thought about little else. The parents and siblings of these people relate how the horse lover seemed to talk about horses and nothing else throughout childhood. Based on personal observation, many, if not most, of these children were from families with no prior horse involvement. Often the families of these children were left wondering, "Where did she come from?"

Horses may be used for ranch work or ridden for competition, therapy, or pleasure (Fig. 9-2). Owners' livelihoods are sometimes dependent on horses; therefore, deep attachments often form when owners and animals work together, often traveling a good portion of the year. In these situations, horses' and humans' lives become intertwined, and their relationships become based on mutual attachment rather than on one-sided exploitation.

The most recent publication of The Veterinary Services Market Survey,[1] prepared for the AVMA by the Charles and Charles Research Group, showed that approximately 2.6 million households owned horses in 1987, with each of those households owning an average of 2.6 horses. From these results, Charles and Charles projected that the estimated horse population in the United States in 1987 was approximately 6.6 million. In addition, they noted that an average of $329.8 million was spent on equine care during that year.

The Charles and Charles survey also showed that most horse-owning households tended to comprise families with children, and these families were more likely to live in rural areas or small towns. In a high percentage of horse-owning households, a woman between 31 and 50 years of age cared for the horses' daily needs and decided whether or not the animals needed veterinary care. Specifically, Charles and Charles stated that 68 percent of women (compared with 32 percent of men) were the primary

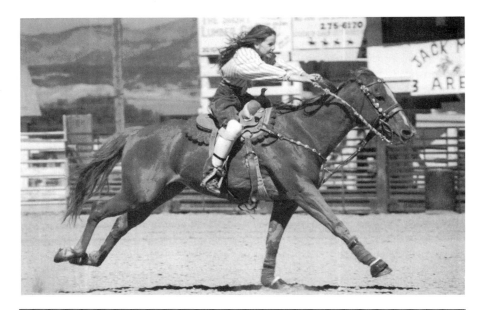

Figure 9-2 A horse owner develops a relationship with her horse that is marked by mutual trust, respect, and affection, much as would be encountered in a relationship between two people who spend several hours every day together doing something enjoyable for both. COPYRIGHT 1992 JEFF BELDEN/JB PHOTOGRAPHY.

caretakers of their horses' needs and that 69 percent of women (compared with 31 percent of men) decided if their jointly owned animals needed veterinary care.

This survey confirms the important role that women play in caring for horses. This information is important because it tells you that many of the veterinarian-client relationships that you will develop with horse-owning clients will be with women.

In general, clinical experience shows that female horse owners react differently to the deaths of their animals than do male owners. A long-time veterinarian told us:

> Most of my clients are women. I work with show horses a lot. Men are quicker to go with euthanasia. Women are slower to accept (euthanasia) and are quicker to cry.

Another veterinarian said:

> Women need to say goodbye. They are generally responsive to a hug or kind words about how special their horse was, an acknowledgment of how well she cared for the horse, or reassurance that

she has made the right decision to help the animal die. Most go
around the corner of the building while the injection is given and
then come back to spend time with the horse once it is down.

In our experience, men, on the other hand, are more likely to work
through their grief privately and to assume supportive roles with their
female partners who more openly express their grief.

Llama Owners

Increasingly, animal owners are sharing their lives with llamas and alpacas. Because these animals have both economic and companionship
value, the veterinarians who care for them are being exposed to the emotions associated with companion animal ownership. Llama expert LaRue
Johnson says:

> Veterinarians must learn to bridge the gap between food animal
> needs, which are primarily economic, and the needs of companion
> animal owners. This is true throughout the entire life of the animal
> and at the time of euthanasia. (Johnson, L., Personal communica-
> tion)

Llama ownership in the United States is gaining in popularity. Experts
say that llamas have gone from being merely zoo curiosities to being the

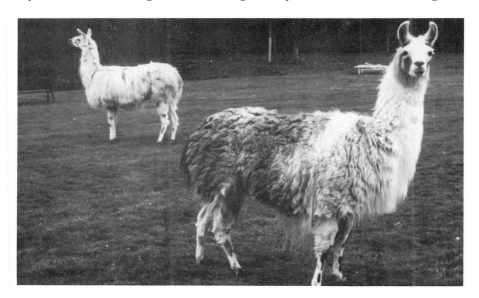

Figure 9-3 In recent years more and more animal lovers have been drawn to the
low-key temperaments of llamas.

focal points of a rapidly growing, multimillion dollar industry.[2] Although their numbers are significantly lower than those of horses, estimates show that approximately 25,000 llamas currently live in the United States and that their numbers are increasing.[2] Most llamas are described as pets by their owners, and most llama owners generally have no previous experience with large-animal ownership. Owners are drawn to llamas because of their adaptability, social natures, and low-key temperaments. These traits make llamas easy to handle, even for novices (Fig. 9-3).

Llamas are generally expensive. Prices range from $500 to $20,000. Because of their emotional attachments to their animals, owners tend to price them high and to be unwilling to negotiate lower prices (Johnson, L., Personal communication). When llamas are sick or must be euthanized, both male and female owners seem to react in ways similar to horse owners.

Food Animal Owners

Most food animal owners are farmers, ranchers, and 4-H members. Food animal owners have a different kind of human-animal bond, but it remains a bond that deserves compassionate understanding during times of loss. As John Herrick said in his column:

> The human-animal bond may not be strong for a group of feeder pigs affected with swine dysentery or a pen of newly arrived feeder cattle with shipping fever. However, there are emotional disturbances among animal producers when they suffer a financial loss because of disease in their animals. If a single animal dies, the economic impact is not great. However, food animal practitioners observe livestock operations as a single entity, and the success or failure of the operation determines whether the operator continues in the operation or pays the loan at the bank, or whether his or her child may remain in college[3] (p. 232).

Many large-animal owners are children who are involved in 4-H projects. In 1990, 1,700,000 children and adolescents, 9 to 19 years of age, participated in animal and poultry projects nationwide (Meier, A., Personal communication). Of that total, approximately 657,000 children were involved with large-animal projects (beef, dairy, horse, pony, sheep, and swine.) A state 4-H specialist told us:

> Every one [each child] has a bond because they raise them from young animals—regardless of the nature of the project. The bond develops due to the child's responsibility to the animal. The bond develops by association and goes beyond economic value. (Meier, A., Personal communication)

Children in 4-H programs routinely give up the animals with whom they have worked—feeding, training, bathing, and brushing—on a daily basis. Because many 4-H members think of their project animals as confidantes, partners, and friends, some young owners feel deep anguish when their animals are sold, are euthanized, or die.

Whether individual food animals die or whole herds are euthanized due to disease, food animal owners experience a wide range of losses. These include the loss of food production, loss of livelihood, loss of security, loss of future hopes and dreams, and even, on some level, the loss of companionship. As John Herrick goes on to say in his column:

> Can you love a pen of hogs, a yard full of feeder cattle, or a string of milking cows? The answer is yes, although it may be a different kind of love. Producers want to take the best possible care of these animals so they will be comfortable.[3] (p. 232)

EUTHANASIA OF LARGE ANIMALS

Whether the large animals you euthanize are horses, llamas, or food animals, large-animal owners (like owners of smaller animals) appreciate it when you extend a caring attitude along with your medical expertise. When clients bring their companion animals to your bond-centered veterinary practice, they want you to attend not only to the medical needs of their animals, but also to their emotional needs. When you strive to meet their needs, you help to relax the social restrictions about what is acceptable when grieving the deaths of large companion animals. This orientation is never more important than during the euthanasias of large animals.

No other medical procedure you perform has as great an effect on you, your staff, and the quality of your veterinarian-client relationships as does the procedure of euthanasia. When euthanasia is performed well, it can soothe and reassure all involved that the decision to end an animal's life was correct. However, when euthanasia is done poorly (that is, thoughtlessly or without compassion and sensitivity), it can deepen, complicate, and prolong grief for everyone.

As Harry Hagstad says:

> Technical competence is a basic requirement for any profession, but some fields require more. A successful veterinarian in private practice can be accurately described as part veterinarian, part pediatrician, and part psychologist. Veterinarians must, first of all, be competent in the technical skills of their profession. In addition, since their patients cannot verbalize their symptoms, veterinarians must, like pediatricians, depend on a third party for an accurate history.

Finally, since the emotional bond between the owner and his or her companion animal is usually strong, sometimes as intense as that which exists between parents and their children, the veterinarian frequently becomes directly involved in a crisis situation and is called upon to assume a counseling role. Some professionals can handle these crises well; others cannot, and try to avoid them.[4] (p. 96)

How can you become one of the veterinarians who handles crises well? To be more specific, how can you be one of the veterinarians who handles the crisis of large-animal euthanasia well? The first step is to change the way you think about client-present euthanasia.

CLIENT-PRESENT EUTHANASIA

In veterinary medicine, human participation in the form of client presence at euthanasia has traditionally been discouraged. Thus, the process has been conducted as a somewhat routine, albeit uncomfortable, medical procedure. Typically, euthanasias have been conducted in sterile or less than ideal environments with only the members of the veterinary staff present. Contemporary veterinary medicine, however, is beginning to see euthanasia in a new light. Because of a new perspective on euthanasia, the procedure is evolving into more than a dreaded clinical task. As we have said before, euthanasia is coming to be viewed more frequently by veterinary professionals and companion animal owners alike, as both a privilege and a gift that can be lovingly bestowed on ill or injured animals.

Modern veterinarians recognize client-present euthanasia as a powerful practice-builder and a potent grief intervention tool. After veterinarians experience the profound effects of conducting euthanasias with both their patients' and clients' needs in mind, most understand why well-planned euthanasias can be effective in building positive relationships between themselves and the companion animal owners whom they serve. Thus, many of the euthanasias performed by today's compassionate, bond-centered practitioners are conducted like ceremonies in which the process itself is treated with the respect and reverence that it deserves.

At some point in your veterinary career, you have probably been told that the term "euthanasia" is derived from two Greek words—"eu" meaning "good" and "thanatos" meaning "death." These words qualify euthanasia as a "good death."[5] Words such as easy, humane, painless, and loving are also associated with euthanasia. Yet, putting these positive attributes aside, euthanasia remains the purposeful act of taking a life. Therefore, the euthanasias of companion animals often affect the individuals involved in intensely emotional ways.

With this in mind, concerned veterinarians, animal health technicians, and grief counselors from across the country have worked together during the last decade to create and perfect euthanasia protocols that have both the patients' and the clients' comfort and well-being in mind. These teams of professionals have considered many variables, including the attitudes of those involved in the euthanasia process, the physical surroundings and aesthetics of the euthanasia site, and the combination of drugs and methods used to induce peaceful and painless death. The ways in which to best prepare clients for their companion animals' deaths and to best help them plan the circumstances surrounding the euthanasia procedure have also been studied. Protocols representing progressive work in this important area of veterinary medicine are described in this chapter.

A NEW PARADIGM

In the old model of euthanasia, the standard operating procedure was to discuss the process as little as possible, to involve clients as little as possible, and to complete the act as quickly as possible. Euthanasia was often mentioned only indirectly or euphemistically, and clients were encouraged to simply "walk away" from their animals so that they would not be burdened by the details of their pets' deaths. It was believed that this impersonal, clinical approach to euthanasia helped to protect both clients and veterinarians from addressing emotions, thus making the process as painless as possible for all involved.

This paradigm probably worked for some, but for others it created different kinds of emotional pain. For many clients and veterinarians alike, it created feelings of guilt, shame, depression, and unresolved grief. The old model of euthanasia was particularly difficult for veterinarians because it placed the bulk of the emotional burden on their shoulders. Usually, with clients' permission, veterinarians were the ones to decide *when, why, how,* and *where* animals should die. In addition, veterinarians usually refrained from formally acknowledging their patients' deaths and from contacting their clients afterward. Thus, the old model forced everyone to grieve in isolation and, in general, did not allow either veterinarians or clients to "finish" their experiences. Many of the veterinarians with whom we have spoken have expressed resentment about this overwhelming responsibility, and many clients have expressed the same emotions about their perceived lack of control over the process.

In the new model of euthanasia, the standard operating procedure stands in direct opposition to that of the old. In the new model, it is more common for veterinarians and clients to discuss euthanasia together, directly, and at length. It is also common to allow as much time for the procedure as is needed and possible, to involve clients in the process as much as possible, and to acknowledge animals' deaths and to talk openly about them afterwards. The new paradigm is much more congruent with what research has told us about both healthy grief resolution and effective practice management.[6,7] Therefore, the new model is both sensitive and pragmatic.

The key word when conducting euthanasias within the new paradigm is *choice*. As much as your clients may love their companion animals, they are probably underinformed consumers of veterinary services. Therefore, they may not always realize that they have choices. For them to make wise and timely decisions when faced with their pets' deaths, they must be provided with information and choices by the veterinarian. In the new paradigm, clients are given choices about as many details as possible. The emotional burdens are shared, and, as a team, veterinarians and clients decide about when, why, how, and where companion animals should die. This paradigm fits well into a bond-centered practice.

When people make conscious choices, they feel empowered;[8] that is, they are more likely to feel that they are making decisions that are right for them. Even in loss-related crises, clients feel that they have an element of control when they are presented with options and choices.

Obviously, we use the new paradigm when making recommendations about how you can conduct large-animal euthanasias in your bond-centered practice. It is important for you to remember, however, that not all of your clients will want or require this kind of time or attention when euthanizing their animals. Our experiences have shown that each client will make different choices. Some will choose total involvement and will orchestrate a fairly complex euthanasia process. Others will choose minimal involvement, opting for only a goodbye nuzzle as they leave the euthanasia site. All of your clients, however, will appreciate being given the option to be as actively involved as *they* choose to be in the euthanasia planning process and in the actual procedure.

THE FIRST CHOICE: DECIDING WHY AND WHEN TO EUTHANIZE

In Chapter 8, we discussed four reasons for deciding to euthanize companion animals. We also discussed several strategies for helping clients decide when to euthanize.

As we said in that chapter, clinical experience has shown that most companion animal owners instinctively know when their animals' battles to recover from disease or injury are over. Experience has also shown that, when you have been honest and straightforward with clients regarding their animals' conditions, you and your clients tend to reach the same conclusions about euthanasia concurrently. Nonetheless, introducing the subject of euthanasia is often uncomfortable. You must, however, inform clients when you feel the appropriate time to consider euthanasia has arrived.

After clients have decided to proceed with euthanasia, you must also take time to prepare them for what lies ahead. Research has shown that longer preparation time diminishes the intensity of grief reactions[9] and that anticipatory grief acts as a mitigating influence on grief after death.[9,10] Successful client-present euthanasias begin with thorough preparation. Preparation minimizes the regrets, the "what ifs," and the "if onlys" that inevitably follow companion animal death.

THE SECOND CHOICE: CLIENT PRESENCE

One of the issues of most concern to large-animal veterinarians is client presence at euthanasia. Harry Hagstad surveyed 100 veterinarians and 100 horse owners.[4] He reported that veterinarians take one of three positions when discussing client presence: (1) discouragement, (2) encouragement, or (3) neutrality. His survey showed that most equine veterinarians do not encourage their clients to be present at euthanasias. In fact, the study showed that only 13 percent of equine veterinarians encouraged owners to be present, 41 percent discouraged owner presence, and that the remaining 46 percent indicated that owner presence was not an issue. (In the study, "not an issue" was not clearly defined.) Hagstad's study also showed that veterinarians were more than twice as likely (55.7 percent) to discourage the presence of adolescent female owners than the presence of adult male owners (24.3 percent). Interestingly, of those who participated in the study, recent graduates were more likely to discourage owner presence than were practitioners with many years of experience.

Common Concerns of Veterinarians about Client-Present Euthanasia

In Chapter 8, we discussed some of the reasons why veterinarians prefer that owners not be present during euthanasias. Large-animal veterinarians who take this position share similar concerns. They want to spare owners emotional pain, and they want to ensure that owners do not associate them with the "negative feelings" that surround death. We asked some of our colleagues to relate their concerns about this issue. Examples of their comments include:

> "Veterinarians fear something will go wrong. We know from experience that it isn't a pretty sight. We discourage owners

from being present to protect them and to protect ourselves. The last thing we want is a client to go out saying Dr. So-and-So euthanized my horse and it was awful."

"No matter how smooth it [euthanasia] goes, it is not a good scene. When it doesn't go well it is a terrible scene."

"If the horse is down, I have no problem with the owner being present. My greatest concern is that I would appear to be hurting the horse or to be doing something wrong because the horse hits the ground so hard."

"Some of the people who want to come in [be present during treatment or euthanasia] have the hardest horses to handle because the horse is spoiled. Sometimes you have to get rough with the horses and clients don't understand and get upset."

"I try to talk clients out of being there. The most important part doesn't have to do with the euthanasia. It has to do with how you handled the case and the notes (condolences) afterwards. But, if the client is present and the euthanasia goes badly, you've lost the case."

These comments reflect the fact that, like small-animal practitioners, the primary reason large-animal veterinarians give for discouraging owners from being present during their animals' deaths is that they feel it will be too upsetting for owners to watch. They know that the odds are high that owners will witness their animals' bodies crashing down, see their horses' heads bouncing hard against the ground, view their llamas' muscles and eyes twitching, watch their animals urinating or defecating, hear their ponies' agonal gasps or whinnying, and endure other somewhat unpredictable body changes. Many large-animal veterinarians believe that no positive value is gained when owners view these final processes.

Some well-meaning veterinarians discourage (and even forbid) owners from witnessing their companion animals' euthanasias, believing that it is best to shield owners from the experience. They may also discourage client presence because they feel that it upsets dying animals or because they fear that, during the procedure, they will become upset themselves. When owners are given the option of being present during their animals' deaths, veterinarians are obliged to place catheters and sedate animals to minimize trauma to the owners. Some veterinarians discourage client presence because it also takes more time, effort, and money.

Large-animal veterinarians have a right to these concerns. Large-animal euthanasias are unpredictable. It is difficult to predict how large animals will react to lethal injections of drugs, regardless of the precautions taken to avoid adverse reactions. Although most animals fall quickly to the ground, some react with excitability and rear up or struggle. Because, with horse deaths, veterinarians confront so many individual variables such as age and a range of medical conditions from broken legs to severe gastrointestinal disorders, it is very difficult to predict animals' responses.

Client safety is another legitimate concern. Because it is difficult to know which way animals will fall during euthanasia, veterinarians fear that their clients may be injured during the procedure. According to the AVMA, the most costly law suits against equine veterinarians are due to personal injury (Dinsmore, J. R., unpublished data). It is easy to see, therefore, why many veterinarians prefer that their clients not be present or, at least, not directly assist with the euthanasias of large animals.

Many large-animal veterinarians say, however, that they feel differently about clients being with their animals during euthanasia. Without question, it is emotionally painful for owners to watch their dearly loved companion animals die; however, clinical experience with owners has shown that being absent when companion animals die potentially increases clients' feelings of pain and distress. Returning to Hagstad's survey, he says:

> Most owners *do* want to be present when their horse or other companion animal is euthanatized, and encouragement is frequently not necessary.[4]

Other veterinarians with whom we talked agreed. Their comments were:

> "Most owners feel the animal needs them to be there."

> "We never try to talk owners out of being present [for euthanasia] if they've come to the decision that they want to be there. We know they had to work hard to come to that decision. We have no right to talk them out of it."

Why Clients Want and Need to Be Present

In Chapter 8, we presented several reasons why small-animal owners want to be present during their pets' euthanasias. Those reasons were:

- To have opportunities to say goodbye.
- To prevent guilt about abandonment.
- To prevent long-term denial.
- To know what death was really like.

These arguments also apply to large-animal owners. Large-animal veterinarians who understand owners' reasons for wanting to be present respect their clients' rights to decide what they need for themselves. They understand that no one else can fully determine what level of emotional pain another person is capable of enduring. They also understand that emotional pain is associated with being denied access to loved ones or in being perceived as unable to handle stressful events.

In regard to this fact, horse owners expressed their thoughts on this issue to us. Examples of their comments include:

> "I was there when he was born. I want to be there when he dies."

> "It was hard to watch but it would have been harder not to be there when Midnight died. I couldn't have lived with myself if I had left him during that time."

> "I needed to know that it went the way my vet said it did. I had to see it for myself."

Many veterinarians who discourage owner presence report that very little discussion is needed to "talk clients out" of being there. These are the veterinarians who most likely say, in discouraging tones:

> "Have you ever witnessed the euthanasia of a horse? It's not pretty! I would not recommend that you see it, but I will leave it up to you."

We believe that very few anxious and confused individuals would be likely to feel that they could handle witnessing the procedure, or that it would be beneficial for them to do so, with this kind of slanted preparation. It can be presumed that, if the option were presented in this manner, most large-animal clients would elect not to attend their animals' euthanasias.

Talking to owners about the impending deaths of their animals is challenging. Preparing owners to be present during euthanasia requires the use of all of the verbal and nonverbal communication skills you learned about in Chapters 6 and 7. During these discussions, it is important for you to remember that you are operating from the TEAM model and, therefore, assuming a helping role. Thus, it is imperative that you speak to your clients with openness and neutrality.

You will be the most helpful to clients when you tell them up front that you will not interfere or take sides either way during their decision-making processes and that you will support them in whatever decisions they make. You will also be most helpful when you present accurate information in nonprejudiced ways. One way to assess your own prejudice toward an overall attitude of discouragement, encouragement, or neutrality is to evaluate how you would respond to the following comment from an anxious client:

> "I would like to be with my horse Red to the very end of his life, but I don't know if I can handle it emotionally."

BOX 9-1

Letter to the Editor

Regarding the article, "There is no good way to euthanatize a horse" (JAVMA, 15 June 1990, pp. 1942–1944,) I can sympathize with the author, but I believe the dilemma can be resolved by following two principles: Prepare the client, and administer the lethal drug as a complete bolus dose.

Here is the way I handle equine euthanasia. First, I tell the client exactly what I am going to do and what will happen. For example, "I will give your horse a sedative that is like morphine to get him calm and pain-free. Then I will administer a large dose of barbiturate—the same drug you take in a sleeping pill—but in this case a lethal dose. About 20 to 30 seconds after I give this in the vein, it will reach the horse's brain and all the little black boxes that control the body—brain waves, heart, respiration—will shut down. He will drop on his side and be dead when he hits the ground. There may be some muscle twitching as long as there is oxygen in the muscles. Sometimes there is still an eye reflex. He will rarely take a breath. But, if he is still alive, he is in such deep anesthesia that he will be dead in a matter of a few seconds."

As for the client being with his horse, I leave this up to the owner. Some like to be there to say good-bye, and I will commonly have the client feed a carrot to the horse when I inject the xylazine. But with the injection of pentobarbital, I have the client step back while I control the horse's collapse. Then the client can pet the horse again after it is safely grounded. . . .

With respect to the procedure itself, I give 200 to 300 mg of xylazine, IV, followed by 120 mL of pentobarbital (6 grains/mL) in a bolus IV dose 2 minutes later; this can be given in about 10 seconds through a 14-gauge needle, using two 60-mL syringes filled with pentobarbital. The horse will collapse on its side about 30 seconds after the beginning of the injection. Its head will hit the ground hard, but the fall can be softened by controlling the head with a good stout lead rope. In 95% of all cases, the horse is dead when it hits the ground, and there is no further movement; however, some horses will have momentary palpebral reflex and some muscle fasciculation.

Reprinted in part from a letter to the Journal of the American Veterinary Medical Association written by James H. Steer, DVM, Petaluma, California, September, 1, 1990. Used with permission from the Journal of the American Veterinary Medical Association.

As you listen to this client's statement, do you place greater emphasis on the first part of the sentence, "I would like to be with my horse Red to the very end of his life. . ." or on the second part of the sentence, ". . .but I don't know if I can handle it emotionally." Where you focus your attention may make a very big difference for the client. You could give more weight to the second part of the statement, taking her words at face value, thus discouraging her from witnessing the death. This approach may also ensure that the euthanasia would be less stressful for you. On the other hand, you could pick up on the wishes expressed in the first part of the client's statement, helping her to explore and possibly resolve her apprehensions about staying with Red. Anxiety about witnessing death is often diminished by simply detailing the euthanasia procedure and the possible side-effects that might result.

Veterinarians who encourage and advocate client presence at euthanasia do so because they see value in the option. Thus, they work to create environments that foster client presence. They strive to make euthanasias meaningful experiences for owners who want to be with their animals to the very end of their animals' lives.

These veterinarians view client presence as a time to show the humane and compassionate side of veterinary medicine. In our experience, when clients are adequately prepared to witness their animals' deaths, their presence at euthanasia leaves them with positive feelings about veterinary medicine instead of horrible images of death scenes that cannot be witnessed by lay persons (Box 9-1).

Explaining the Procedure

In terms of large-animal euthanasia, you can best prepare clients by offering them accurate, detailed information about what will occur. With their permission, owners should be informed about what occurs during euthanasia, regardless of their choice about presence or nonpresence. To begin, you should review the procedure in a step-by-step fashion. For example, owners should be told what drugs will be given and where and how they will affect their animals. They should also be told that the drugs will take effect in several seconds and that their animals may fall (perhaps hard) to the ground. You should be honest, specific, and thorough in your descriptions of death by euthanasia because this is the only way owners can make informed decisions about whether or not to be present. You should also focus on the fact that death is quick and painless.

At the CSU-Veterinary Teaching Hospital, when clients are offered the option of being present at large-animal euthanasias, the veterinarians' or counselors' preparatory descriptions are similar to the following (Box 9-2). These statements are not delivered in long, dry monologues. In general, the topics take about 10 minutes to cover, and clients often have questions and comments along the way.

> "Mrs. Green, we understand that your horse Chief is very important to you. Therefore, we want you to feel you have

had the opportunity to say goodbye to him in whatever way is right for you. We realize that this may include being present, if possible, when Chief is euthanized. Because you need information to make an informed decision about being present, with your permission, I would like to provide you with that now."

With the client's permission, the veterinarian continues:

"The first thing we will do is place a catheter in Chief's neck. This will make it easier for us to administer the drug when the time comes. If necessary, we may also give Chief a mild sedative. When he is actually euthanized, Chief will die from the injection of a very strong barbiturate. The drug will cause his brain to stop functioning so he will feel no pain. Soon after, the rest of Chief's body will shut down until his heart stops. I want to repeat, no pain is associated with this procedure.

"After the injection is given, Chief will stand for several seconds, collapse, and then fall. He will not know what is happening, and will be dead by the time he hits the ground.

BOX 9-2

Preparing Clients to Be Present at Equine Euthanasia

If owners want to be present during their horses' euthanasias, it is important to prepare them for what they may see during and after death. Although equine euthanasias are unpredictable, owners should be prepared to witness all or most of the events mentioned below. They should also be told that death by humane euthanasia is painless. During or after death, a horse may:

- Appear excited
- Seem to struggle
- Rear up
- Buckle and fall hard
- Hit the ground hard with both his body and head
- Exhibit muscle twitching
- "Paddle" or "run in place" on the ground
- Exhibit leg stiffening
- Urinate, defecate, flatulate
- Release several gasps after death
- Bleed from the nose, mouth, or catheter or needle insertion sites
- Have his eyes open
- Have a heartbeat for several minutes after death has actually occurred

He may hit the ground very hard. For a few seconds, he may move his legs a bit or stretch them out stiffly. In addition, Chief may take several deep gasps, but he will not be aware of this. You may see his eyes moving back and forth for several seconds, and his eyes will remain open after death. Generally, no blood comes from the nose or mouth (unless a particular disease is present that would cause this). Chief will most likely urinate, defecate, or pass gas within a few minutes. He may also have a heartbeat for a couple of minutes, but generally no respiration. Chief will be completely unaware of what is happening during this time, but I still want to prepare you that this may be difficult to watch."

The veterinarian continues by saying something like:

"It will be impossible for us to fully control Chief's collapse; therefore, we cannot predict which direction he will fall. In some instances, we have had horses rear up or kick. Therefore, it will be important that you stand away from your horse until he is on the ground. If you wish to soothe, pet, brush, or talk to him again, you will be able to in a few minutes after I have pronounced him dead. Then, you will need to come in on the safe side of his body, away from his legs. Under no circumstances should you come close to Chief during the procedure. This is for your safety and for Chief's benefit. I can't perform euthanasia in the most humane way if I am distracted by your presence. Remember, you should not try to intervene even if it appears I need help. If I need help, my technician will step in."

Veterinarians close the description of what will occur by reassuring owners that they will support them whatever they decide. They say something like:

"You will need to decide what is best for you based on everything I've told you. We want to ensure that your needs are met, so I will respect your decision whether or not you want to be there."

These explanations are greatly enhanced when conversations are conducted in private, quiet settings with both veterinarians and owners sitting or standing at the same eye level. It is also enhanced when veterinarians show their sense of compassion by offering tissues or gentle touches to owners who cry or openly express their feelings.

If clients are interested, you can also provide them with a description or, if possible, a tour of possible euthanasia sites. This information should be given whether or not the site is aesthetically pleasing. At CSU, for example, horses are often euthanized on the concrete pavement behind the hospital near necropsy or in an induction stall. For clients to make informed decisions about witnessing their animals' deaths, these sites should be seen or least described. The clients we know who have toured possible euthanasia sites tell us that they have found these visual representations extremely helpful. Knowing what to expect helped to calm their anxieties about being present at their animals' euthanasias.

Regardless of clients' decisions, you should ask them if they would prefer to lead their horses to the euthanasia area. They should also be assured that they can have time alone with their animals to say goodbye before and after the procedure.

Although client presence has value, encouraging client presence must be done with care. You should never talk clients into being present at euthanasia. Some clients very clearly decide to leave their animals in their veterinarian's hands to be euthanized. This option is as acceptable as any other, and clients should not be deterred from this decision.

THE THIRD CHOICE: EUTHANASIA LOGISTICS

The third component of euthanasia preparation is planning and agreeing on the logistic details of the procedure. For example, appropriate times and settings must be determined. Whether you are in a hospital, clinic, or stable, remember that the timing of euthanasia may be somewhat flexible. Whenever possible, try to schedule the euthanasia during a relatively quiet time of the day so that animals and clients can have your undivided attention, particularly when you are planning to euthanize an animal at a public place where other owners may be present. Suggest that clients avoid feeding times or other high-traffic times.

Owners must also decide who else, if anyone, is to accompany them to the euthanasia. For example, with proper preparation, children often choose to be present when their companion animals die. It is a good idea to encourage owners to ask someone to attend their animals' euthanasias with them, given that even sensitively conducted deaths are difficult to bear alone.

Regardless of where and when euthanasia occurs, procedural matters should be addressed before the euthanasia, if possible. Consent forms should be signed, and arrangements for payment should be made. If the owner is a trusted client, a bill can be sent after the event. However, the bill should *never* be included in a condolence card!

Location

Across the country, new protocols for facilitating client presence at large-animal euthanasias are under consideration. Much thought and preparation is going into the development of these protocols in hopes of minimizing the physical distress for animals and the mental and emotional distress for humans. Because numerous methods and sites are available for large-animal euthanasias, safety and financial considerations are high priorities.

Financial considerations are important to discuss before euthanasia for the benefit of both you and your clients. Because some of these protocols involve considerable amounts of time and resources, you should charge for them accordingly. By the same token, clients have a right to decide how much they can afford to spend on euthanasia. When they understand the different options and why the costs vary, they can make informed choices that are right for them.

Regardless of the methods and sites that your clients choose, they should be reassured that their animals will die without pain. They should also be prepared for the event in much the same manner as described in Chapter 8.

Recommended Methods for Large-Animal Euthanasias in Veterinary Teaching Hospitals and Surgery Practices

If client-present euthanasias are done in veterinary teaching hospitals or large-animal surgery practices, an ambulatory animal can be moved into a surgery preparation room for euthanasia. There, an intravenous catheter can be placed, usually without much discomfort to the animal, and a mild sedative can be given to calm the animal before moving him or her into an anesthesia induction stall.

The anesthesia induction stall we use at CSU is padded (walls and floor) and is approximately 9 by 12 feet in size (Fig. 9-4). It is equipped with a padded wooden gate, which is used to keep the animal safely against the wall during the administration of the euthanasia solution. The gate swings up against the animal and pushes him or her into a space approximately equal to an adult horse's length and width. At this time, a lead rope is loosely looped through a wall tie or iron ring to partially control the animal's movements. The animal may show brief excitability when gently pushed against the wall, but this is momentary because the euthanasia solution is injected into the catheter immediately.

In seconds to minutes, as the animal goes down, the lead rope is loosened, and the gate is slowly moved back, allowing the animal to fall onto the padded floor. A thick strap with loops at each end (a cargo strap like those used in the shipping industry works well) is placed on the floor before the gate is opened and before the horse falls. Later, the strap is

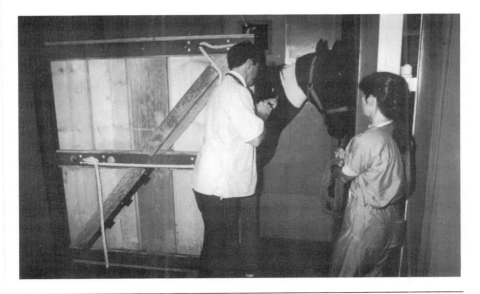

Figure 9-4 An anesthesia induction stall can be used to bring a horse down safely and in a more aesthetically acceptable manner, particularly when clients are present.

attached to a hoist for moving the horse onto a cart and then to the necropsy or body disposal area.

Animals can also be euthanized in an anesthesia recovery stall. At CSU, this room is approximately 14 by 14 feet in size (Fig. 9-5). Like the induction stall, the recovery room is padded but does not have a swinging gate. After the animal is in the stall, the lead rope is loosely attached to a wall tie or iron ring to partially control the animal's movements. The veterinarian and technician then ensure that they are safely positioned while working with the animal. If possible, they attempt to guide the animal down slowly. The veterinarian may also try to push the animal toward the wall so that the animal can lean against it. This way, the animal slumps down rather than falling with full body weight onto the mat. An animal may still fall hard, but a fall onto a recovery pad is more aesthetically pleasing to witness than one that occurs on concrete. The recovery room also has a hoist that allows an animal to be lifted up onto a cart for transport to necropsy or other body care areas. If an animal needs to be transported through a client area, the body should be draped.

We want to emphasize that clients can observe these euthanasias but should not be directly involved with the procedures. They should stand a safe distance from their animals (to be determined by the veterinarian on a case-by-case basis), perhaps in the doorway of the anesthesia induction or

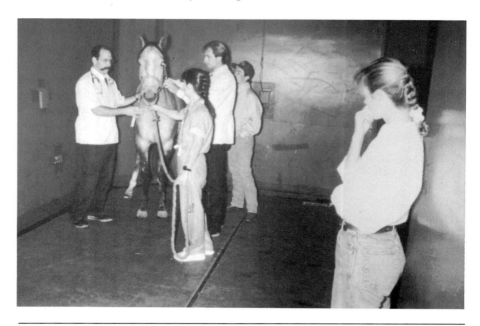

Figure 9-5 The padded walls and floors of a surgery recovery stall provide a more protective and private setting for equine euthanasias.

recovery stall (Fig. 9-5). Clients can enter the stall to spend time with their animals after they are down. Again, they should be given time to say goodbye to their animals and then escorted out before the hoist is used to move the animal. If possible, a staff member should stay with the animal's body at the euthanasia site. Almost every owner whom we have assisted during euthanasia takes one last look back at their companion animal before they actually leave. When they see a friendly, familiar face next to their animal, they feel reassured that their companion animal will not be forgotten or treated with disrespect once they leave.

It should be noted that neither of these rooms are used if animals are suspected to have contagious conditions such as strangles or salmonellosis. If this is the case, the situation is fully explained to the owner, and an appropriate place (based on convenience, safety, and privacy) is used for the euthanasia with or without the owner's presence.

On some occasions, the decision is made to euthanize large animals during surgery. If the decision is made to euthanize on the surgery table, or if animals die unexpectedly on the table, owners are sometimes given the opportunity to see their companion animals one last time to say goodbye. In these cases, owners are dressed in surgery scrubs, and the surgical incisions are adequately draped so that owners are not overwhelmed by the medical aspects of the scene. If it is impossible to bring owners into the surgery room, incisions can be quickly closed with sutures and covered with a blanket or drape. Animals can then be moved onto a cart, out of the surgery room, and into a suitable visitation area.

Because surgical environments are sterile, it is not advisable to routinely allow clients to enter the surgery room. Other measures can be taken, however, to both sensitively acknowledge owners' bonds with their animals and to attend to the emotions that accompany the severing of those bonds. For example, before inducement, regardless of how minor the surgery is, owners can be encouraged to spend a little time with their animals. Allowing clients to use a viewing window into the surgery room can also give them the feeling that they are still connected to their animals.

Recommended Methods for Large-Animal Euthanasia in Private Practice

If you do not have access to facilities like those described above, you may have no choice other than to euthanize large animals outside of your veterinary clinic (Fig. 9-6). In these situations, you must ensure that clients

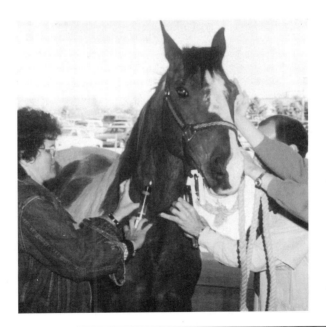

Figure 9-6 The most convenient euthanasia sites often lack privacy. This one, across from a faculty parking lot, yet directly behind the necropsy building, facilitates immediate removal of the body after death.

understand why the procedure is being done in this location. Although the location is different, the preparation for euthanasia remains the same (for example, educate clients, use catheters and sedatives, and allow clients time to say goodbye), and, even if the location is not aesthetically pleasing, owners should be allowed to decide whether or not they want to be present. As before, for safety reasons, clients must stand away from their animals during the procedure at a distance that is deemed appropriate by their veterinarian.

You may be tempted to euthanize large animals in a stall, especially if clients choose to be present; however, it may be hazardous to you and your staff to perform euthanasia in a stall that is not specifically equipped for the procedure. Obviously, you should never compromise your own safety. In addition, it is very difficult to remove a large animal's body after euthanasia has been completed. Stalls should therefore only be used when animals are already down or are unable to be moved due to illness or injury.

To protect animals during euthanasias that are conducted in stalls, you can pad concrete areas with hay or other protective padding; however, use caution because this material can become slippery. The padding can be easily moved after the procedure is completed. Most owners will understand when you explain why stalls are not the most practical areas for euthanizing large animals. They, too, are interested in using areas that will later facilitate the most efficient disposal or rendering of their companion animals' bodies.

Recommended Methods for Large-Animal Euthanasia on Ambulatory Services

The most common place for large animals to be euthanized is in clients' pastures and stables. Obviously, in these cases, you do not have access to well-equipped surgery induction stalls or padded recovery rooms. Under most conditions, you also do not have the benefit of support staff or excessive amounts of time in which to help clients make life and death decisions. It is therefore helpful to try to mobilize clients' support systems before arriving at their homes. For example, after receiving your clients' calls for euthanasia, you can encourage owners to bring friends or family members along with them to the euthanasia site to help them with their decision-making. If the euthanasia is planned, you might also ask clients to determine whether other family members or friends might want or need to say goodbye to the animal. Having extra support helps you and your clients because it allows you to focus on medical procedures while clients receive comfort from others.

When large animals are injured or in distress, you need to act quickly and practically. Also, on ambulatory services, you often do not have the luxury of euthanizing sick or injured animals in privacy. Emergency euthanasias are often done in pastures, stables, arenas, show rings, or race tracks. The presence of others sometimes puts more pressure on you to "perform" with compassion and sensitivity; therefore, you must have a repertoire of euthanasia and communication techniques that can be used quickly and efficiently. These methods must be as aesthetically acceptable to untrained observers as possible. In such situations, time for precautions against the possible side-effects of the euthanasia drugs is limited. Thus, in many emergencies, catheters and sedatives are not used because the goal is to help animals die as quickly and painlessly as possible. Sometimes, however, it is worth a few extra minutes to ensure that large animals' euthanasias go smoothly. Within reason, you should take time to use catheters, sedatives, to explain any intervening variables to clients, and to prepare them for what they may observe. For obvious reasons, clients' goodbyes to their animals before death may be shortened. Therefore, time with their animals' bodies should be offered afterward.

Body Care

Whenever possible, decisions about body care should also be made before euthanasia. Owners should be offered all of the options available to them, and each should be explained with honesty and sensitivity. The cost of each option should also be disclosed. It is helpful to use visual aids during this explanation. For example, if you have brochures about pet cemeteries and crematories or if you make urns available for owners to purchase, samples can be shown to them. Do not underestimate large-animal owners' needs for this information. Increasingly more horse and llama owners are choosing to bury or cremate their companion animals, despite the expense of these procedures.

Body care options can be explained by you or by your technician. Again, it is important to emphasize that this information is not delivered in the form of a dry, continuous monologue, given that owners often respond by crying or by asking several questions. When offering body care options for large animals, say something like:

> "Mrs. Green, we can offer you three options for taking care of Chief's body after he dies. The first option is that you can take him with you and bury him at home, in a pet cemetery, or in another appropriate place. If that is your choice, we encourage you to make proper arrangements for transporting his body. We have a local pet cemetery that may be able to help you with this.
> "Second, we can cremate Chief's body and either dispose of the cremains for you or return them to you, if you so desire. If you want them returned to you, you may want to

choose an urn or another kind of container to keep them in.
Some people like to keep their animals' cremains, and some
like to spread them in an appropriate location. Because so
many people today move quite often, many owners choose
cremation so they can take their companion animals' cremains
with them.

"Your third option, Mrs. Green, is to have us take care of
Chief's body for you. Although I wish I had a more aesthetically pleasing option to offer you, my only option is _____."
(Veterinarians should fill in the blank with whatever is accurate, usually delivery to or pick up by a rendering company.
It may also be helpful to ask clients if they understand what
rendering means and, if they do not, to explain it to them.
Ways to explain rendering to both adults and children are
given in Chapters 10 and 12, respectively. If clients want information about rendering, provide them with names and
telephone numbers of services that are familiar to you.)

There *are* pet cemeteries and crematories who will bury or cremate
horses, llamas, and other large animals. These are labor-intensive procedures, however, therefore the cost usually runs into hundreds, and even
thousands, of dollars. Therefore, during the explanation of body care options, the expense involved with large-animal burial and cremation should
be made clear to owners. If owners do choose to bury their animals on their
land, explain that the most efficient method involves digging the grave
before the euthanasia and then carrying out the procedure at the grave site.

Most owners have no choice but to render their animals; however, many
may feel that it would be more meaningful to bury or cremate them. When
clients express this dilemma to you, you can help them to devise creative
solutions. For example, you may suggest that they take the horseshoes or
hair from the tail or mane with them and bury them on their property. Or,
as is done with some racehorses, suggest that they bury the legs and heart
of the horse, and send the remains to be rendered. There are numerous
other creative solutions to this problem. The idea is to give clients permission to take action that is meaningful to them.

FACILITATING CLIENT-PRESENT EUTHANASIAS

Owners who arrive for euthanasia appointments should be given priority
over everything except medical emergencies. They should also be immediately escorted to wherever the euthanasia will occur.

Whenever possible, it is recommended that all client-present euthanasias be conducted by a team of at least two veterinary professionals. This

approach allows whoever is assisting the veterinarian to focus on owner needs and allows the veterinarian to concentrate on the medical aspects of the euthanasia procedure. Pagers should be turned off during the actual procedure to avoid unnecessary distractions.

It is highly recommended that, if owners have elected to be present, the use of both a catheter and a sedative be carefully evaluated. Catheters and sedatives are not always necessary, and they do not always improve the medical procedures involved with euthanasia. They are often an enhancement to the emotional side of euthanasia, however, because they provide extra insurance that animals die peacefully, without adverse side-effects. Let us look at each individually.

Catheters

If you use a catheter, it should be placed in the jugular vein. This approach allows easier and safer access to the animal. A catheter not only facilitates rapid administration, but also ensures direct injection into the vein without multiple attempts. Large animals are given local blocks (1 mL of lidocane) subcutaneously, just over the vein, to anesthetize a small area of their necks and ease placement of a catheter into their jugular veins. Most large animals will feel no discomfort with the insertion of the catheter. If you are concerned about the added cost of using catheters for euthanasias, non-sterile, previously used catheters can be placed. Make sure that used catheters are in working condition before you attempt to use them with an owner present.

If a catheter is not used, a 14-gauge needle should be inserted into the jugular vein. The needle should be loosely attached to the first syringe so that it can be removed and the second syringe attached without delay. Be sure to explain to the owner that blood will be seen flowing from the needle as the syringes are exchanged. If an assistant is available, the solution from both syringes can be injected into both jugular veins simultaneously.

Drugs

Because client-presence during euthanasia has been infrequent in large-animal medicine, drug combinations that would reliably produce deaths that are both humane and psychologically acceptable for owners have not been methodically tested. Successful methods are being developed for minimizing the side-effects of euthanasia which make the dying process *appear* difficult to owners (vocalizations, reflexive muscle contractions, and agonal gasping). With various methods now in use, unconsciousness is reached rapidly, death occurs quickly, and the process appears to be pain-less for the animal. (Authors' note: Because we are not veterinarians, we wish to make it clear that we are not making recommendations about how you should use any of the drugs listed in this chapter. Rather, we are simply reporting what several large-animal practitioners in both private and university practices and veterinary pharmacists have told us.)

When clients are present, carefully evaluate the usefulness of sedatives or tranquilizers before euthanasias because they may calm animals and smooth the way animals fall. Several drugs, in various combinations, can be used to sedate or tranquilize animals before euthanasia. According to several veterinarians whom we consulted, a tranquilizer such as acepromazine or sedatives such as detomidine or xylazine [Rompun (Miles Inc., A Division of Animal Health Products, Shawnee Mission, Kansas)] can be used. Xylazine, for example, is a short-acting sedative-analgesic that is often used for pain in colicing horses. Ketamine, an anesthetic, can also be used, but only in combination with a sedative such as xylazine. Butorphanol, a narcotic agonist-antagonist analgesic, can also be used to calm animals before euthanasia. The amount of drug used varies based on the type of drug, the nature of the situation, and the needs and disposition of the animal. It is important to remember, however, that when using sedatives and tranquilizers before euthanasia, it may take longer for the euthanasia solution to take effect, particularly for animals suffering from cardiovascular problems, other serious illnesses, or old age.

Pentobarbital sodium, a Class Two barbiturate, is most commonly used for euthanasia of large animals. The recommended dosage is 40 mg per pound of animal. The drug is administered intravenously and as rapidly as possible. It is important to be accurate when preparing the dosage because clinical experience has shown that underdosing animals usually causes them to die slower. An inadequate dose, or even slow delivery of the dosage, can result in extreme excitement in the animal. At a client-present euthanasia, such excitement will cause the animal, the owner, and you more distress.

In special circumstances, some veterinarians recommend adding an appropriate dose of succinylcholine, a paralytic agent, to the second syringe of pentobarbital. This eliminates gasps, "running in place," and other residual effects associated with euthanasia. This drug should be added *only* to the euthanasia solution so that animals are unaware of its paralyzing effect. The 1993 Report of the AVMA Panel on Euthanasia summarizes some of the unacceptable agents and methods for euthanasia. It condemns the sole use of succinylcholine, or any other neuromuscular blocking agent, for the purpose of euthanasia without use of a sedative[11] because it causes death by suffocation. We can assume that suffocating an animal that is fully aware of what is occurring would produce great distress and severe anxiety.

Saying Goodbye

Before the procedure begins, owners should be given the opportunity, if they so desire, to spend a short time alone with their companion animals. If owners are left alone to say their last goodbyes, you should state when you will return. For example, you may say, "I will be back in about 10 minutes." If more time can be allowed for clients to say goodbye, it should be provided.

Alternatively, you may ask owners to somehow signal you or a member of your staff when they are ready to proceed. If owners are asked to signal, the task must be made as simple as possible. It is a good idea for at least one member of your veterinary team to remain close by so he or she can watch for the summons.

If owners are still saying goodbye after the agreed amount of time, you can approach them and gently say, "It is time for us to proceed. May we begin?" Most owners will indicate their answer by either nodding or shaking their heads. If their answer is "no," it is appropriate for you to give them 5 or 10 minutes more. Any statement to this effect, however, must be made in a calm, quiet voice with no detectable overtones of impatience. Owners often report that they felt rushed through the euthanasia process by their veterinarian and feel that this negated the other positive aspects of their experience.

When owners are ready to proceed, it is normal for you and the members of your veterinary team to feel somewhat awkward as you enter the environment in which the euthanasia is to be done. You may wonder what you should say or do to comfort your grieving clients. Sometimes, no words are necessary. A touch on an owner's arm or a hug around their shoulders communicates support and understanding quite well.

Euthanizing Horses

Before you begin the lethal injections, you should again tell the owners that you are ready to begin. Whenever possible, you should keep syringes out of sight and handle them very discretely because some people become very alarmed at the sight of needles.

After the procedure has begun, the drugs should be injected as quickly as possible. During this time, the owner should stand away from the horse, and your full attention should be given to bringing the horse down as safely and gently as possible (Fig. 9-7). During this time, it is natural for you to talk to the horse, calming it and guiding it down safely.

After the animal has actually died, it is very important for you to use a stethoscope to listen for a final heartbeat. Then, when you can do so with certainty, the animal should be pronounced dead. You should do this by

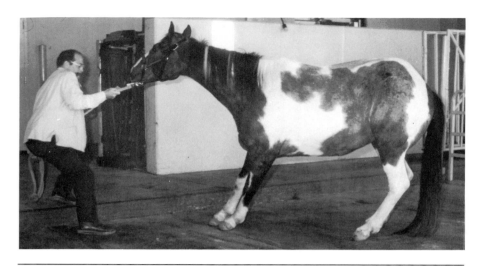

Figure 9-7 Generally the horse begins to collapse within seconds of the injection of euthanasia solution. The veterinarian must use all of his or her concentration and physical strength to bring the horse down as quickly and safely as possible.

walking over to where your client is standing and saying a clear, simple statement such as:

> "Mrs. Green, Chief is dead. If you want to, you can go in on the safe side of his body, away from his legs, and spend time with him."

At this time, owners may gasp, cry, sob, or sigh with relief. They may make remarks about how quickly death came and about how meaningful the experience was to them. This is a good time for you to reassure owners about their decisions to euthanize their animals. It is also a good time for you to express your own feelings of affection and respect for their animals. For example, you might say, "I'm going to miss Chief, too. He always nuzzled me when I came into his stall." These statements may prompt owners to begin a review of their animals' lives. They may share special or funny stories. Many owners appreciate the opportunity to talk a bit about their animals and to reminisce about the life that has just ended.

Euthanizing Llamas

For the most part, llamas are easier to euthanize than other large animals, primarily because of their size. Adult llamas weigh an average of 250 to 500 pounds and grow to 40 to 50 inches high at the withers.[2] Their small size, compared with horses, allows veterinarians and owners to stay close to llamas throughout the euthanasia procedure. In addition, llamas are more easily controlled and more easily guided to the ground as their legs begin to knuckle under them. During euthanasia, llamas' collapse onto the ground can be softened by euthanizing them on a large pad or a bed of straw and by using a rope around their necks to control their heads.

Currently, the exact amount of drug necessary to euthanize llamas has not been "fine-tuned." For the most part, veterinarians use 400 mg/mL of concentrated pentobarbital injected intravenously. This solution has been shown to be consistently effective in producing death. In addition, at this time, many food-animal veterinarians working with llamas do not use sedatives before injecting the euthanasia solution. It is recommended, however, that if clients are present to use an appropriate dose of butorphanol intramuscularly before the intravenous injection of the euthanasia solution.

When clients are present, the worst that can happen is injecting the sedative or the euthanasia solution into the common carotid artery when attempting to hit the jugular vein. The carotid artery and the jugular vein are in very close proximity in the llama (more so than in other animals), and the two can be easily confused even by an experienced practitioner. If the needle is inserted into the carotid artery, the pressure in the syringe will automatically push the plunger out (unless the animal's blood pressure is low), indicating that the needle is incorrectly placed. Injection of solutions into the carotid artery can cause convulsions for several minutes, and these are very disturbing. Because of the close proximity and, therefore, the potential for adverse reactions, it is highly recommended that you use intravenous catheters when clients are present. Use of an intravenous

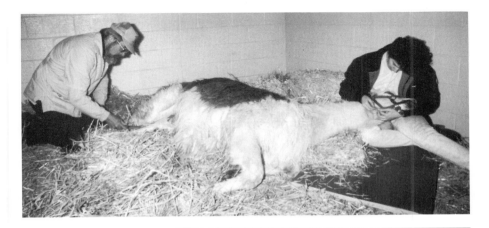

Figure 9-8 A client-present euthanasia of a llama.

catheter extension set provides an added advantage in that llamas can move without disrupting the injection of fluid. Because intravenous catheter placement can be difficult, an alternative is to initially use an appropriate dosage of ketamine plus Rompun intramuscularly followed by injection of pentobarbital intravenously through the medial saphenous vein (Fig. 9-8).

You should prepare llama owners for what will occur before, during, and after their llamas' deaths in much the same way you prepare horse owners. For example, you should explain that death will occur within seconds and that their llamas will become limp and lay over onto the ground. Owners should also be told that gasps, some muscle twitching, urination, defecation, or expulsion of stomach contents from the nose and mouth may occur. Again, you should emphasize that their animals will not feel any pain.

As they are injected, each drug should be named so that owners are kept abreast of how the procedure is progressing. For example, you might say, "Marcia, I am giving Brownie a sedative that will make him sleepy." With the next injection, you might say, "Now I am injecting the final drug." Aside from these statements, it is best for you to remain silent. Most owners want to focus on saying goodbye to their animals and find comments, questions, and chatter distracting to their concentration.

Some llama or alpaca owners may want to keep their animals' wool for economic or sentimental reasons, especially in the case of neonates. Therefore, owners may want their animals' hides tanned and may ask you to skin their animals. Because most veterinarians do not have the time necessary to devote to this task, it is good to know people in your community who will agree to complete this process at a reasonable fee. Alternatively, if owners are skilled at shearing, they may want to shear their animals themselves either before or after death. Before they begin this activity, however, owners should be warned that it could be emotionally painful for them to do so. As with other elements of client preparation, you should ask owners about their wishes before their arrival at the clinic. This approach ensures that they will bring the tools they need with them. It also helps to avoid confusion and saves time.

AFTER-DEATH FOLLOW-UP

After euthanasia, some clients want to leave the veterinary facility or euthanasia site quickly, whereas others need more time alone with their companion animals. Because many owners have invested so much in the physical care of their companion animals, even after death, their animals' bodies remain important to them. If you have appointments waiting and owners want to spend time with the body, you can tell owners that you will be back in 10 minutes or in whatever time frame is reasonable. Alternatively, you or your assistant can ask your next clients if they would mind waiting a few extra minutes past their designated appointment times to allow another owner to finish saying goodbye to an animal who has died. Almost everyone is gracious under these circumstances.

Sometimes, family members who have not been present at the euthanasia may also want to view an animal's body before it is buried, cremated, or sent for rendering. It should be stressed that, if animals are soiled due to urination, defecation, treatment, or surgery, they should be cleaned or brushed before presenting them for owners to see. In addition, all catheters and tape should be removed. When owners are ready to leave, they should be escorted out a side or back door, if possible, so that they do not have to exit through busy areas.

Contacting owners after their companion animals have died is a crucial part of retaining their trust. Sending clients personalized condolence cards or letters should be standard procedure. The content of a condolence should include your personal comments about the companion animal who has died. You should also point out that the owner's decision to euthanize the animal was both timely and humane. In addition, it is also helpful to mention any preliminary necropsy results that serve to validate the owner's decision. More about after death follow-up is discussed in Chapter 10.

CONCLUSION

Much can be learned as we search for better methods for euthanizing large companion animals. For example, the ideal drug and dosage has yet to be found, although veterinarians are gathering ideas on what is needed. According to Donald Buelke, the ideal euthanasia solution would have the following characteristics:[12]

- The product would induce an artificial state of somnolence or relaxation that would allow the horse to become recumbent in a somewhat natural manner.
- The product would be easy to administer. It would be effective in a small dose that could easily be administered through a small-gauge needle.
- The product would be lethal in a single dose, thus precluding repeated venipunctures and handling. It would not require special, phased injection procedures.
- The product would be reasonably safe to the people administering it.
- The product would work consistently in all instances, not just 95% of the time.

- The product by itself would not create undesirable side effects such as twitching, vocalizing, or gasping.
- The product would be economical.

In addition, ideal euthanasia sites and circumstances conducive to client presence are also yet to be found. However, rather than continuing with the old paradigm, which discourages client-presence, we suggest that you work with your clients, support staff, other practitioners, and human service professionals to develop more progressive and emotionally acceptable methods and equipment. For example, we would like to see the development of a portable large-animal euthanasia apparatus that incorporates features such as padded sides and a swinging gate. This structure would operate much like the anesthesia induction stall described earlier and would be particularly useful on ambulatory calls.

Do not wait for ideal circumstances to arise, however, before you offer clients the option of being involved, in some way, in their animals' euthanasias. Even if owners are not present during death, you can at least allow them to say goodbye to their animals before euthanasia and to view their animals' bodies afterward. With the honest and detailed preparation described in this chapter, clients can decide for themselves what they do and do not want to witness regarding their companion animals' deaths. Then, as long as the methods you use are humane (Box 9-3), client presence does not need to be your choice; it can be theirs.

BOX 9-3

Helping during Large-Animal Euthanasia

This checklist can be used to facilitate client-present euthanasias.

- Discuss all possible side effects, scenarios, and behaviors.
- Mobilize clients' own support systems.
- If possible, schedule euthanasias during more quiet times of day.
- If possible, conduct euthanasias in private areas.
- Give clients time to say goodbye to companion animals before and after death.
- Evaluate the advisability of sedating or tranquilizing animals before euthanasia.
- Ensure needles are not screwed on too tightly. This approach allows syringes to be changed easily when giving two injections of pentobarbital.
- Use stout lead ropes to control horses' heads as they fall.
- Using a stethoscope, pronounce companion animals dead.
- Offer clients horse shoes, pieces of mane or tail, or llama wool.
- Team cases whenever possible.
- Cover your costs.

251

REFERENCES

1. Troutman, C.M.: The Veterinary Services Market for Companion Animals. Overland Park, Kan., Charles, Charles Research Group and the American Veterinary Medical Association, 1988.
2. Ebel, S.: The llama industry in the United States. *In* Johnson, L., ed.: Llama Medicine. Vet. Clin. North Am. [Food Anim. Pract.], 5:1–20, W.B. Saunders Company, 1989.
3. Herrick, J.B.: Helping the "hurting" client. J. Am. Vet. Med. Assoc., 189:232-233, 1991.
4. Hagstad, H.V.: Equine euthanasia and client grief. *In* Kay, W.J., Cohen, S.P., Fudin, C.E., Kutscher, A.H., Nieburg, H.A., Grey, R.E., and Ostman, M.M., eds.: Euthanasia of the Companion Animal: The Impact on Pet Owners, Veterinarians, and Society. Philadelphia, The Charles Press, 1988, pp. 90–96.
5. Fogle B.: Attachment—euthanasia—grieving. *In* Fogle, B., ed. Interrelations Between People and Pets. Springfield, Mo., Charles C. Thomas, 1981.
6. Rando, T.A: Grief, Dying, and Death: Clinical Interventions for Caregivers. Champaign, Ill., Research Press Company, 1984.
7. Lagoni, L., Hetts, S., and Withrow, S.J.: The veterinarian's role in pet loss: Grief education, support, and facilitation. *In* Withrow, S.J., and MacEwen, E.G., eds. Clinical Veterinary Oncology. Philadelphia, J.B. Lippincott, 1989, pp. 436–445.
8. Gershon, D., and Straub, G.: Empowerment: The Art of Creating Your Life As You Want It. New York, Dell Publishing, 1989.
9. Ball, J.F.: Widow's grief: The impact of age and mode of death. Omega, 7:307–333, 1977.
10. Parkes, C.M., and Weiss, R.S.: Recovery from Bereavement. New York, Basic Books, 1983.
11. Andrews, E.J., Bennett, B.T., Clark, J.D., Houpt, K.A., Pascoe, P.J., Robinson, G.W., and Boyce, J.R.: 1993 Report of the AVMA Panel on Euthanasia. J. Am. Vet. Med. Assoc., 202:229–249, 1993.
12. Buelke, D.: There's no good way to euthanatize a horse. J. Am. Vet. Med. Assoc., 196: 1942–1944, 1990.

10

Grief Follow-up and After Care

In a bond-centered practice, your professional involvement with clients does not end when companion animals die. In fact, your patients' deaths will often bond clients to you in ways that are more profound than if you had cured their pets, especially when clients feel you truly helped them through the difficult times. Emotionally intense veterinarian-client relationships demand that you continue to have contact with clients after the deaths of their pets. This contact can be maintained by implementing a case follow-up and client after-care plan.

Follow-up after patient death helps everyone involved to draw closure to the human-human and human-companion animal relationships that develop during the course of treatment. There are many ways you can follow-up and continue to help clients, staff members, and yourself after companion animal death. The most obvious and important ways are described in this chapter.

CONDOLENCES

In a bond-centered practice, all clients should receive condolence cards or letters from you after their pets' deaths. The only exceptions to this rule are in cases of clients who have caused their pets' deaths through abuse or convenience euthanasia. In many of these cases, your condolences would probably be wasted.

Offering condolences to clients after pets die can take various forms. Cards specifically addressing pet loss are available from many companies (*see* the Resource Appendix for the addresses of some of the many condolence card companies in the United States). These cards can be purchased in large quantities and kept on hand for your use. You can also type or write a brief personal letter to clients. When you send written condolences, it may be helpful to use the following guidelines:

- Establish a standard policy about sending condolences. That is, if you send written condolences to one client, send them to all of your clients (with the exception of those situations mentioned previously). It is difficult to judge your clients' needs for support based solely on outward appearances. Sometimes, those who appear to be unaffected by pet loss need and appreciate your support the most. In addition, if you practice in a small community, word of mouth is important to your continued success. Clients will be confused and offended if, while talking with one another, they realize that one received your condolences and support and another did not.
- Begin by addressing each member of your client's family by name if you have had contact with them (or if your client has mentioned them frequently as sources of support). It is especially important to include children in your condolences.
- If you are sending a card or typed letter, sign your name rather than typing it or using a stamped or embossed signature. In addition, add a brief hand-written note. When clients receive presigned, impersonal condolences, they often view them more as marketing tools than as sincere gestures of support.
- Use the pet's name (spelled correctly) and be certain to refer correctly to the pet's age, breed, gender, and so forth.
- If appropriate, reassure clients that they did everything they could for their pets both medically and emotionally and that, in the end, they made timely and appropriate decisions about their pets' treatments, euthanasias, or deaths.
- Recall something special or unique about the pet who died and refer to it in concrete, specific terms. This approach lets clients know that you are referring to *their pets* rather than sending them a form letter or offering a version of a standard cliché.
- If preliminary results about postmortems are available and if they *confirm or reinforce* clients' decisions about treatment or euthanasia, they can be included. If the results of postmortems are likely to cause clients to question or doubt their

decisions, they should first be discussed face-to-face or by telephone so that clients have a chance to ask questions.

- Take advantage of this opportunity to educate clients about normal grief. In your own words, normalize some of the manifestations of grief, and give clients permission to experience them. It is also appropriate to include educational and supportive written materials (Box 10-1).
- Invite clients to contact you if they have further questions or concerns. If appropriate, offer referrals to local pet loss support groups or pet loss counselors and include their brochures or business cards.

Two examples of effective condolences are shown here. The first is a brief note suitable for a condolence card, and the second is a longer, more detailed note suitable for a letter.

Dear Roger, Jill, and Matthew,

  I have thought of you often since Toby's death. I really believe that your decision to help her die was the right one. You did everything you could for her and, in the end, spared her any further pain and suffering.

BOX 10-1

Condolence Packet

When sending condolences, you can customize educational packets by including such information as ways to contact local pet cemeteries or crematories, ways to help children with pet loss, adopting new pets, and dealing with behavior changes in surviving pets. The following list represents items appropriate for inclusion with condolence cards and letters.

- Handout: The Manifestations of Grief (Box 2-1)
- Handout: A Loss and Grief Bibliography (Resource Appendix)
- Handout: Memorialization (Box 10-6)
- Handout: How to Help Yourself (Box 10-9)
- Brochure: Death of the Family Pet: Losing a Family Friend (Available from ALPO Pet Foods, Inc.)
- Brochure: Pet Loss & Human Emotion (Available from the American Veterinary Medical Association)
- Brochure describing local pet loss support groups
- Business cards of local pet loss counselors

The next few weeks are bound to be hard. I'll check in with you next week to see if I can be of any further support.

Warmly,

Jeanette Willis, DVM

Dear Roger, Jill, and Matthew,

Please accept by sincere condolences regarding Toby's recent death. She was a gentle, loving dog and I can only imagine the empty space her death has left in your daily lives. Toby was special to me, too. She always cheered me when she came through the door holding her tennis ball in her mouth. I loved to see her stubby, little tail wag in greeting to me and I was always touched by the trust that I saw in her eyes. All of us here at The Pet Clinic will miss her, yet I know that you, her family, will miss her most of all.

I want you to know that the preliminary postmortem results that I have received confirm that Toby's cancer was advanced and that her quality of life was deteriorating rapidly. You did everything you could for her. Even though I'm sure that the decision to help her die last Friday was one of the hardest you have ever made in your lives, I believe it was a timely and humane one. As I told you last week, I am 100% supportive of your decision.

I am enclosing some information about pet loss and grief. It takes a very long time to adjust to the loss of a family member. I believe that being aware of the normal symptoms of grief and knowing that you are likely to experience many of them over the next several weeks and months can help. I work with a pet loss counselor who is available to support any or all of you through your grief. Should you ever want to contact her, I have enclosed her business card. By the same token, if I can be of further help to you, please don't hesitate to call or to stop by the clinic.

Warmly,

Jeanette Willis, DVM

Many clients are grateful for your condolences but find it difficult to acknowledge your kindness. In fact, at CSU, it is not unusual for clients to contact us weeks, months, and sometimes years after their pets' death. Usually, clients begin their thank you notes to us by apologizing for not getting back to us sooner. They go on to say that they were deeply moved by our condolences and had tried to write to us many times but simply could not. Also, you may occasionally hear from clients who are disturbed by your condolences because they "remind" them of their pets' deaths. We urge you to acknowledge these clients' complaints regarding condolences but not to be intimidated by them. If you have established a practice policy about sending condolence cards to all clients who lose their pets, continue to do so. Most clients are sincerely moved by the condolences they receive from their veterinarians, and it is unfair to deprive them of your support.

CONDOLENCES BY TELEPHONE

Many of the clients with whom we have worked also appreciate and bene-fit from follow-up telephone calls. We realize that, for the most part, it is unrealistic to expect you or your staff to have time for comprehensive follow-up conversations. Nonetheless, you will encounter clients who, for one reason or another, require more than a brief, casual follow-up call. Clients in this category may include your most valuable, long-term clients, clients who were highly attached to their companion animals and who were relatively unsupported by others, or clients who reach out to you, initiating a call for help. Whenever possible, it is important for you to take time to talk with and listen to your clients because these conversations can represent the successful or unsuccessful culmination of all your helping efforts.

We realize that the thought of talking to clients after their pets' deaths may be intimidating. You may wonder what you could possibly say that would be helpful to clients during this time. Also, it is logical for you to assume that, because grief is a predominant feature of life, your clients will understand and have access to information regarding normal grief. Grief researchers Arnold and Gemma[1] suggest, however, that this is not the case. They reported that bereaved persons live with a sense of confusion regarding what is normal and what is crazy and that, unfortunately, most are surrounded by others who offer little support or understanding of their grief.

Grief therapist and educator Therese Rando[2] has noted some of the main types of support that grievers need most from others:

- Acceptance.
- Nonjudgmental listening.
- Assistance in blending memories of the past with the present and the future.
- Help with releasing the emotional ties they have to the rela-tionships they have lost.
- Help in subsequently "replacing" the relationships they have lost.

As stated previously, you may be the most available and effective source of this kind of support for many of your clients, especially immediately after their pets' deaths. Most grievers simply need to talk with others who accept pet death as a significant loss and who will listen to the details of their stories without judgment. Many clients have never reviewed the circumstances of their pets' deaths from beginning to end. Also, they have not had the opportunity to reminisce at length about their pets' lives and personalities. These opportunities can be created via telephone. Telephone conversations can provide clients with the encouragement they need to let their grief flow normally.

During such calls, the most important kind of support you can give clients is through listening. You can also extend your condolences, assuage clients' doubts, answer questions that have arisen, and take care of any "unfinished business" regarding the pet loss experience. Also, because clients are in the midst of grief and are actually experiencing the pain of loss, it is a prime time to ensure that they are well-informed and educated about the normal course and manifestations of grief. In fact, in the Changes Program we make a practice of pointing out several important aspects of grief. These points comprise our grief education "spiel" described in Chapter 7. For example, we point out that, during grief, it is not unusual to experience visual, auditory, or olfactory "hallucinations" about pets who have died. We also remind clients that, when they are grieving, it is normal to have vivid dreams in which pets who have died appear and perhaps say goodbye or relay some kind of message. We introduce this information ourselves rather than waiting to see whether clients bring it up. In our experience, most pet owners do experience some form of dream, vision, or hallucination after pet loss; yet, these particular manifestations of grief often make clients feel that they are "losing it" or "going crazy." Clients can therefore be reticent to tell anyone about these feelings. Reassuring clients that these manifestations are normal greatly helps to facilitate healthy grief outcomes.

When talking with clients about grief, we suggest that they give themselves a full year to grieve for their pets. Our reasoning behind this time frame is that, during the year after their pets' deaths, clients encounter many anniversaries and "first times" that trigger the painful feelings associated with pet loss. For example, depending on their level of attachment, some pet owners feel "down" and depressed each month (or even each week) on the date or day that their pets died. Other clients have strong grief reactions during the holidays, family vacations, summer camping trips, and so forth, depending on the activities that pet owners most often shared with their pets. When clients are able to put their lives into the context of grief, they are also better able to make sense of the ongoing, painful, and sometimes disturbing, symptoms that they continue to experience.

Some clients may seem unreceptive to your efforts to follow-up. These clients will usually respond to your questions with brief, polite comments

BOX 10-2

Follow-Up Telephone Tactics

Beginning a Call

Beginning a follow-up call is easier when your clients expect that you will contact them. It also helps to think of calls as scheduled appointments, allowing yourself to fully attend to them. Begin a call by clearly stating the purpose of the contact and your time limitations. Remember that voice tone is important.

When you initiate:

"It was an emotional time when you were last here and we made some difficult decisions. I was wondering if you have any questions or concerns that I could help you sort through during the next few minutes."

"I have a few minutes between appointments and I wanted to see how you've been doing since JoJo died."

When your client initiates:

"I have about ten minutes now. Is this something I can help you with in that length of time or should we schedule a time when I can talk longer?"

"I'm glad you called. I'd be happy to talk with you for about fifteen minutes."

During a Call

It's helpful to encourage clients to talk long enough for you to gather the information you need. You can do this by using the various verbal communication techniques discussed in Chapter 7. For example, you might make use of paraphrase, minimal encouragers, and direct or open-ended questions.

"Uh-huh. . ."

"Go on. . ."

"Take your time. . ."

"So you're feeling confused about when to euthanize JoJo."

"I can hear the sadness in your voice. You miss JoJo a lot."

"You sound exhausted. . ."

"Tell me more about JoJo's accident. What actually happened?"

"JoJo died so unexpectedly. How have you said goodbye?"

Ending a Call

Ending a call is always easier if you have clearly stated your limits and boundaries regarding time, fees, services, and so forth up front. You can also cue clients that the conversation is coming to a close by summarizing the content of your conversation or by asking them what they would like to have happen next. When drawing conversations to a close, it can be helpful to you to physically stand up when you are attempting to finish a call. Sometimes clients ignore your attempts to end a conversation and you have to be blunt, rather than tactful and polite. The last of the following statements is an example of a blunt closure to a conversation.

> "As I said at the beginning of the call, I have an appointment in five minutes. What do we need to cover in order to wrap up our conversation?"

> "We've talked about all of your medical options, body care options, and gone through the euthanasia process step-by-step. If you realize you need more information, please contact me again."

> "You've been very honest with me about your feelings of guilt and anxiety. Is there anything else you feel you want to tell me about before we end our conversation?"

> "How shall we proceed from here?"

> "How shall we leave it between us? Would you like to call me in a week or so, or would you feel more comfortable if I called you?"

> "I need to finish this conversation with you now. I hope this call was helpful to you."

or with effusive reassurances that they are "fine." Their responses may catch you off guard, especially if you know that they were very upset the last time you saw them. Remember, however, that people deal with loss and grief in many different ways and that your clients' willingness and readiness to accept help will make all the difference in follow-up interactions with them. If clients are not ready and willing to talk when you call them, simply offer your condolences and support and keep the door open for any future contact that they may wish to have (Box 10-2).

OWNERS OF NONTRADITIONAL PETS

When we think of companion animals, we most often think of dogs, cats, or horses. Less common, but generally accepted, companions are birds, rabbits, small mammals, and other more exotic animals (Figs. 10-1 and 10-2). Species of fish and reptiles also serve as companion animals to some. In the United States, only 8 percent of exotic pets are ever seen by a veterinarian.[3]

We have already discussed the ways in which trivializing the deaths of companion animals contribute to difficulties in grieving. Owners of less common or nontraditional pets may find this trivialization magnified to a greater degree. If clients have developed strong attachments to animals such as ducks, fish, or iguanas, it may be difficult for you and your staff to understand their attachments and to be empathetic to them. At such times,

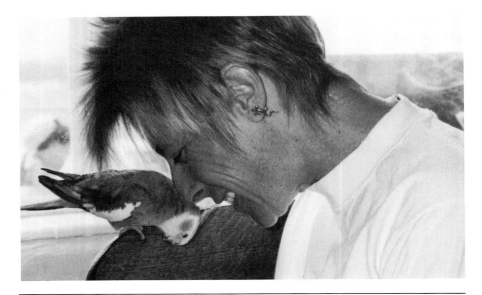

Figure 10-1 Many people feel as close to their pet birds as they do to their dogs and cats.   PHOTO COURTESY OF MEG OLMERT AND PAULA BIRD COHEN.

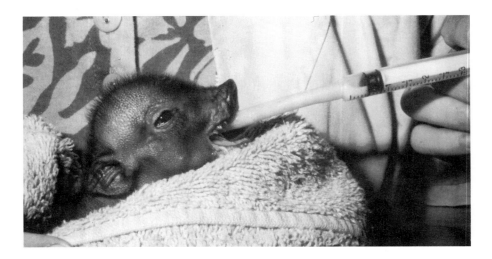

Figure 10-2 Vietnamese pigs are becoming more popular as companion animals.

however, your bond-centered practice philosophies and basic helping skills can truly come into play. Whether *you* could ever become attached to a snake or a goat is not the issue. The fact is that your clients have developed these attachments, and that should be your frame of reference for helping.

Because humane euthanasia procedures for nontraditional and exotic pets vary, client presence during companion animal death may be contra-indicated. Regardless of client presence, however, you should follow-up with owners of nontraditional pets just as you would with other clients. Send condolences and make follow-up telephone calls. In some cases, owners of nontraditional pets are in greater need of your help because the support and understanding that they find among family and friends may be limited.

PICKING UP BODIES OR RECEIVING CREMAINS

One very important, and most often overlooked, aspect of case follow-up and after-care concerns remains retrieval. Remains retrieval refers to the time at which clients return to your office to pick up either their pet's body or the cremated remains. We have heard very sad and disturbing accounts of this event from clients. Many have described the occasion as heartless, cruel, insensitive, and degrading. We have learned that these feelings arise when clients have certain expectations about how the event will be handled, only to experience something completely different and less fulfilling. For example, one client told us that, after being notified that her pet's cremains were available for her to pick up, she agreed to pick them up at 4:30 on her way home from work. She *assumed* that by "making an appointment" she would be able to see and talk with her veterinarian, thereby receiving some desperately needed comfort. Instead, the receptionist (whom she barely knew) handed her pet's cremains to her as soon as she walked through the door, dismissing her with a comment about "calling if she had any questions." When she asked about seeing the veterinarian, she was told that the doctor was not in the hospital and would not be available until the next day. The client was deeply disappointed and felt that, because she no longer had a pet who was alive, she had been "brushed off."

In this case, nothing could have been farther from the truth. After hearing about her client's experience (from the client herself), the veterinarian quickly took steps to rectify the situation. She modified the way in which clients were informed about remains retrieval, giving clients a choice between simply stopping by or setting up an appointment. She also trained her staff to understand the importance of offering clients warm support and sincere condolences during this difficult time. In this case, neither the

BOX 10-3

Cremation Letter—Cremains Returned

Dear Friend,

These are the cremains of your beloved pet. Receiving them may stir up painful emotions within you as the finality of your pet's death is fully realized. Feelings of sadness, anger, guilt, and even relief are normal. They represent the healing process that naturally follows loss.

What you do with your pet's cremains is a personal decision. Some pet owners are comforted by keeping their companion animals' cremains nearby. Others choose to scatter or bury them outdoors. It often helps grieving people to have a memorial service or funeral ceremony at the time they receive their pets' cremains. We encourage you to talk with family and friends to decide on the most meaningful way for you to honor the memory of your pet.

If you allowed the Colorado State University Veterinary Teaching Hospital to perform a postmortem examination on your pet, your contribution to our better understanding of disease is gratefully acknowledged. Many advances in veterinary medicine are made due to the knowledge gained from studying the effects of disease, trauma, and treatment on companion animals.

This is your time for grieving and we can only partially appreciate your feelings of grief. Perhaps there is comfort in knowing we at CSU share in your sense of loss. If you would like to talk further about your pet's death, Changes: The Support for People and Pets Program is available to you. The Changes Program is a free service and offers grief education and support to people who are adjusting to the illness or death of their companion animals. If you would like to find out more about The Changes Program or talk with a Changes counselor, contact them Tuesday through Friday from 9:00 A.M. to 5:00 P.M. at 491-1242.

Respectfully,

A.W. Nelson, D.V.M.
Professor and Hospital Director

veterinarian nor her staff were malicious in the treatment of their client. It was simply a case of miscommunication and oversight on the part of the veterinary team.

When notifying clients that their pets' remains are available to be picked up, it is helpful to let them decide whether they want to take time to sit down and talk with their veterinarian or technician. Given the choice, some clients will prefer simply to pick up their pet's body or cremains, leaving immediately afterward. Regardless of the way in which clients want the event to be structured, some overture of acknowledgment, condolence, and support should be provided, especially if clients have re-

BOX 10-4

Cremains Letter—Cremains Not Returned

Dear Friend,

Our condolences to you upon the recent death of your pet. We can only partially appreciate the grief you must be feeling. Perhaps there is comfort in knowing we at the Colorado State University Veterinary Teaching Hospital understand the important role your companion animal played in your life. We share in your sense of loss and sincerely wish to help in any way possible.

As you requested, your pet's body was cremated on the date noted below. From experience, we realize that knowing choices for body care are promptly carried out helps grief proceed in healthy, normal ways. We hope you, too, find it helpful to know your wishes were respected.

If you have further questions about your pet's death or cremation, please contact us in the Hospital Director's Office at 221–4535, Ext. 268. If you would like to talk about your pet's death, please contact one of the counselors who work with Changes: The Support for People and Pets Program. The Changes Program is a free service for clients of the veterinary hospital. The program offers grief education and support to people who are adjusting to the illness or death of a companion animal. Counselors can be reached Tuesday through Friday from 9:00 A.M. to 5:00 P.M. at 491–1242.

Respectfully,

A.W. Nelson, D.V.M.
Professor and Hospital Director   Cremation Date:_____

ceived little or no personal contact. At CSU, we developed a letter that accompanies pets' cremains when they are returned to our clients. In addition, we developed a letter that is sent to clients when they request cremation but do not wish to have their pets' cremains returned. These letters are reprinted in Boxes 10-3 and 10-4, respectively.

If clients wish to handle the occasion of remains retrieval like any other appointment, it is important to set a time for an office visit. Given the sensitive nature of this meeting, it is probably best to not charge clients for this appointment. (See Chapter 13 for a discussion of the ways in which financial arrangements can be handled in these situations.) When clients arrive, it is helpful to take them into a private room—your office, an examination room, or the visitation-euthanasia room—and gently present the pet's body or cremains to them with kindness and reverence. If possible, do not use the same room in which clients' pets died or were euthanized. As always, if clients are picking up their pets' bodies, prepare them for what they will see and feel, and have the body positioned so that it is relatively pleasing to look at and ready to transport. If clients are picking up their pets' cremains, you also need to prepare them for what they will see and feel. Pet owners often needed to be supported while they assimilate this phase of the grief process because, for many, the difference in form, size, volume, and weight between a furry body and a mound of "ashes" can be shocking and emotionally overwhelming (see the reading at the end of this chapter).

When clients finally confront their pets' remains, spiritual concerns can also arise. Clients may ask you about your own religious beliefs, ponder the existence of "pet heaven," or attempt to engage you in a debate about animals' souls. These discussions can be uncomfortable for both you and your clients, particularly if you find that you disagree. Because it is your role to educate, facilitate, support, and refer during your clients' grief, it is probably most helpful to direct your clients' questions to an appropriate member of the clergy.

MEMORIALS

Just as many ways exist in which to offer your condolences to clients, many ways also exist in which you can help clients to memorialize their pets. Some veterinarians send their clients flowers or make donations to animal organizations or to special service groups in the names of their clients' pets (*see* the Resource Appendix for a sample list of these organizations and groups). Such gestures are certainly appreciated by clients. Obviously, however, the expenses associated with monetary contributions can add up quickly and, ultimately, cost you hundreds (and even thousands) of dollars each year. For this reason, most veterinarians find that they need to impose some criteria on the memorials that they create for their clients' companion animals. In many cases, these criteria are based on financial considerations. For example, one veterinarian whom we know donates $10.00 for every $100.00 that his clients spend on treatment after their pets die of terminal illnesses or injuries. He makes his donations to animal charities, research foundations, or service organizations, depending on each of his client's interests and patient's cause of death. Another veterinarian uses social support as her criterion for memorializing. She sends flowers to clients if they live alone and had only their pet for emotional support. She also sends flowers to any of her clients who choose to be present during their pets euthanasias. She believes that this gesture not only acknowledges the courage required for clients to stay with their companion animals during death but also reinforces her offers of support.

Veterinarians can also give clients permission to create their own memorials. Pet owners do this in many ways (Figs. 10-3 and 10-4). Some collect their memories in scrapbooks, in photo albums, or on videotape. Some

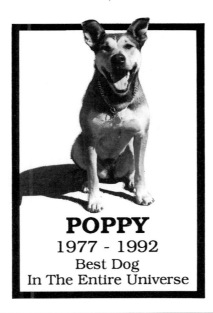

POPPY
1977 - 1992
Best Dog
In The Entire Universe

Figure 10-3 This tribute to Poppy was created by the dog's owner and published in a local newspaper.

frame favorite pictures or write poems or letters to their pets (Box 10-5). Other pet owners record their feelings, thoughts, and specific recollections into a journal, whereas others plant memorial trees or flower gardens in their yards. Many pet owners plan and carry through with memorializing pets on their own, but others need you to suggest some ideas (Box 10-6). A few suggestions can often act as a catalyst for them to develop their own ideas for memorials.

Some pet owners find it meaningful to have an object that links them to their pets. This object may be something that belonged to or was used by a pet, such as a dog's collar, a cat's toy mouse, a bed, a special blanket, or even a food or water dish. The object may also be part of the actual animal, such as a feather, a piece of fur, the wool of a llama, part of a horse's mane or tail, or even a paw print set in clay or stamped in ink. It is helpful to tell clients that, if they feel comforted by keeping these objects with them or in plain view, they should do so. Pet owners too often are advised to get rid of or to put away anything that belonged to their pets because keeping such items is thought of as representative of a morbid connection to a dead animal. In general, we have not found this to be true. Most of our clients have been comforted by the various transitional objects that they have chosen to keep and have put them to creative use. For example, one young client made her dog's tags into a necklace and wore it as a good luck charm

WHIZ KID "WHIZZY" LITTLE

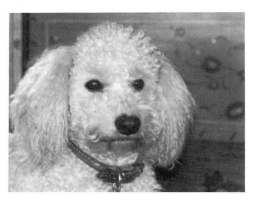

1975-1989

Your pain in life is over my dear friend — only transferred to me in my suffering for your loss. As caretaker of our memories together I accept this pain and I promise you will never be forgotten.

Figure 10-4 Whiz Kid's owner placed this announcement in her local newspaper as a way of honoring her pet and notifying others of the death.

during her track meets. Another client clipped some fur from her cat and slept with it under her pillow for months. Because her cat had slept beside her in bed for seventeen years, she found that having tactile access to some of her fur helped her to complete her grieving process.

As a helper, you should be aware that this type of memorial can be associated with one drawback, that is, if you extend the offer, you must, to the best of your ability, maintain a nonjudgmental attitude and grant your clients' requests, despite your own personal responses to them. Sometimes, maintaining such an attitude can be difficult. We had a client who requested the hide of his dog (to be tanned), one who wanted the shell of her turtle (to be shellacked and used as an urn for the turtle's cremains), and others who took the skin of their snake (to be nailed up on the side of a shed—by the way, they told us that we were welcome to the snake's meat)! We even had one client who requested one of his dog's canine teeth and a sliver of his dog's heart. With the exception of the dog's hide (we could not find a taxidermist who was willing to tan it, so the client settled for keeping the dog's tail), we granted all of these requests, simply because they were important to our clients.

BOX 10-5

Dearest Winston

I am writing this as the hours of
your time with us draw to a close.

What words can express the gratitude
for all that you brought to us. . . .

Your exuberance at the end of a
long day;

The happiness we shared as we rode
together as a family;

The peace of sitting in fresh
green grass.

. . . all of these things became
monumentally important because of
you, Mr. Bear.

Remember that you will always be
with us . . . our guide, our
inspiration, our teacher. Thank you
for opening our lives to the
absolute true beauty in simplicity.

Goodbye. Sleep peacefully.
We
love you.

This poem is a memorial to Richard and Laura Hill's Sheepdog Sir Winston. It was written by Laura on the day Sir Winston was euthanized, August 18, 1991.

Many clients also choose to commemorate their pets by conducting funerals or memorial services for them. These funerals run the gamut from simple, private ceremonies designed to honor pets' memories and pay tribute to their lives to elaborate, public goodbye rituals, sometimes costing hundreds (or even thousands) of dollars. Some clients conduct their own memorial rituals, whereas others take advantage of the funeral services offered by pet cemeteries and crematories.

According to grief therapist J. William Worden, funerals have four important functions:[4]

BOX 10-6

Memorialization

Dedicated to and in loving memory of Barney by Dr. Leah M. Hertzel, Class of 1991, UC Davis School of Veterinary Medicine

Below are a variety of ideas for memorializing a pet. The ideas were contributed by volunteers of the Pet Loss Support Hotline at the University of California at Davis, School of Veterinary Medicine. I was inspired to create this when I learned of the impending death of my beloved cat Barney. Barney died on June 30, 1990. This is intended to be a living document such that ideas can be continually added to it.

- Take lots of photographs and, when you think you've taken enough, take some more. Use the photos to fill an album, place them in your pet's favorite spots in the house, make a collage with them, fill a multi-picture frame with them, carry pictures in your wallet.
- Write a poem, story, or song about or dedicated to your pet.
- Write down your special memories of your pet. Add stories or anecdotes from friends and family. Alternatively make a tape recording of the same thing.
- Chronicle your pet's life with photos or by keeping a journal.
- Write a letter to your pet expressing feelings you may be struggling with.
- Videotape your pet doing anything and everything—eating, sleeping, playing, or just sitting there.
- Make something that reminds you of your pet (for example, a drawing, a clay sculpture, or a needlework project).
- Have a professional portrait, sketch, or sculpture done of your pet. This can be done after the pet's death from a photograph. You can also have a photo of your pet transferred to a T-shirt, clock, button, or mug. (Check advertisements in magazines like Dog Fancy and Cat Fancy for sources)
- Keep baby teeth, whiskers, fur (from shaved areas) and place them in a locket.
- For horses, save shoes, tail, and mane hairs.
- Have fur spun to make yarn in order to knit/crochet something in memory of your pet (see article in March, 1990 Dog Fancy). Pet needs to have medium-to-long hair.
- Keep pet tags. Place these on a key ring so you will always be carrying the memory of your special friend with you.
- Have a plaque made to honor your pet. Place it in a special place—next to your pet's ashes, on a tree near where your pet was buried, in the hospital where your pet was cared for, etc.
- Volunteer your time at a humane organization or help find homes for strays and unwanted pets.

- Help your veterinarian and pet loss counselor start a pet loss support group in your area.
- Plant a bush, shrub, tree, or flowers over or near location where body or ashes are buried.
- Place a bench with an engraved nameplate or an inscription beside where your pet is buried.
- Place ashes in a potted houseplant.
- Collect pet's collars, tags, bowls, blankets, etc. and place them in a special area in honor of your pet. You can also place ashes, sympathy cards, and so forth with them.
- Send out announcements of your pet's death to those who were close to you and your pet.
- If your pet is not buried near you, take pictures of your pet's grave and place these in a special spot, which you can "visit."

1. To make real the fact of loss.

2. To provide an opportunity to express thoughts and feelings, both positive and negative, about the one who has died.

3. To reflect on and pay tribute to the life of the one who has died.

4. To draw social support to the bereaved person or family shortly after a loved one's death has occurred.

We have met both veterinarians and pet owners who scoff at funerals for companion animals. It is, however, important to point out that, in our society, funerals serve as primary facilitators of grief. Not only do funerals provide socially sanctioned ways to dispose of a loved one's body, they also acknowledge that death has occurred. Funerals provide a setting in which both private and public sorrow can be expressed and shared,[5] thus providing an important way for grievers to garner some much-needed social support. In fact, one study indicated that people's grief responses are positively affected when they realize, or even imagine, that others are also mourning for their loved ones who have died.[6]

Sometimes, clients invite their veterinarians to their pets' funerals. You may want to attend some of these ceremonies as a way for you to say goodbye to a special patient, particularly if you are conducting a home euthanasia. Whether you choose to attend pets' funerals is up to you. We advise you to accept clients' invitations with caution, however, because attending every funeral or memorial service can become exhausting and time-consuming. Also, if you only attend some ceremonies and not others, clients can be hurt or offended by your choices. As with sending condolences, if you practice in a small town, offended clients can translate into negative publicity for you and your practice. It is probably best for you and your staff to establish a practice policy regarding animal funerals. This way, you can accept or decline your clients' invitations in accordance with a previously established follow-up plan.

OTHER PETS' GRIEF

It is a well-known fact that animals form attachments to other animals, including humans.[7,8] It is also clear that animals in the same household can become attached to each other. When animals become attached to one another, they behave in ways that keep them in close proximity. For example, animals in the same family may sleep with each other, play together, and follow each other around (Fig. 10-5). The more social the species (that is, species living in structured groups), the more likely that individuals within that species will be to form attachments to each other. For example, dogs, horses, and birds will be more likely to form close attachments to other pets than will cats. (Not to say that cats never become attached to each other, as obviously they do.)

When animals are attached to one another, separation can result in distress reactions. During these reactions, young animals may respond with high-pitched distress vocalizations, whereas adult animals may show various behaviors. For example, dogs who have an unreasonable fear of being left alone may become destructive, housesoil, or refuse to eat or drink when separated from their owners.[9]

Specifically, the ways in which companion animals respond to the death of another family pet has not been scientifically studied; however, a great many anecdotal accounts have been reported, based on observations of both wild and domesticated animals reacting to the death of a social com-

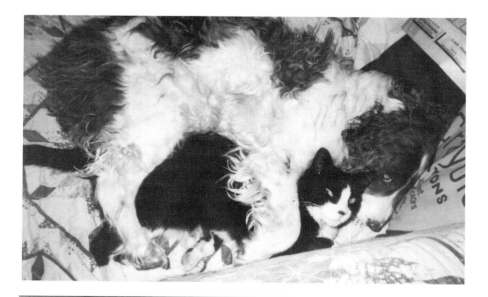

Figure 10-5 Cinda and Freebie share the couch.

panion or a mate.[10] If pets in the same family are attached to each other, a separation reaction to the death of one pet should not be surprising. Likewise, behavioral changes in surviving animals may also be reactions to owners' distress and to any changes in routine that may accompany loss.

Many of the manifestations that animals display appear to be similar to those of human grief. For example, anxiety, restlessness, depression, sighing, and sleeping and eating disturbances also have been reported. After the death of one pet, surviving animals can also appear to search for the pet who died, be less interested in their usual activities, or want to be with their owners more. However, these types of reactions do not always occur. For example, while we were writing in this textbook, Suzanne had to have two of her dogs euthanized due to illness and old age (Brandy was 16½ and Blaze was 13 years old). Their deaths occurred within 8 months of each other, but Suzanne and her husband Dan did not notice any behavioral changes in their third surviving dog, who had grown up with the dogs who died. This absence of reaction may have been due to the fact that Katie was more attached to the human members of her family than to her canine companions. For this and many other reasons, the separation reaction in animals is probably not the exact equivalent of human grief.

When their pets show signs of separation reactions, owners may come to you for advice about how to help their surviving pets. Not much documentation exists regarding which methods are (and which are not) effective. Thus, the following suggestions are based on what is known about separation reactions and animal behavior.

- Owners should be encouraged to keep their pets' daily routines as unchanged as possible. The more predictable, familiar, and consistent the environment, the better.
- Owners should be careful not to inadvertently reinforce their pets' negative behavior changes, such as loss of appetite or lethargy. If pets learn that not eating results in their owners encouraging them with special treats and tidbits, the animals may become less likely to eat their regular meals. Temporary problems can then become long-term difficulties because owners in fact reward their animals' refusals to eat. Therefore, owners should be encouraged to keep their surviving pets on their regular diets.
- Similar to the second suggestion, if pets receive more attention and petting when they are depressed and inactive, these behaviors can become a way for them to obtain attention. Instead, owners should find ways to provide their pets with attention and affection when pets are behaving in desirable ways. Opportunities to provide positive reinforcement can be created by keeping surviving pets active with

toys, games, or exercise. These activities may also help owners to feel better.

- Owners may notice a change in the dominance hierarchy between the surviving pets, particularly if the pet who died was the dominant animal. Again, such reactions will be more likely in species that form rigid dominance hierarchies (such as dogs, horses, and birds) than those with more flexible social systems (such as cats). Whenever members are added or lost from groups of social animals, the relationships between the remaining members are likely to change and to be temporarily unstable. During this time, it is common for remaining animals to compete for the vacant spot in the "pecking order." Such competition may consist of skirmishes and conflicts involving growls, hisses, posturing, and even some inhibited attacks that do not result in injury.

  For the most part, owners need to allow animals to work out their own relationships. The more that owners interfere, the more likely the hierarchy is to remain unstable, thus prolonging and possibly intensifying conflicts until one of the animals is injured. Owners should not attempt to punish animals and instead should either let animals end skirmishes on their own or, if possible, distract them with food or toys. If conflicts continue to occur or if fights intensify, you may want to refer clients with the problem to a certified applied animal behaviorist.

- Some owners ask about letting their surviving pets see, and even smell, the body of a pet who has died. In fact, we have worked with several owners who have brought their surviving pets to the veterinary teaching hospital so they could attend their dying animal's euthanasia along with the rest of the family. Although no evidence suggests that this practice is helpful or has any effect on surviving animals, it is sometimes helpful to the owners. Thus, if owners want to involve their pets in this way, they can be encouraged to do so.

Sometimes, owners may feel that they should obtain new pets to help their surviving pets cope with loss. Unless owners are emotionally ready for new animals, however, this strategy is likely to backfire. Losses cannot be replaced for animals any more than they can for people, and no assurances exist that surviving pets will form close, friendly relationships with new animals. Only new relationships are possible. Maximizing the chances for successful relationships to occur between animals requires commitment, time, and patience from all human family members. Families who are still grieving will probably not have the energy, desire, or time required to train new pets and to help them adjust to their households. In these cases, if it is best for the human family members to wait before obtaining new animals, it is probably best for the surviving animals as well.

ADOPTING NEW PETS

When to adopt a new pet after a much-loved pet has died is a dilemma for many clients. For many, the processes of grieving and bonding are diametrically opposed; therefore, many pet owners find it difficult to grieve fully for one pet while attempting to "get to know" or bond with another. For this reason, it is almost never helpful for veterinarians, friends, or family members to push former pet owners into adopting new pets right away. In fact, even the suggestion implies that pet death is a relatively insignificant loss and that pets are easily replaced.

This "replacement philosophy" commonly surrounds the death of a pet. Unfortunately, many grieving pet owners get used to hearing various versions of:

> "Are you still upset about Tiger? After all, he was only a dog and there are plenty of dogs who need homes. Let's go out right now and you can get another one! That will make you feel better."

In their attempts to help, well-meaning friends and family members may also take it upon themselves to buy or adopt another animal for someone they know who is grieving. Quickly replacing a pet is rarely helpful, however, and reflects a lack of empathy and understanding regarding pet loss.

Sometimes, pet owners themselves quickly adopt other companion animals. This approach works for some. For example, some pet owners have had long periods of anticipatory grief before their pets' deaths and, for the most part, have prepared themselves to begin a new relationship with another companion animal. Other pet owners have needs that must be met fairly soon by another companion animal. Owners who are blind, deaf, or disabled and who make use of service animals are in this category.

All too often, however, pet owners adopt new pets in an attempt to avoid or distract themselves from fully experiencing the sadness and loneliness of grief. If pet owners are motivated to adopt new pets as a way to circumvent the grieving process, they will often make comments like:

> "I want another golden retriever just like Bear."

> "I'm going to get a white, female kitten and name her Muffy too."

> "I'm going to get another bird who will sing to me all after-
> noon."

These comments should alert you to the possibility that clients may be trying to "bring their dead pets back" in the form of new companion animals. Obviously, they should be cautioned that this approach almost never works. Animals are as individual as people. They have different personalities, temperaments, habits, and needs.

In our experience, when pet owners attempt too soon to replace pets who have died, they complicate the grieving process by adding the burden of guilt. In most cases, the new pet is nothing like the one who died. For example, although the old and new dogs may be of the same gender and breed, the pet who died may have been older and more mellow in temper- ament, whereas the new pet may be young, untrained, and immature. Also, although clients may have thought of the pet who died as a best friend, confidante, protector, or even as a parental figure, the new pet may seem more like a dependent, needy child. When pet owners expect or need one thing from a pet but get another, they often fail to adequately bond with the new animal. In addition to grief, they then feel guilty for not loving the new animal. If they finally decide that they cannot keep the new animal, they also feel guilty for not providing it with a loving home.

When your clients themselves ask or begin to talk about getting new pets, you can help them in several ways to choose the appropriate time for adoption and the appropriate type of companion animal. First, listen for comments like:

> "I miss having a furry critter in my house."

> "I've always been intrigued with Great Danes. I might be
> interested in trying that breed this time."

> "I'll always love Niko, but I'm ready to love another cat too."

These comments imply an interest in, rather than a desperate need for, a new pet. They tell you that clients have reached a stronger, more confident place in their grief and are now ready to *explore the possibility* of adopting a new pet.

At this point, it is your responsibility as a helper to assist clients in considering the consequences of adopting a new pet. For example, if your clients were accustomed to the habits of an old dog, are they ready for a puppy? If they have other surviving pets, or if they have children, have they thought about the effects that a new animal will have on them? If other people (especially children) live in the same home, have they dis- cussed the possibility of adopting a new pet with them? If they want a pet who fulfills the role of peer or companion, would they be more satisfied with an adult animal? Are they anticipating lifestyle changes or special circumstances that might make it more practical to adopt a new pet now as opposed to later? Have they researched the various species and breeds of animals to ensure that they will adopt a pet who is right for them? Perhaps most importantly, if their current pet is still alive but is very old, ill, or injured, is it fair to bring a new pet into their home?

Even when all of these consequences have been considered and clients have begun the process of bonding with new pets, problems may yet arise. Again, that problem may be guilt. It is not uncommon for pet owners to feel guilty after they realize that they are capable of loving and dedicating themselves to new pets. The intensity of their feelings for a new pet often makes them feel disloyal to the pet who has died. Pet owners may also feel guilty that they are once again happy and enjoying life when the pet the loved is no longer able to do so. Consequently, this time of breaking old bonds and creating new ones might make some pet owners wonder how they can "so easily" let go of their former companion animals and bond with their new ones. They may also question whether they really loved their pet who died, given that their hearts now belong to another.

It is important to help clients sort through these loyalty conflicts. You can help by letting clients know that love is not limited and that human beings are capable of loving more than one being at a time, both living and dead. Clients also need to understand that they do not have to "choose" between loving their new pets or the pets who have died. Instead, they can choose to love them both. When the pet owners with whom we work begin to seriously discuss or to search for new companion animals, we often predict that this loyalty conflict may occur. When we predict that it may happen, it does not seem to be as disturbing to them if it arises. We also find that, when we predict that loyalty conflicts may arise, they often do not, perhaps due to the fact that we have educated them about the possibility and, thus, removed the power of the phenomena.

When clients decide to adopt new pets, we suggest that they mark the occasion with some kind of symbolic ritual. For example, we might suggest that they get a picture of their former pet and show it to the new pet, in effect, introducing them to one another. We might also encourage clients to take their new pet to the park where they used to walk or on a trail where they used to ride, meanwhile "talking" to both the former and the new pet, recalling the good times they had as well as planning for the good times that are now ahead. At first, these rituals may sound silly or morose, but, to grieving pet owners, they are neither. When we suggest these activities, many pet owners tell us that they have either already done them, or that they have been wanting to do them, but were too self-conscious about following through. Either way, our suggestions give them permission to grieve in ways that are meaningful for them.

To conclude this section, it is not unusual for veterinarians to hear clients make comments like:

"I'll never get another pet again."

or

"This is my last pet. It's too hard when you lose them like this."

In these cases, your first reaction is probably to say something like:

"You don't mean that! One day soon I know you'll be in here with a new puppy, wanting him to be vaccinated."

or

"Think of all the animals out there who need good homes. There's probably one waiting for you right now."

Such comments, however, are not helpful. They ignore your clients' feelings and serve to shut down any further conversation, thereby making clients feel even more isolated and alienated in their grief. Usually, these comments do not represent clients' true feelings about pet ownership. Rather, they reflect the sadness and grief they feel about their pets' deaths. If you acknowledge and support your clients' feelings and grief rather than try to refute or deny them, you will contribute to a more positive grief outcome. Thus, it is more helpful to simply paraphrase your clients' comments, saying something like:

"It sounds like this loss is especially sad for you."

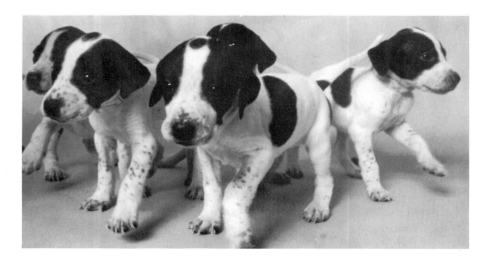

Figure 10-6 When pet owners are ready, many form new human-animal bonds.

or

> "I can hear that the thought of a new pet is not very comfort-
> ing right now."

After pet owners have had a chance to grieve, most do share their lives
with companion animals again (Fig. 10-6).

MAKING REFERRALS

When it is impossible for you to meet some of your clients' needs for
ongoing grief education and support, you can refer them to one or more of
the various resources designed to provide these services. Again, referrals
are easier to make when you work from an established case follow-up and
client after-care policy.

The first step in establishing a client after-care policy is to decide which
of your clients, and under what medical or emotional circumstances, you
will refer. These guidelines can vary widely. For example, some veterinarians inform each client who experiences pet loss about local support
groups, pet loss counselors, and pet loss support hotlines, usually by
providing clients with a packet of written materials at the time of their pets'
deaths. With referral names, addresses, and telephone numbers in hand,
clients are informed of the resources available to them and can choose for
themselves which, if any, they want to use. Other veterinarians make
referrals on more of a case-by-case basis. They assess which of their clients
may be in need of extended support-based services by examining several
factors. These factors may include the strength of their client's human-
companion animal bond, the circumstances surrounding their patient's
death, their client's personal social support system, and their client's ability to cope. When one or more of these factors seem to complicate a client's
grief, the client is considered to be a good candidate for referral.

Some veterinarians have developed close working relationships with
specific mental health professionals in their communities. Together, they
have created interdisciplinary teams that can be very effective when intervening in pet loss-related crisis and grief. So far, these teams are most
likely to exist as part of veterinary teaching hospitals or large, specialty
practices. Interdisciplinary teams are ideal for promoting positive grief
outcomes for clients because they allow clients to get help during many of
the difficult times that precede the death of a pet. For example, pet loss
counselors often provide assistance during decision-making and euthanasia preparation. They can also provide help when children are involved in
cases.

Finding an interested, qualified counselor or therapist with whom to
work, however, can be difficult. It is not as simple as picking a name from

BOX 10-7

Interview Questions

When conducting interviews with potential pet loss counselors, the goals are to assess the ways in which they would support your clients during times of loss and those in which they would facilitate your clients' adjustment and growth processes during grief. The following list represents some of the key questions you might ask during an interview.

Professional Background

- What is your educational and experiential background?
  (Ask for a resume or vitae. This should include information about where and when they graduated and how long they have been in practice.)
- Are you certified or licensed? If so, by whom?
  (Many states have licensing boards governing or directing the field of human services. Contact your state's psychological association.)
- Have any grievances or lawsuits been successfully filed against you?
  (Again, check with the state association.)
- What are your basic fees? Will you work on a sliding fee scale? Do you take insurance?
- What specific training do you have in the area of loss and grief counseling?
  (Here you are looking for some education and training that extends the interviewee's knowledge and skills beyond the classic works of Elisabeth Kubler-Ross.)
- What is your experience facilitating support groups?

Personal Background

- How do you view pet loss? Are you familiar with the specific issues that effect clients?
- Are you a pet owner? Have you personally experienced a pet's death? If so, how did you handle it?
- How do you feel about veterinarians? What have your veterinarian-client relationships been like?
- What kinds of community activities are you interested in or involved in?

Program Development

- How do you suggest we begin to develop a pet loss education and support service designed to meet client needs?
- How do you suggest you begin to work with me, my colleagues, and our veterinary staffs in terms of trainings, debriefings, and so forth?
- Are you willing to work on an emergency or crisis intervention basis? Both on-site at our clinics and on the telephone with clients?
- Are you willing to facilitate a pet loss support group?

- How do you suggest we structure our financial arrangements?
- Would you be willing to be involved in fundraising projects to raise money for the service?
- Would you be willing to develop written materials (brochures, job descriptions, service guidelines, client handouts, grant proposals, and so forth)?
- Do you have experience in program or materials development?

the Yellow Pages. Many different kinds of mental health professionals exist, and they are referred to by many labels. These groups include psychiatrists (doctors of human medicine who specialize in psychiatry), psychologists (those holding doctorates in psychology), EEDs (those who hold doctorates in education), licensed social workers (often represented as LSWI or LSWII—those who hold at least master's degrees in social work or a related field), marriage and family therapists (often represented as MFTs—those who hold at least master's degrees in human development and family studies or a related field), and psychotherapists or counselors (degreed or not degreed, depending on their training). To date, no official credentialing or licensing body specifically certifies mental health professionals as grief counselors or grief therapists. In fact, very few university-based graduate programs offer specific training in the techniques of grief therapy.

Therefore, simply because someone is a mental health professional does not mean that they understand or are skilled in working with issues of grief. It is also important to remember that, even if someone is knowledgeable about working with grief, they may not necessarily be sympathetic to issues of pet loss and pet owner grief. Thus, if you are interested in teaming with a mental health professional, it is important to screen your potential candidates and to choose wisely. As with any job, the best way to accomplish this task is through an application and interview process. During an interview, you should ask several important questions, many of which are included in Box 10-7.

Before interviewing, it is a good idea to advertise for a pet loss counselor and to require that interested professionals fill out an application as well as submit a brief proposal regarding their ideas for creating a pet loss counseling team. During the interview, it is important for you to clearly state any expectations you may have regarding the pet loss counselor's role, conduct, and the ways in which you would like to work together as a team. When making your final selection, check out any references that may have been given to you but, ultimately, trust your instincts. Sometimes relatively young, inexperienced human service professionals are the best ones to take on new projects because they are motivated toward creating a unique market niche for themselves in their communities.

After you have selected an appropriate person to be the pet loss counselor on your team, you should establish a method by which you can evaluate whether the therapist's help is effective. One way is to telephone clients whom you have referred to the therapist to see whether they would be willing to provide you with both positive and negative feedback. You might also want to send clients a brief questionnaire. It is also important for you to understand that, ethically, therapists cannot talk to you about clients whom you have referred to them. In fact, without the client's permission, they cannot even confirm or deny that a client has contacted them because such statements would breach therapist-client confidentiality.

The next step when working with a pet loss counselor is to agree on financial arrangements. Several ways exist in which to work financially with pet loss counselors. One is to simply find a therapist to whom you feel comfortable referring your clients. In this scenario, the therapist charges clients according to his or her regular fees, and you keep your business affairs entirely separate. This way is by far the easiest for you; however, it is much more difficult for your clients. Very few clients seem to feel comfortable about entering into long-term, therapeutic relationships and paying full fees solely to deal with the deaths of their pets. Although they know in their minds that the death of a pet is a life event worthy of seeking professional help, few can justify spending $90.00 per hour or more in seeking such help.

Another way to arrange finances is to team with veterinarians from several other practices to hire a pet loss counselor on a retainer basis. In this scenario, each practice might contribute a previously agreed sum each month toward a pet loss counselor's salary. In exchange for the salary, a counselor would offer various services, such as client support, telephone crisis intervention, staff trainings, weekly staff debriefing sessions, or educational materials development. The amount of work a counselor would do for each practice would depend on the amount of the retainer and the needs of each practice. Counselors who work within these arrangements report that it is best to rotate through each veterinary practice on a day-to-day basis. In other words, they have found that, with the exception of intervening in situations involving crises or decision-making, they can set client appointments and facilitate staff debriefings for one clinic on Monday, another on Tuesday, and so forth. Many counselors also report that, within the parameters of the retainer, they must limit the number of client after-care sessions that they offer free of charge. By after-care sessions, we mean appointments that are scheduled by pet owners after the deaths of their pets for the specific purpose of receiving pet loss counseling. Pet loss counselors say that they most often limit these sessions to two or three. After clients have reached this number of sessions, they are offered the option of continuing in therapy with the pet loss counselor, but they are transferred to the counselor's private practice. Within this setting, clients are free to explore personal issues other than pet loss.

A third way to work with a pet loss counselor is to hire a mental health professional using money raised through your local veterinary medical association. This money often comes from membership dues. The most common scenario in this case is for the counselor to facilitate a pet loss support group rather than see clients on a one-to-one basis. Any local veterinarian can then refer clients to this group free of charge. Many of these support groups are springing up across the country.

As discussed in Chapter 3, support groups can normalize the grief experience for pet owners. They can also provide a forum for pet owners to become educated about the grief process and to express their feelings of loss. After you decide to offer a group to your clients, you must connect with one or more persons who are willing to facilitate it.

When working with groups, it is important to know how to provide structure, diffuse anger, address issues of suicide, and so forth. For these and other reasons, veterinarians who try to facilitate groups themselves can easily become frustrated and quickly find themselves "in over their heads." Also, clients who attend support groups sometimes want and need to discuss both their positive and negative feelings regarding how their veterinarians handled their cases. If veterinarians are facilitating these groups, clients may be intimidated about discussing any negative feelings. In addition, if veterinarians are present when their colleagues are being discussed, it can become very uncomfortable for them as well.

Support groups are therefore, perhaps most effective when they are facilitated by trained, experienced mental health professionals. Ideally, these professionals know how to work with group dynamics, understand issues pertinent to pet loss, and have strong backgrounds in providing grief education and counseling. It is also to your advantage to work with a professional because they should carry their own malpractice insurance. Whenever possible, it is also a good idea to have groups offered or cofacilitated by both male and female therapists because some clients feel more comfortable working with one gender or another.

Occasionally, former pet owners who have themselves experienced the grief associated with pet loss volunteer to run pet loss support groups. Although this arrangement can work, we do not recommend it. Unless pet owners make a true commitment to complete their own grief work and to learn how to help others move through the grief process, it is often difficult for them to remain objective enough to truly assist others with their feelings of loss. When facilitators use the group forum to resolve their own grief rather than to provide objective help to others, it does not reflect well on you or your practice. When clients attend a group expecting to get help, but instead spend their time listening to the facilitator's experiences, they

BOX 10-8

Letter to the Editor

Recently, a woman was directed by a friend to visit the Denver Area Veterinary Medical Association (DAVMS)-sponsored Pet Loss Support Group following the death of her pet. She returned to her veterinarian to ask why he/she hadn't recommended that she attend the group. Her veterinarian replied, "If your husband died, the hospital wouldn't pay for your therapy," and went on to angrily condemn the use of his/her dues to fund the group.

How different was the above scenario from the one I recently experienced. One of my elderly clients had been present for the euthanasia of her 15-year-old dog. When I told her about the Pet Loss Support Group, she said, "Well, how nice! When my husband died, do you know that there were no groups available for me?"

The DAVMS-sponsored Pet Loss Support Group is just that—a support group. It is not therapy. It is facilitated by a professional through the DAVMS members' dues at a cost of approximately $10.00 per year per member. It is a service that we offer that perhaps puts us one step above "Real Doctors" and what they provide for their patients in need following the death of a loved one.

Whether each of us would attend a support group or not, and whether or not we think it is a legitimate use of funds, it is perceived as a positive service by our clients. If you don't use your brochures or recommend the group, you'll never know—unless, as the first veterinarian found out—one of your clients hears about the group and questions why you didn't recommend it.

I would be happy to discuss the group with any members who would like to call.

This letter was written by Dr. Paige Garnett, former chair of the Denver Area Veterinary Medical Association's Human-Animal Bond Committee. It was published in the Association's newsletter *The Bulletin*, 1991.

---

usually feel cheated. Needless to say, in these cases, groups are not viewed as helpful, and clients most often do not return.

When trained, ethical, committed facilitators for the group have been selected, operating money must be obtained. Often, pet loss support groups are funded jointly by local veterinary medical associations, humane societies, pet cemeteries and crematories, and private donations. Some groups also hold fund raisers or apply for small grants from animal-oriented organizations. Experience has shown that, when pet owners are asked to pay to attend a pet loss support group, attendance is much lower.[11] Depending on the size of the veterinary association, if the group is to be offered free of charge to pet owners, a yearly budget of several hundred to several thousand dollars is usually needed. This money pays the salaries of the facilitators and also pays for brochures, advertising, educational materials, and mailing costs regarding follow-up communication. In some cases, money is also needed to cover rental costs for meeting space. One note of caution: It is common for humane societies to graciously offer their facilities for pet loss support group meetings; however, many clients do not feel comfortable with this arrangement. They say that they feel even sadder when they leave their support meetings knowing they are also leaving many animals who are in need of good homes. Additionally, they say that, by meeting in these facilities, they feel pressured to adopt new pets long before they are ready.

In general, the veterinarians and clients who have made use of pet loss support groups seem to find participation to be a positive experience.[11,12] In one study, approximately 80 percent of veterinarians surveyed rated the value of their support group as positive. When asked about their clients' reactions to being told about their group, the same veterinarians rated their reactions as positive 60 percent of the time.[12] In this same study, approximately 80 percent of the clients surveyed rated their support group as having positive value. In addition, those referred to the group by their own veterinarians reported that they were now more likely to refer friends to their veterinarians. Even more important, those clients who attended the group due to referrals from friends or from the media, but who were not referred by their veterinarians, reported that they were now less likely to refer friends to their veterinarians (Box 10-8).

Pet loss support groups can be run on various schedules. Some meet once a month, whereas others get together once a week. Some are open, ongoing meetings in which attendance and attendees fluctuate from meeting to meeting. Other groups are more structured, with the same members attending each meeting for a specified amount of time. However you decide to organize your pet loss support group, remember that it takes time for community awareness to grow. It also takes time for veterinarians to become comfortable when referring clients to groups.

The Delta Society offers a state-by-state directory of pet loss support groups. They also offer a packet of materials describing how to establish a support group in your community. The Delta Society's telephone number and address are included in the Resource Appendix.

If you and your clients do not have access to a pet loss support group, several pet loss support hotlines are available for your clients to call. The pioneer among these is operated by the School of Veterinary Medicine at the University of California, Davis. It is staffed by trained, student volunteers who are involved with the university's Human-Animal Program. The telephone numbers of this and other pet loss support hotlines are listed in the Resource Appendix.

As you can see, you can design and implement support programs for your clients in many ways. Making support available to clients does no good, however, if you are uncomfortable making referrals. When we teach and train veterinarians and veterinary students, we are consistently asked to provide them with the appropriate words to use in making referrals. We do this because we believe it is important for you to have two or three ways in which you can smoothly and confidently let clients know about the resources available to them. A sampling of these referral techniques and statements follow. We hope you can adapt some of them for your own use.

- *Self-disclosure:* This normalizes the need for help and puts you and your client "in the same boat."

  "I know how hard Grover's death has been for you. I work with a person who specializes in helping pet owners deal with the grief they feel after their pets die. Many of my clients talk with her, at least once or twice, and it seems to help a great deal. My staff and I talk with her about our tough cases too. I'd like to give you her name and number."

- *The illusion of choice:* In most cases, this referral gets clients connected with a counselor in one way or another, yet still gives clients some feeling of control as they decide whether to call the counselor themselves or have the counselor call them.

  "You've been struggling with this decision for quite some time now, Bonnie. I'd like to have you speak with a member of our team who specializes in helping people who are faced with your situation. Would you like to call her to arrange a time to talk or would you prefer that I ask her to call you?"

- *The one-down approach:* This places clear boundaries and limits on your helping capabilities without making clients feel that you are brushing them off or implying that they are abnormal, "crazy," or in great need of help. To do this, you need to be honest about your limitations, but avoid making statements like:

  "I'm in over my head here and I think you need some professional help."

  A statement like this is likely to hurt or offend clients. It is better to say something like:

  "It sounds like some factors are complicating your grief. I know they can be worked out, but I'm simply not trained in this area. I would be doing you a disservice if I tried to be the one who helped you sort through them, but I do know someone who can help you. I know her well and recommend her highly. She sees appointments here every Wednesday. Shall we see if she has some time free?"

- *The medical analogy:* Most clients are familiar with the process of being referred to a specialist because it is common in human medicine. This referral often works well with clients who are "stuck" in the grief process and who need structure and guidance regarding how to proceed.

"Paul, if you had a broken arm, you wouldn't walk around for weeks without having it looked at. The same is true with a broken heart. I know someone who can help you with the process of healing. Let's call him now and see if he can set up an appointment to see you today or tomorrow."

- *The back door approach:* This is usually less threatening for clients because they do not perceive it as being aimed directly at them. Many adults will seek help for their children or for another member of their family even if they are reluctant to ask for help for themselves:

"Joan, I know you and Miles have children. Have you thought about how you might involve them in or tell them about Juicy's illness?"

Pause here for their answer. Sometimes clients will quickly say something like:

"Oh, I don't think they should know about this at all."

or

"I don't want them to have to deal with this every day. I think we'll just tell them after he's gone."

Some parents may even ask you to lie to their children, asking you to tell them that you found another home for their pet. Working with parents and children is described in detail in Chapter 12. In terms of referring parents to a pet loss counselor, however, you might continue by saying:

"I can understand that you want to protect your children from this sad news. However, in my experience, it's often more painful for children to be kept in the dark about their pet's death. There are some very effective ways you can help children deal with pet loss, and I work with a woman

who can provide you with this information. Would you like
to have her name and number?"

You may have to refer clients to a pet loss counselor several times before
they are ready to talk with one. For many people, talking to a counselor
makes their pets' deaths seem more real. Thus, they avoid the encounter
for as long as possible. Clients who are reluctant to seek professional help
often continue to ask *you* to help them with their grief. It is important for
you to continue to abide by the policies that you have set and to work with
the limits and boundaries that you have established regarding your helping role. You need to sensitively, but consistently decline to provide them
with further help and refer them to the counselor with whom you work,
regardless of whether they actually follow through with seeking help.

UPDATING FILES AND TERMINATING CASES

After pets have died, remember to update your patient records. Record the
date and manner of the animal's death. Also, record any significant information regarding your clients' grief reactions. You might also make note of
which room was used for euthanasia so you can avoid the space during
your client's next visit. Be sure to also purge the animal's name from your
mailing lists. Owners can be offended if they receive vaccination or annual
check-up reminders in the mail regarding pets who have died.

In some cases, it is a good idea to offer clients the opportunity to be
involved in an "exit interview" with you and your staff. Such a meeting is
particularly important if, during the course of an animal's treatment, you,
your staff, and your client formed a close-knit team, bonded by your devotion to the client's companion animal. During an exit interview, you should
briefly review the medical procedures and decisions pertinent to the case.
Everyone should then have an opportunity to express their emotions,
grief, or gratitude about the process. In some cases, the exit interview
provides clients with the opportunity to give you feedback regarding the
ways in which their cases were handled. They may tell you what you did
that was (and what was not) helpful. This opportunity allows you to receive reinforcement for what you did well and to learn from your mistakes.

Occasionally, you may encounter a case in which one or more of your
staff members need an exit interview more than your client. These are the
cases in which, for one reason or another, staff members have gotten
emotionally "hooked" by the client, the patient, or both. These cases can
be especially painful for veterinary professionals because they stir up old
losses and hurts. You will recognize these cases because they will be the
ones that get everyone "mobilized" and upset. They will also be extremely
difficult to terminate or to detach from emotionally. We talk about stress

and the concept of emotional detachment in Chapter 11. In this section, we want to focus specifically on creating a plan for staff debriefing.

Critical incident stress debriefing, usually referred to as "debriefing," refers to a new and specific form of crisis intervention. It is often used to help people deal with large-scale disasters such as hurricanes, airplane crashes, or war, but it can also be effective when applied to personal crises. According to Leonard Zunin and Hilary Stanton Zunin, authors of *The Art of Condolence*, the goal of this approach is "to eliminate, or at least minimize, delayed stress reactions and their physical and psychological toll."[13]

Jeffrey T. Mitchell, originator of the term and the process, clarifies debriefing's central theme:

> The tone must be positive, supportive, and understanding. Everyone has feelings which need to be shared and accepted. The main rule is—no one criticizes another; all listen to what was, or is, going on inside each other.[14] (p. 33)

Debriefing is effective when used one-on-one or in groups. It is usually not effective in the hours immediately after a death, but can be used in the days or even weeks that follow. Anyone familiar with the basic tenets of helping can facilitate the debriefing process. All you have to do is follow the four basic steps involved in the process:

1. Ask about the facts. In the early stages of grief, it is easier for most grievers to talk about facts rather than feelings. Conversations about facts seem less invasive and threatening, require less trust, and help set loss in a realistic perspective.

2. Inquire about thoughts. Areas to explore during this phase of debriefing include grievers' first thoughts, their current thoughts, and any repetitive thoughts that they may be having.

3. Acknowledge and validate feelings. People are more likely to share their feelings, even the ones they may think of as crazy or abnormal when you have proven yourself to be patient, accepting, nonjudgmental, and ready to listen.

4. Reassure and support. Even the most general understanding of grief and how it personally impacts you or a member of your staff can be validating and reassuring.

Whenever you take on the role of helper, some emotional interplay is bound to occur within the reaction. If you are a sensitive helper, you may take on and experience the moods and feelings of your clients. Thus, their anger, loneliness, irritability, sadness, emptiness, helplessness, and frustration may be directly felt by you. In addition, involvement with grieving clients can also rekindle your own memories and feelings of loss. It may

BOX 10-9

How to Help Yourself

Gail Bishop

- **Give yourself permission to grieve.** Only you know how much this relationship meant to you and only you know how much you hurt because of the loss. Allow yourself the time and space to grieve.
- **Rest-Relax-Exercise.** Grief is an exhausting experience emotionally. Allow time to replenish yourself. Listen to your inner voice . . . what do you need right now? A hot bath, a long walk, a nap, a trip, or even a short diversion are all ways in which to nurture yourself.
- **Surround yourself with people who understand.** Now, more than ever, you need to have supportive, loving people around you. Allow others to care for you. It's their way of helping and it can be healing for you.
- **Educate yourself about the grief process.** A little education can go a long way. Knowing *what* you are experiencing helps "normalize" an experience that feels anything but normal! You wouldn't get behind the wheel of a car before you educated yourself about how to drive, would you?
- **Acknowledge your feelings.** Talk or write about your feelings as this can help sort them out. Some people have difficulty discussing feelings with others. If this is the case, writing a journal or letter can be helpful.
- **Allow yourself small pleasures.** Sometimes, it's the everyday, little pleasures that serve as small steps in your healing process. Sunsets, a favorite food, an accomplishment, or helping someone else are all ways in which you can begin to enjoy life again.
- **Be patient with yourself.** Grieving the loss of a significant relationship takes time, much more time than society sanctions, so go easy on yourself!
- **Give yourself permission to backslide.** The nature of grief can be compared to riding on a roller coaster or to waves crashing on the shore. One day you may be feeling good only to wake up the next day in the depths of despair. This is normal! Holidays, anniversaries, memories, and smells can trigger tears, sadness, and other feelings of grief. Again, be patient with yourself.
- **Seek professional assistance if necessary.** If you feel suicidal, "stuck" in your grief process, or uncomfortable with how you are handling your loss, seek assistance. Many people, groups, and organizations are available to help, sometimes at no cost to you. Please do not feel like you have to work through this alone.
- **Get in touch with your higher power.** Many people derive an enormous amount of support from their religious or spiritual beliefs. This belief alone can often sustain you when other support systems cannot.

- **Identify what has helped you in the past.** You already have a
  wealth of coping mechanisms that you have been using all your
  life. Identify and implement them now.

Gail Bishop is a grief counselor and Director of Family Services at the Allnut Funeral
Service in Fort Collins, Colorado.

also be helpful to rely on two of the basic concepts underlying emotional
detachment when it becomes difficult to distinguish between grief that
belongs to you and that belonging to your clients:

- To avoid thinking of yourself as a rescuer and treating your
  clients like victims. Grieving clients often resent being
  treated like victims because they feel that it is demeaning.
- To avoid becoming so identified with grieving clients that
  you grieve *for* them instead of with them. It is vital to recognize that, as much as you want to help, it is not your responsibility to grieve *for* your clients. A surrogate griever,
  no matter how well intended, cannot and will not accomplish anything. To remain emotionally healthy, each of us
  must do our own, and only our own, grief work.

Some weeks, you and your staff will deal with several patients' deaths.
You may even deal with several during any given day. When patient
deaths seem to pile up and "get to you," it may be time to find someone
who is willing to help you or a staff member debrief. You might also want
to schedule debriefing sessions on a regular basis. Talking about cases and
the patients you lose can help (Box 10-9). Knowing that others feel stress
and grief similar to yours can help a lot.

CONCLUSION

You can't judge which clients may need help simply by looking at them.
Many factors come into play when loss is involved. For example, sometimes clients who appear to be best able to handle crises—those who have
intelligence, self-confidence, family support, and adequate income—seem
to be hardest hit by them. Perhaps people who are accustomed to feeling a
sense of mastery in their lives are most shaken by uncontrollable events
like death.

As a bond-centered practitioner, you want to be ready and willing to
support all of your clients to the best of your abilities. The rewards of
helping pet owners through the grief associated with pet loss are many. As
veterinarian Doreen John wrote us:

Would you believe that I have received numerous "thank you"
cards, some flowers and plants, and even chocolates for putting

different clients' pets to sleep. A fellow veterinarian made fun of me one day about those things, but you know, they make me feel even better than when I receive a gift from a client with an animal which I made healthy again. I just feel that the client dealing with the euthanasia decision is much more vulnerable to pain and emotional damage and the receipt of a 'thank you' makes me know I caused no further trauma for them and maybe helped to make it a little easier. (John D., Personal communication)

The following excerpt from a letter written by a former client illustrates the power of "saying goodbye" to companion animals who have died.

Saying Goodbye
Laura Brumage

I've just returned to Los Angeles after spending a week in Colorado Springs visiting my mom and dad. On a particularly emotional afternoon, I found myself possessed by the need to "find Socksy" in the hall closet where her ashes have been stored for over a year. Tearing the closet apart, I found a small box in a dark corner. Nobody wanted to deal with her remains. I pulled the box out and went hysterical when I realized that my once beautiful, vibrant dog was in a 3 × 3 box and even more hysterical when I opened it to see a labeled bag of ashes. Bone chips.

Clutching the bag to my stomach, I took a walk through the parks and streets of downtown Colorado Springs, pulling Kleenex after Kleenex out of the jumbo box I held under one arm. I just walked and sobbed and walked and sobbed.

We wound up at a home and gift shop where Socks and I chose a beautiful clay urn decorated with pink and white yarn, feathers, and Indian beads. We agreed that this would be her new home. After leaving the store, we went to the park where Socksy ran so often with all the members of the family and in the shade of a big maple tree, I sat with her in my lap. It was calming and beautiful. Her spirit danced with me and licked my face. Socks always did love salty tears!

Piercing the bag and pouring her ashes into the urn was easier than I'd ever thought it could be. I ran my fingers through them, marveling at the varied textures and colors. She is beautiful even in death.

We walked home and I had a new lilt in my step. I had been released and Socks really wasn't gone at all, just transformed. Her vase sits on the mantel overlooking her favorite park and the Rocky Mountains. I can walk by, lift the lid, and say hello to her everyday. It's the greatest. I know that when Lynn and Karen go home, they, too, will be enriched when they lift the lid and see "Our Miss Socks."

REFERENCES

1. Arnold, J.H., and Gemma, P.B.: The loss of a child and parental grief. Adv. Thanatol., 6:23–27, 1987.
2. Rando, T.A.: Grief, Dying, and Death: Clinical Interventions for Caregivers. Champaign, Ill., Research Press Company, 1984.
3. Troutman, C.M.: The Veterinary Services Market for Companion Animals. Overland Park, Kan., Charles, Charles Research Group and the American Veterinary Medical Association, 1988.
4. Worden, J.W.: Grief Counseling and Grief Therapy: A Handbook for the Mental Health Practitioner. New York, Springer Publishing Company, 1982.
5. Fulton, R.: Death and the funeral in contemporary society. *In* Wass, H., ed.: Dying: Facing the Facts. New York, Hemisphere Publishing Corporation/McGraw-Hill Book Company, 1979, pp. 236–255.
6. Fulcomer, D.M.: The adjustive behavior of some recently bereaved spouses: A psychosociological study. Doctoral dissertation, Northwestern University, 1942, p. 182.
7. Scott, J.P., Stewart, J.M., and DeGhett, V.J.: Separation in infant dogs: Emotional response and motivational consequences. *In* Scott, J.P., and Senay, E., eds.: Separation and Depression: Clinical and Research Aspects. Washington, D.C., American Association for the Advancement of Science, 1973, pp. 3–32.
8. Cairns, R.B.: Attachment behavior in mammals. Psychol. Rev., 73:409–429, 1966.
9. Borchelt, P.L.: Separation-elicited behavior problems in dogs. *In* Katcher, A.H., and Beck, A.M., eds.: New Perspectives on Our Lives with Companion Animals. Philadelphia, University of Pennsylvania Press, 1983, pp. 187–196.
10. Iliff, S.A., and Albright, J.L.: Grief and mourning following human and animal death. *In* Kay, W.J., Cohen, S.P., Fudin, C.E., Kutscher, A.H., Nieburg, H.A., Grey, R.E., and Osman, M.M., eds.: Euthanasia of the Companion Animal: The Impact on Pet Owners, Veterinarians, and Society. Philadelphia, The Charles Press, 1988, pp. 115–132.
11. Garnett, P.: Local VMA offers pet loss help. Trends Magazine, 9:43–44, April/May 1993.
12. Hart, L.A., Mader, B., Rivero, C., and Hart, B.L.: A pet loss support group: Evaluation of the first year. Calif. Vet., 41:13–15, 26, March/April 1987.
13. Zunin, L.M., and Zunin, H.S.: The Art of Condolence: What to Write, What to Say, What to Do at a Time of Loss. New York, HarperCollins Publishers, 1991.
14. Mitchell, J.T.: When disaster strikes. J. Emerg. Med. Serv., January: 33–36, 1983.

11

Stress

This chapter addresses a practice reality: stress. Stress can potentially affect every aspect of your bond-centered practice and your feelings about yourself, both professionally and personally. It makes the difference between veterinary professionals who say, "I am glad I stuck it out in veterinary school. I love my work!" and those who say, "I never realized how much I would give up to practice veterinary medicine. If I knew then what I know now . . ."

Stress management is a broad topic. Numerous books and seminars address the subject and tell us of the literally thousands of ways to reduce stress at work and at home. Yet, truly learning to manage stress is a therapeutic issue. The ways in which you deal with stress depend on your values and philosophies, the way you feel about yourself, the way you were raised, and your repertoire of stress management skills. Thus, it is impossible to change the way you handle stressful events without evaluating your motives for behavior, your personal needs, and your subconscious commitment to change (or to staying the same).

Although true stress management begins with self-exploration, stress management experts say that most people will never directly address the root causes of their stress.[1] Thus, this chapter makes no demand for extensive personal evaluation or for a leap into psychotherapy. Rather, this chapter seeks to simply plant seeds for future cultivation and to make suggestions for improving your work style and your environment.

The first half of this chapter provides foundational information about stress, its definition, the common symptoms, and its negative effect on the ability to communicate. Stress in the medical professions, specifically in veterinary medicine, and the unique stressors related to loss and grief work are also examined. An antecedent condition called codependency, which contributes heavily to stress, is also explored.

The second half of the chapter introduces you to specific techniques for managing the stress that is related specifically to loss. The need for reviewing your own loss history is presented, and tips for developing a work style of "detached concern" are given. Helpful ways to take care of yourself on a case-by-case and on a day-by-day basis are presented.

The material in this chapter is important to you. You are a veterinarian because you have a strong desire to help people and animals. You have also invested much time and money in veterinary medicine; therefore, you want to stay in the profession. Yet, people are not going to see you as helpful if you are erratic, overwhelmed, and burned-out. You cannot help others if you cannot help yourself. You want to enjoy a long and happy career, and learning how to manage your stress will allow you to do that.

UNDERSTANDING STRESS

Stress is a response to a demand. It may come from major life events or from the cumulative effects of minor, everyday hassles. According to Lazarus and Folkman, educators at the University of California at Berkeley:

> The definition of stress emphasizes the *relationship* between the person and the environment, which takes into account characteristics of the person on the one hand, and the nature of the environmental event on the other. This parallels the modern medical concept of illness, which is no longer seen as caused solely by an external organism; whether or not illness occurs depends also on the organism's susceptibility. Similarly, there is no objective way to predict psychological stress without reference to properties of the person. Psychological stress, therefore, is a the relationship between a person and the environment that is appraised as taxing or exceeding his or her resources and endangering his or her well-being. The judgment that a particular person-environment relationship is stressful hinges on cognitive appraisal.[2] (p. 21)

Stress can be positive or negative. Positive stress, or "eu-stress," results when you must adapt to positive life changes. Eu-stress (from the word euphoria) is experienced, for example, when moving into a larger office or home, planning a wedding, or becoming a parent. Negative stress, or "distress," is experienced when unwanted adjustments must be made. Distress (from the word dis-ease) is experienced, for example, with the death of a loved one, the loss of a job, or the loss a valuable possession.[3] Some situations combine both eu-stress and dis-tress, such as giving an important lecture, engaging in a technical climb up the side of a mountain, or helping a suffering animal to die by euthanasia.

A stressor is the person, place, activity, or event that causes stress. The most common demands or stressors are change, fear, overload (for example, overcommitment), underload (for example, boredom), uncertainty, and a perceived lack of control. When any or all of these stressors are present in your life, you adapt in three major ways. First, when a stressor is recognized, your brain sends forth a biochemical messenger to the pituitary gland, triggering the secretion of adrenaline, resulting in a general readiness to "fight" or to "flee." Your system stays alarmed until a decision about fight or flight has been made. When the immediate threat dissipates or is overcome, your system adapts to the new circumstances in a second way. It builds resistance to the stressor by shifting into a "higher gear" to meet the extra challenge.[3] If the stressor continues, the ability to adapt, adjust, and resist is eventually lost, and exhaustion sets in. If this third adaptation called exhaustion is unduly prolonged, physical or emotional damage occurs. New crises, such as loss or death, retrigger the alarm phase and the whole cycle begins again on an even more dangerous level (Fig. 11-1).

Under threatening conditions, the stress response is desirable because it enables you to meet extreme challenges. When present too often or for too

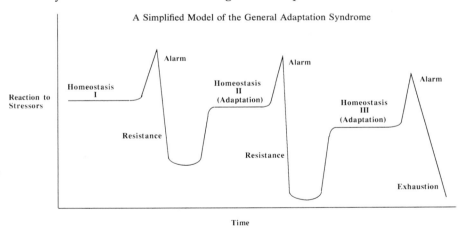

Figure 11-1 Homeostasis is defined as a state of balance and equilibrium. This state of balance can be disrupted by stress. Everyone encounters stressors throughout life. Together, the alarm and resistance stages allow adaptation to stress. Repeated alarm and resistance stages can lead to exhaustion if the stressors persist and stress management plans are not implemented. Depending on the severity of the stressor and the characteristics of the individual, adaptation (or subsequent exhaustion) can occur immediately after a stressful event or can be the result of cumulative effects occurring over days, weeks, or even an entire lifetime. This syndrome can eventually result in death.

BOX 11-1

Stressful Job Conditions

Most veterinary professionals receive very little training on how to establish clear and realistic practice policies, set personal limits, manage staff conflict, or give appropriate feedback to clients or colleagues. A lack of training in these areas contributes to stressful job conditions. Stressful job conditions include:

- Unrealistic work deadlines
- Heavy workloads or not enough work
- Frequently on-call after regular business hours
- A gap between what you *must* do and what you *want* to do (for example, convenience euthanasia)
- Role ambiguity (confusion about roles in clinic hierarchies or in certain situations)
- Having a lot of responsibility, but very little authority (for example, technicians, receptionists, new veterinarians, students)
- Having responsibility for people versus tasks or things
- Personality conflicts and communication difficulties among staff
- Lack of feedback regarding job performance
- A tense (or apathetic) atmosphere within the organization

long, however, the stressor causes your body to remain in a state of permanent mobilization, resulting in chronic tension. Worse, the hormones that are secreted in abundance during prolonged stress can ultimately cause damage to the vital organs and to the nervous system itself.

In addition, when symptoms of stress are untreated for long periods, "burnout" results. Edelwich defined burnout as the progressive loss of idealism, energy, and purpose.[4] Elkins and Elkins referred to burnout as a state of emotional exhaustion in which work becomes routine and mechanical.[5] In a 1987 nationwide survey of 1,000 veterinarians, they reported that 50 percent of the responding veterinarians reported clear-cut signs of burnout, with the highest burnout scores reported by veterinarians who had been in practice for 10 to 14 years.[5]

Experts agree that it is difficult to recover from burnout. After you have reached that point, you may need to leave the situation entirely or seek help from a trained mental health professional. Additional information about burnout can be found in the books listed in the Bibliography section of the Resource Appendix.

Stress Symptoms

Along with the pressures of the work environment (Box 11-1), frequent involvement with patient death and client grief can create stressful job conditions for veterinary professionals. Stressful job conditions provide fertile ground for stress symptoms.

BOX 11-2

Stress Symptoms

Physical Health Problems

Headaches, fatigue, insomnia, neckaches, backaches, aching muscles, hypertension, rapid heart beat, allergies, overeating, undereating, nausea, ulcers, diarrhea, lowered resistance to infections

Emotional Difficulties

Depression, apathy, feelings of powerlessness, feelings of forboding, worrying, anxiety, hyperventilation, angry feelings, irritability, outbursts, defensiveness, chronic complaining, cynicism, hostility toward others, withdrawal, alienation, paranoia, strained relationships, sexual problems

Substandard Job Performance

Lack of concentration, poor judgment, increased errors, lapses in routine procedures, inability to complete tasks, crisis-orientation, indecisiveness, withdrawal, negative attitude, blaming, viewing conflicting opinions as threats, a tendency to work harder and longer just to stay on top of things

Substance Abuse

Over-indulging in alcohol, drugs, caffeine, nicotine, sugar

Note: The level of debilitation associated with each of these stress symptoms differs from one person to another.

Stress symptoms are bodily messages that indicate that something needs to change. They tell you that something is wrong or that something needs attention. They also tell you to slow down, to ask for help, and to find healthy outlets for your thoughts and feelings. Symptoms are most commonly experienced in physical or emotional difficulties, in substandard job performance, or in substance abuse. Box 11-2 lists general stress symptoms.

If stress symptoms are not addressed, they tend to multiply. Minor problems often become major ones. It has been said that stress-related symptoms are analogous to warning lights in automobiles. For example, just as the oil warning light in your car lights up when the oil is low, a stress symptom acts in the same way, telling you that its time to replenish yourself. Failure to address these symptoms is analogous to ignoring your body's "oil light." Worse yet, medicating your symptoms with alcohol or drugs is like taking a gun from the glove compartment and shooting out the oil light, just so you will not have to look at it anymore! Although this approach might bring short-term relief, your car's engine will eventually burn out. So will you.

BOX 11-3

Negative Forms of Communication

Stress affects you and influences your interactions with clients and staff. Stress is often manifested in negative forms of communication.

Physical withdrawal: When people are stressed, they may isolate themselves or quit talking to others. This behavior can be confusing and can strain relationships.

Avoidance of emotional situations: People who withdraw from emotional situations often do so because they lack confidence in their abilities to provide assistance and are unclear about how they can be helpful. Some people avoid involvement with others who are emotional because they are uncomfortable with their own emotions and do not want to cry or become upset in front of others.

Selective inattention: Some issues are easy to deal with while others are not. People who engage in selective inattention push conflictual situations out of their minds and hope they will go away without intervention. This approach usually creates more barriers to communication.

Indirect communication: This occurs when people are unwilling to openly confront conflict and instead engage in gossiping or complaining about one another. Indirect communication undermines team building and does not lead to problem resolution.

Cynical or sarcastic comments: Some individuals reduce stress by laughing or teasing about issues of loss or death. They do this to lighten the mood or to distance themselves from painful feelings. Although this is not uncommon or unhealthy, stressed individuals frequently make these comments at the wrong place and time.

Exaggerated anger: People who are stressed often appear angry. They may use anger to "blow off steam." Anger is often a mask for hurt, sadness, or frustration. Anger is often used to distract from the pain of loss and grief.

Unnecessary risk-taking: When people are stressed, they are not very discerning. Therefore, they take risks that they should not and fail to take those that they should. They also say things that they should not and fail to say things that they should.

The Negative Effects of Stress on Communication

Stress affects you, and it affects your relationships with those around you. Not only does it contribute to the development of the stress symptoms listed in Box 11-2, it also significantly influences your communication patterns. In fact, evidence suggests that heavy workloads may impair communication skills.[6] These findings are significant because, as we discussed in Chapter 5, the ability to communicate plays a significant role in the success or failure of veterinary practice.

Many of the common communication difficulties that arise under stressful conditions are listed in Box 11-3. As you read through the list, identify the negative forms of communication that you use when under stress. Determine which forms you use with clients, with staff, and with your family. By acknowledging your tendencies to withdraw, to become angry, or to make jokes inappropriately, for example, you take the first step toward changing the behavior. A staff discussion of problem communication patterns in your clinic can prepare staff members for what to expect from one another during stressful periods.

STRESS IN THE HELPING PROFESSIONS

In the helping professions, you work with others in emotionally demanding situations over long periods. You are exposed to your clients' (and patients') psychologic, social, and physical problems, and you are expected to be both skilled and personally concerned. A job in which you help others involves a certain degree of stress.

All of the helping professions have unique pressures, anxieties, and conflicts inherent to the work itself and to the context in which the work is done. The specific degree and type of stress depends on the particular demands of your job and on the resources available to you. Occupations like veterinary medicine, which expose you to loss and grief, are potentially highly stressful.

Stress Related to Veterinary Practice

Stress is inevitable in veterinary practice. Much results from attempts to balance the provision of quality care for pets and pet owners with your own personal needs and limitations—not an easy task. Veterinary medicine is an intellectually, emotionally, and physically demanding profession. During typical work weeks, you solve numerous complex medical problems. You also provide medical treatment and emotional guidance to clients who are dealing with the illnesses, injuries, and deaths of their pets. Providing this level of care is a "given" in your profession. According to Cecelia Soares:

> The veterinarian is *expected* to be concerned, which is almost a forgotten quality in most service-oriented professions today. If the veterinarian is void of altruistic characteristics, he is likely to get creamed by clientele.[7] (p. 522)

As a veterinary professional, you must meet the challenges inherent in simultaneously responding to the medical needs of patients and the emotional needs of clients. Simultaneously, you must handle your personal feelings about cases while helping others. Each of these performance expectations has the potential to produce stress. In addition, euthanasias and personality traits are also common stressors.

Euthanasia

Even when procedures go smoothly and clients are compassionately supported, the taking of a life remains a profound and, at times, a distressing process. A survey of 130 veterinary students and practitioners conducted at the University of Georgia College of Veterinary Medicine showed that 18 percent of those surveyed had observed severe long-term emotional effects after euthanasia.[8] In the same study, survey participants reported their physical and emotional reactions to performing euthanasia. Sixty-one percent felt a lump in their throat, 57 percent felt depressed, 48 percent felt anger, 46 percent felt like crying, 41 percent felt a sense of failure or inadequacy, and 35 percent felt the need for solitude.

During discussions with University of California-Davis researchers, small-animal veterinarians said that frequent performance of euthanasia is one of the primary reasons for their burnout.[9] Suvey participants consisted of 14 veterinarians reputed to be quite effective in dealing with clients during euthanasia. They were queried to learn more about the ways in which they handled the various challenges associated with euthanasia. The veterinarians in the survey had been in practice for a median of 9 years and reported performing a median of eight euthanasias per month. The veterinarians commonly reported that they had not been prepared in college for dealing with euthanasia, but rather had learned various strategies from personal experience for dealing with euthanasia.

To reduce the stress associated with euthanasia—for the client and for themselves—the veterinarians took great care when handling the animals, used gentle and respectful touches, tranquilized the animals, catheterized the veins, and presented the animals attractively. They reported that they avoided problems during euthanasia by communicating clearly, using sensitive and comforting language, expressing compassion, acknowledging the client's feelings, allowing the client to be present during euthanasia, offering a soothing environment, and sharing experiences with colleagues.

The peak stressors cited included accidental deaths in their hospitals, dealing with long-term clients' losses, and the needless euthanasia of healthy animals or those that could have been saved by veterinary care.[9]

Personality Traits

Another source of stress stems from personality traits found in most veterinary professionals. Experts who study veterinarians at work report that veterinarians are "people-pleasers" who espouse idealistic philosophies. Thus, veterinarians tend to feel that no task is too big to accomplish. Therefore, when something does go wrong, veterinarians have a tendency for self-deprecation.[7] Ellen Whiteley, a private feline practitioner and coauthor of *Women in Veterinary Medicine: Twenty Profiles of Success* says sometimes veterinarians do not allow themselves the things that they need. She says:

> We are a profession of stress, mainly because we are overworked,
> but also because if you look at the kinds of individuals who become
> veterinarians, you can see that sometimes we're our own worst en-
> emy. We're achieving, loyal, and gaol oriented, and when you get
> the type of individual who is a driver and achiever and a perfection-
> ist, you have the kind of individual who's already set up for stress.[7]
> (p. 522)

Unfortunately, these attitudes are pervasive in veterinary medicine. They encourage veterinarians to ignore their physical, mental, and emotional fatigue and to keep a "stiff upper lip." With the demands of contemporary veterinary practice however, these attitudes are unrealistic and burdensome. Yet, because such attitudes are so deeply ingrained, efforts to depart from them most often go unsupported.

A "giving philosophy" and a strong work ethic are the norms in veterinary medicine and are maintained by the university professors teaching in the nation's veterinary schools and by the clinicians and technicians working in private practice. It is very difficult however, to uphold a giving philosophy while protecting your own health and well-being. It is especially difficult to achieve a balance between giving to others and protecting yourself when you have not been taught how to do so.

Stress Related to Helping during Times of Loss

By choosing a career in veterinary medicine, you will get your share of exposure to loss and grief. As we said in Chapter 2, because you perform euthanasia, you will witness your clients' acute responses to grief. Along with your clients' grief reactions, you will also have your own.

Many students and practitioners are beginning to acknowledge this fact. Most of the veterinary students who enroll in CSU's elective courses on client relations report that they take these classes to learn how to cope with their own emotions during stressful times. One student told us, "I didn't take this class to learn how to care for pet owners. I care too much! I'm here to learn how to keep realistic perspectives on my cases and how to handle my own emotions." A practicing veterinarian told us, "I had so many self-imposed rules about how I had to hand my emotions during euthanasias that I couldn't fully attend to my clients . . . I didn't encourage my clients to be present because I was afraid I would start to cry."

You can expect, from time to time, to feel your own grief during patient death. Such reactions are normal and should be expected. Research has shown, for example, that the grief reactions of professional caregivers are similar to those experienced by the families with whom they work, although they are usually of lesser intensity and of shorter duration.[10] Research and clinical experience have also shown that, as professional caregivers increasingly attempt to respond to the needs of the dying, stronger attachments to patients are made, leaving helpers even more vulnerable to experiencing grief (Fig. 11-2).[11] Fulton notes that this increased vulnerability can be accentuated in the absence of strong family support for the dying.[12] Researchers say that this sociologic trend is contributing to the development of a "surrogate griever" role for the caregiver; that is, one who grieves in place of family members.[11] This phenomenon may be especially pronounced in humane society and "shelter" staffs (Fig. 11-3).

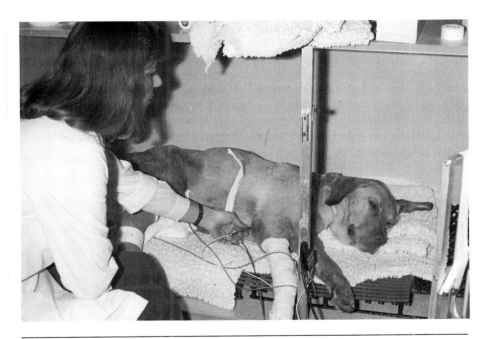

Figure 11-2 Veterinary professionals provide care for critically ill or injured animals and may experience their own feelings of grief when animals cannot be saved.

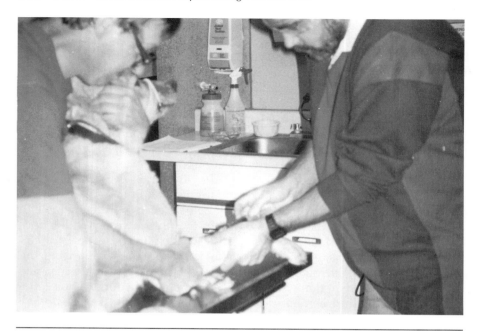

Figure 11-3 Humane society and shelter staff members, who have the unenviable task of euthanizing unwanted healthy animals, often feel isolated in their grief.

Some stressors are specifically related to helping during loss and and uniquely associated with the care of terminally ill patients and their families. Researchers Vachon,[13] Lazare,[14] and Cook and Oltjenbruns,[11] identified some of the common stressors that arise when working with the dying. With some adaptation to veterinary practice, those stressors are:

- Difficulty accepting the fact that the patients' physical and psychosocial problems cannot always be controlled.
- Frustration at having invested large amounts of energy in caring for a patient who then dies, taking this investment with them.
- Disappointment if expectations for patients to die a "good death"—however this may be defined—are not met.
- Difficulty ending a life you once saved.
- Difficulty establishing a sense of realistic limitations on what veterinary care, which is expected to be all-encompassing, can actually provide.
- Difficulty deciding where to draw limits in involvement with patients and their owners, particularly during off-duty hours.

- Feeling overwhelmed by the frequency of losses (sometimes several patients die within a short period).
- Holding on to unresolved guilt concerning patient care, especially when a misdiagnosis or mistake is made.
- Difficulty with the social negation of the loss (when the impact of the loss on the caregiver is not acknowledged by others).
- Belief in the assumption that one has to be strong because of a given occupation or role.

Most veterinary professionals will experience at least some discomfort when addressing these issues. It is normal to be touched by the pets and pet owners in your care and to occasionally struggle with the feelings that arise in practice. As a loving, compassionate person, you want to retain access to these feelings although, at times, they may be painful.

You get into emotional trouble, however, when your feelings of responsibility begin to overpower all of your other feelings. Grief educator Alan Wolfelt[15] says that you are in trouble if you:

- Think of yourself as indispensable.
- Constantly worry about patients and clients even when away from work.
- Neglect your own relationships.
- Have a tendency to overcommit yourself.

He says that, if you are having those feelings, you are "confusing caregiving with caretaking" and are most likely a "codependent bereavement caregiver." This common psychologic condition called codependency is reviewed next.

Stress Related to Codependency

An antecedent condition called codependency contributes to stress in all helping professions, including veterinary medicine, and undermines effective helping during times of loss. Codependency is usually defined as an ongoing pattern of thinking, feeling, and behaving that stems from an *excessive need to please others*. According to Tim Cermack, MD, a leading figure in the field of codependency, the condition manifests in persons who feel that they are responsible for meeting others' needs to the exclusion of meeting their own.[16] Codependents *always* put other people's needs before their own. Codependency, therefore, is a condition in which people's behaviors and feelings are externally, rather than internally, driven and in which their search for approval is outer-directed rather than inner-directed.

Codependency is most closely associated with the area of chemical dependency. As codependency theories have been tested and applied, however, researchers and clinicians have found that the condition also manifests in people who are not directly affected by drugs or alcohol. It is now generally accepted that codependency is a condition that affects millions of people from diverse family backgrounds, varying degrees of education, and differing life experiences. It is also generally accepted that most codependents come from, what are called in the literature, dysfunctional families. Dysfunctional families are those in which roles are not clearly defined, boundaries are blurred, and individual identities are not respected or nurtured. Codependency results from dysfunctional familial and societal conditioning. Codependency characteristics are so prevalent in dysfunctional families and societies that they are adopted, accepted, and viewed as "normal" ways of functioning.

The classic role played by codependent persons is that of "caretaker." Caretakers try to meet everyone's needs, to make everyone happy, and to orchestrate positive outcomes for all situations. They regularly give time and effort well beyond their actual abilities and capacities, often sacrificing personal needs to achieve "approval" from others. Many people in the helping professions, including those in veterinary medicine, are codependent caretakers.

Psychiatrist Charles Whitfield is a leader in the codependency recovery field. He has postulated that 80 percent of people in helping professions are codependent.[17] Educator and addictions expert Sharon Wegscheider-Cruse further suggests that a staggering 96 percent of persons in the general population experience difficulty in life due to codependency.[18] Although codependency is statistically normative in our society, it is not a "normal" state. Humans do not achieve their full potential or function in the most efficient, effective ways when they are codependent.

Some good news about codependency does exist, however. It is not terminal! Recognition of the problem, a desire to change, and the development of new interpersonal skills alleviate codependency and result in higher levels of functioning, both at home and at work. Recognition of the problem begins with identification of codependent characteristics.

Codependent Characteristics

Cecelia Soares and Bonnie Mader, who teach classes on client relations at the University of California-Davis, base some of their lecture material in codependency theories. They enlighten veterinary students and practitioners about codependency's effects on the practice of veterinary medicine.[19] Drawing on their work, and on the extensive pioneering work of psychotherapists John Bradshaw,[20] Janet Woititz,[21] and Melody Beattie,[22] we elaborate on seven codependent characteristics in the following section.

Blurring of Boundaries.   A boundary is a predetermined or pre-established limit. It defines the extent of your flexibility. Everyone has personal and professional boundaries or limits that regulate their behaviors and their responses to others' behaviors. The problem is that most professionals are unaware of their boundaries.

Veterinarians need to become aware of their boundaries and to allow themselves to abide by them. When veterinarians' boundaries are clearly defined, others know what to expect from interchanges with them. They understand how far they will (and will not) go toward accommodating the needs of clients, staff, and family. For example, when your clients and staff know that Saturday is your "Family Day," they know not to ask you to take nonemergency cases or do extra work at that time.

Difficulty Saying "No."   Codependent persons have difficulty saying "no." They feel that they must do whatever is asked of them, regardless of the nature of the request. This behavior stems from a desire not to let anyone down. Setting limits by saying "no" sometimes throws codependents into states of turmoil as internally they struggle to meet their own needs and those of others. The desire to be "all things to all people" is overwhelming and often results in codependents taking on more than that which can be comfortably managed. Codependents' abilities to say "no" to others' requests may be further complicated by a tendency to perceive all circumstances as having equal value. Prioritizing tasks becomes impossible when all tasks are viewed with the same degree of importance.

Many veterinarians struggle with overcommitment and lack of prioritization. Consider, for example, the veterinarian who is often asked to bury clients' pets and to attend pets' memorial ceremonies. If she views all of these requests as equally important and regularly agrees to accommodate them (even though she does not have time and clearly sees this degree of responsibility as beyond her role), she will eventually feel great resentment as having to complete these tasks.

Constant Seeking of Approval.   Most people agree that they would rather have, than not have, the approval of others. With codependents, however, the need to gain *everyone's* approval *all of the time* is a significant motivating factor. Codependents expend great amounts of energy courting those whose approval is desired or whose approval status is unknown. Conversely, those whom the codependent believes can be safely disappointed are often neglected. Unfortunately, the people who can most often be safely disappointed are those who are closest to the codependent. This group usually includes family and close friends. Because their approval is already a known commodity, it is assumed that time with them can be forfeited because they will understand and will continue to hold the relationship in high esteem.

Veterinarians who are approval-driven may agree to stay after hours on routine, nonemergency cases to accommodate their clients' schedules while simultaneously disappointing their families by missing planned dinners or special events. They act in this way because accommodating clients, even at their family's expense, assures veterinarians of their clients' approval.

Acting on Suppositions.   This behavior occurs when actions and internal dialog are governed by suppositions about what other people think and feel. For example, nonverbal and verbal behaviors are frequently misinterpreted by codependents to mean "I did something wrong," or "I am not appreciated." Facial expressions, gestures, and comments are often internalized by codependents in a negative, self-deprecating manner without verbally confirming the intended message.

For example, a veterinarian's client scowls as she writes a check to cover her bill. Her veterinarian observes the scowl and assumes that she is unhappy with him for charging too much. This belief, in turn, fosters unsettling, disruptive thoughts in him. If the veterinarian calmly inquires about the meaning of the facial expression, he might discover that the client is not upset with him at all. For example, he might discover that the client's scowl is due to the realization that she forgot to record her previous check. Codependent veterinarians do not "check out" their suppositions, however, because they do not want to offend or upset anybody. Checking out assumptions often spares veterinarians unnecessary, self-inflicted feelings of anxiety.

Over-Identifying with Professionals Roles.   This condition exists when codependents overlap their personal and professional roles to such a degree that little distinction exists between the two. Thus, they have difficulty differentiating what is central to the them as individuals and what is central to their careers. Those who define themselves by their careers, without acknowledging other life roles, exhibit this trait.

Great social reinforcement exists for those who define themselves as highly skilled, highly educated veterinary professionals. Thus, it is particularly difficult for veterinarians to break the habit of overidentification. Yet, it is important to do so because veterinarians who overidentify with their work experience decreases in self-esteem when they perceive that others are not in complete agreement with their professional values. For example, a thought process that reflects veterinarians' overidentification is, "If you want a second opinion, it means you don't agree with *my* professional opinion and don't value me personally."

Being Hyper-Responsible.   This characteristic surfaces when codependents feel responsible for every aspect of their own lives and for the lives of those around them. They expect perfection and chastise themselves for the most minute infraction, allowing no room for oversight or human error. Codependents with this characteristic fail to acknowledge their personal accomplishments. Author Janet Woittiz succinctly describes this misguided thought pattern as, "Anything that goes wrong is my fault. Anything that goes right, of course, is the result of fate, luck, or chance"[21] (p. 41).

Examples of hyper-responsibility in veterinary medicine are veterinarians who refuse to take or cancel vacations, those who are unable or unwilling to take a team approach to cases, or those who refuse to turn over responsibility for cases to specialists or to equally competent colleagues when situations demand it. These veterinarians are in the "Super Vet" trap and are often unaware of the toll this codependency characteristic takes on their lives.

Becoming Negatively Invested in Work.   When codependents become negatively invested in their work, the job is never far from their thoughts. In terms of veterinary medicine, this condition has been described as "the case having the veterinarian rather than the veterinarian having the case."[19] Examples of a veterinarian's negative investment in work include:

- A high degree of involvement with a particular animal or owner, which elicits a negative emotional response.
- Overinvestment in the outcome of a case beyond the normal limits of professional concern.
- Overstepping professional bounds and using personal influence to sway a client's decision.
- Continually having thoughts of a case invade one's mind, even during "off time."
- Difficulty "letting go" of a case even though the case has been terminated medically.

The codependent characteristics described above represent some of the ways in which you can lose your abilities to emotionally detach from cases. Lack of emotional detachment leads to stress and burnout. When you use effective detached-concern strategies, however, stress is reduced and job satisfaction is increased. Now let us turn to the second half of this chapter, in which you will learn about exploring your personal reasons for helping, how to emotionally detach from cases, and how to take care of yourself on a day-to-day basis.

STRESS MANAGEMENT STRATEGIES

All successful stress management plans rest on a foundation of attitude change. Attitude change calls for a solid commitment to self-exploration and to approaching tasks and situations in new ways. It involves a thorough history-taking, a discarding of some of your deeply held values and beliefs, and an incorporation of new ways of thinking and behaving. Obviously, this level of commitment to attitude change is often difficult to achieve.

Attitude change for the purpose of stress management in veterinary practice has two aspects. Both are based on knowledge of the ways in which to emotionally detach from cases. The first aspect involves an evaluation of the personal factors that influence your helping abilities during times of loss. This kind of evaluation is necessary to ensure that the way in which you handle cases is not based on inaccurate information of childhood or from socially imposed norms and values. In other words, personal evaluation helps you to ensure that your interventions are client-motivated rather than personally motivated. This form of self-evaluation is particularly important if you strongly identify with the characteristics of codependency discussed earlier.

The second aspect of attitude change involves the development and incorporation of a helping philosophy and work style called "detached concern." This concept is discussed in detail later in this chapter. For now, let us begin by looking at your personal reasons for helping.

Personal Factors That Influence Helping During Loss

In their book, *Helping the Bereaved: Therapeutic Interventions for Children, Adolescents, and Adults,* Alicia Cook and Daniel Dworkin ask helpers to explore three areas when preparing to work with grieving clients.[23] With some adaption on our part, these areas are the helper's:

- Personal background with loss, death, and grief.
- Current issues, values, and beliefs regarding loss, death, and grief.
- Motivations for wanting to help.

Drawing further from Cook and Dworkin, let us look at these three areas individually.

Your Personal Loss Background

The losses that you experienced throughout your childhood have influenced you, perhaps more deeply than you realize. For example, you may have experienced many kinds of losses as a child and young adult. On the other hand, you may have experienced relatively few. Also, your loss experiences may be confined to the deaths of loved ones or they may be related to the effects of war or natural disasters. Your family, culture, and society have also affected the ways in which you think about and cope with death. You grew up with influences that are unique to you. The degree to which you have been able to accept, integrate, and resolve your own losses affects your ability to help others with grief. Therefore, continuing to look inward and to be aware of your own feelings about and responses to death is critical to effective helping.

To understand how you have been influenced in your life and to assess your own attitudes about death and grief, consider the answers you would give to the following questions:

- What were your first experiences with loss and death? What were your needs at that time and how did others respond to your needs? What are your strongest emotional impressions of these situations? Do you feel sadness, anger, confusion, a sense of security? How have the most significant of these losses affected your life and ability to help others during loss?
- What are your personal experiences with pet loss? How were companion animals' deaths treated in your family? Was the truth of a pet's death ever kept from you? Were you allowed to see your pets' bodies and to conduct burials or memorial services for them?
- How was crying addressed in your family? Were tears ignored or encouraged? Was crying viewed as a sign of weakness or as one of healthy vulnerability and sensitivity?
- What do you think people need during grief? What do you think is helpful to offer or provide for them?

Your Current Issues, Values, and Beliefs about Loss, Death, and Grief

As a growing, changing human being, you constantly encounter new experiences and situations that further influence your life. Often, the ongoing events of your life make it easier or more difficult to help others. For example, if you are experiencing the terminal illness and dying process of one of your own family members, you may find it difficult to attend to the grief of others, especially if you personally value human life over animal life. On the other hand, experiencing the death of a loved one may enhance your ability to empathize with clients who have lost their pets because you are more easily able to relate to their feelings and to their situations.

Insights regarding your own issues of grief are frequently accompanied by emotional intensity. For this reason, primarily, most people avoid personal examination of their issues. They want to protect themselves from their own painful feelings. Ironically, however, continuous self-examination can actually build a higher tolerance for emotional pain, thereby lessening the intensity of feelings.

As a helper, you can better assist clients with grief when you periodically monitor yourself in regard to it. It is a good idea to occasionally ask yourself the following questions:

- How do you feel when you listen to someone describe the details of their loss experience? Sensations like warmth, empathy, and a feeling of connectedness indicate a willingness to nurture, care for, and help another person, whereas feelings like depression, impatience, and anger often indicate high levels of stress and warn of impending burnout.
- Which cases do you have the hardest time handling, and how do they remind you of your own losses or potential losses? What do you do when you are confronted with these cases?
- Which of your values "get in the way" when working with grieving clients? In other words, under what circumstances are you most likely to judge or to develop negative attitudes about clients and their situations?
- What grief work of your own do you still have to do? What personal losses are unresolved? What actions do you need to take to continue or begin your own grieving process?
- Have you thought about your own death? How much reflection have you given it, and how does it make you feel?

Your Motivations as a Helper during Loss

People develop a desire to help others for many reasons. Both healthy and unhealthy motivations exist, and it is worthwhile to examine your own. If your own experiences with loss have enhanced your life and have helped you grow personally, you probably have a fairly high level of self-esteem and sense of well-being. These characteristics are necessary if you are to allow clients to focus on their own needs without feeling compelled to have your own needs met at the same time. If, however, your own losses continue to diminish your self-esteem and sense of well-being, you may seek to "help" clients because you hope to create opportunities for your own loss-related needs to be met. In the latter situation, you may not purposely create these interchanges or consciously know that you are helping others as a way of helping yourself. It is not uncommon for inexperienced helpers to have difficulty separating their own needs from those of their clients. The greatest danger in helping others in an attempt to help yourself is that you may assume that what you would want or need in any given situation is also what your clients want and need in the same situation. Such assumptions are almost always erroneous.

By virtue of your occupation, you experience a great deal of loss as you watch animals whom you care about die. You probably have grief accumulated inside of you that has never really been addressed or acknowledged. As you begin to develop skills to help others with grief, you will, in fact, be helping yourself. This is fine. Helping is never a totally unselfish act.

During your helping endeavors, however, you may find that particular cases touch you and cause you to react more strongly than you would imagine. Look closely at these cases. Is the animal similar to one you lost? Does the client remind you of someone you loved and lost or someone toward whom you have animosity? Does the decision at hand remind you of a dilemma you faced previously in your personal life?

Getting "triggered" or "hooked" by cases is nothing to be ashamed of—it happens to everyone who works with people who are experiencing emotional pain. When you find yourself triggered or hooked by cases, however, you do not have to fix the situation or find a way to make your feelings disappear. You need only to notice your discomfort and then let the realization of your own personal losses explain your unexpected response. When you have this conscious awareness, separate the case at hand from the situation you are remembering, and, if you can, proceed to provide care for your client. Later, use what you have learned, and allow yourself to grieve. When you are aware of your own losses and of the ways in which they affect you, you are more likely to take time to care for yourself. As stated earlier, when you care for yourself, you are more able to care for others.

A large part of caring for yourself involves learning from your experiences. Malenik and colleagues[24] interviewed 14 adults whose parents had died during the 2 years preceeding the study. About 50 percent of the participants reported that they had experienced a beneficial outcome from the experience, despite the fact that the deaths of their parents had been very painful. For example, individuals reported such benefits as increased emotional strength and self-reliance, greater caring for friends and loved ones, and deepened levels of appreciation for life. Another positive outcome they reported was that they now placed more value on the present rather than investing so heavily in the future.

Benoliel noted that experiencing significant loss can encourage people to search for meaning in life.[25] For example, some create music, poetry, or art based on their experiences. Others find meaning through enhancing their relationships with other people.

Based on their need to draw on your energy, some clients will occasionally make requests of you that are beyond your capabilities or desires to grant. When you feel the boundaries of your personal and professional responsibilities being stretched, it is helpful to be prepared with answers that release you from agonizing decisions. These answers come from formal practice policies and philosophies that are designed to protect you from added stress. You are not truly helping anyone if you are stressed and are feeling resentful about your caregiving agreements. It is often more helpful in the long-run for you to say "no." Facing difficult situations without you can prompt clients to seek help from their friends, family, or human service professionals, thus providing a possible stimulus for personal growth and development. The idea of caring for others while caring for yourself is reviewed in the following pages.

DEVELOPING DETACHED CONCERN

You will find a balance between caring too much and caring too little through the development of a work style called "detached concern." Detached concern, according to researchers Lief and Fox, is defined as detaching from cases sufficiently to maintain sound medical judgment and equanimity, while simultaneously maintaining enough concern for patients and clients to provide them with sensitive and understanding care.[26] In other words, a work style based on detached concern allows you to give yourself fully to the situation at hand while concurrently preserving yourself physically, intellectually, and emotionally. When you practice medicine with detached concern for patients and clients, you are able to maintain appropriate boundaries between your personal and professional lives and between the cases you see during the course of your day. The ability to maintain appropriate boundaries preserves your energy and enthusiasm and prevents you from "burning-out" on your profession.

You can learn to reduce levels of professional stress by achieving a healthy balance between emotional attachment and emotional detachment. This balance *is* detached concern. Detached concern is difficult to achieve because, as a veterinarian, you are challenged by it on a case-by-case basis. In any given day, you must quickly form attachments to clients and to their pets as you examine, diagnose, and treat medical problems. Just as quickly, however, you must detach from the circumstances and emotions that have arisen on that case and move on to the next one. For example, you are often expected to euthanize a special client's beloved pet and then address the next client's anxiety about the change in scheduling caused by the euthanasia. Dealing with anger immediately following sadness and grief is taxing. Compartmentalizing emotion in this manner takes great insight, skill, and a lot of practice.

All too often, when you are faced with the "emotional roller coaster rides" of practice, you stop attempting to compartmentalize and detach altogether. Mentally, you may form firm rules about not expressing your emotions with clients, show disinterest in case outcomes, and fail to follow-up with clients after they leave your office. Excessive detachment jeopardizes case management and is a classic sign of burn-out. A work style based on excessive detachment presents an attitude of aloofness and indifference to clients. In the long-run, this form of detachment is as damaging to you as is overinvolvement in cases.

As you can see, a work style based on detached concern brings a healthy balance to your practice. When this philosophic foundation has been established, you can develop a stress management system that helps you to maintain it on a day-to-day basis. In the pages that follow, stress management philosophies and techniques that are helpful to all medical professionals are presented. Each of these strategies helps to maintain a philosophy of detached concern and supports the incorporation of positive coping styles.

Four General Stress Management Categories

As discussed in the beginning of this chapter, information about stress management theories and practices abound. Thousands of ways exist in which to cope with life's hassles. You probably already know about many of these approaches. Taking action is the difficult part.

For the purposes if this chapter, we have grouped the selected stress management strategies into four categories: replenishing activities, personal and professional development, time management, and drawing closure. As you read through the chapter, select one form of stress management from each of the four categories. Be sure that your selections are realistic, convenient, and right for you—and then begin to use them today!

Replenishing Activities

Replenishing activities are activities that simply *make you feel better*. Replenishing is defined as restoring to fullness or completeness something that has been wholly or partially emptied. It is analogous to refilling your automobile's gas tank or recharging a battery. Replenishing leaves you feeling renewed, refreshed, and restocked, thus giving you an energy supply on which to draw so that you can handle the challenges that come your way. The replenishing activities we have chosen to discuss include: relaxation techniques, humor, health care, and time in natural settings.

Relaxation Techniques. A relaxation routine can happen anywhere and anytime. It allows the mind to slow down, to let go, and to be at peace. The core component of any relaxation program is deep and rhythmic breathing. Deep breathing has both calming and revitalizing effects. Noticing your breathing pattern and changing it from one that is tension-producing to one that's relaxation program is deep and rhythmic breathing. Deep breathing has both calming and revitalizing effects. Noticing your breathing pattern and changing it from one that is tension-producing to one that's relaxation-producing is one of the most crucial—and simplest—relaxation techniques. As little as 5 minutes of deep breathing can refresh you on even the most difficult days.

Other forms of relaxation include spending time alone, sitting quietly, listening to music, massage, guided visualizations, yoga, meditation, and systematic muscle relaxation routines (Fig. 11-4). All can be learned from

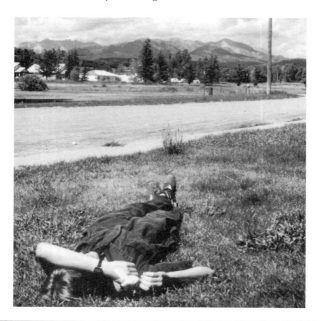

Figure 11-4 To effectively manage stress and prevent burnout, veterinary professionals should try to find a few minutes each day to relax. This can be done simply, while sitting at a desk or walking outdoors. This student decided to "take five" outside.

various accredited instructors. Numerous audiocassette tapes are also available. All relaxation programs should be drug-free.

Humor.   Laughter is good for you. It is a great stress reducer. In fact, the study of humor and its effects on the human body has a name: gelotology. According to William F. Fry,[27] a psychiatrist at the Stanford School of Medicine and a well-known gelotologist who has written three books on humor and health, a good laugh:

- Gives the heart muscles a good workout.
- Improves circulation.
- Fills the lungs with oxygen-rich air.
- Clears the respiratory passages.
- Stimulates alertness hormones that stimulate various tissues.
- Alters the brain, diminishing tension in the central nervous system.
- Counteracts fear, anger, and depression; all negative emotions linked to physical illnesses.
- May relieve pain.

A good sense of humor is important for another reason. Potential employers look for it.[28] According to two recent studies of executives and personnel officers at two large American corporations, 84 percent of those surveyed at one company thought that employees with a sense of humor do a better job than do those with little or no sense of humor,[29] and 98 percent of those surveyed at the other company said that they would hire people with good humor over people who seem to lack humor[30] (Fig. 11-5). It seems that people who have a well-developed sense of humor tend to be regarded as more creative, less rigid, and more willing to consider and embrace new ideas and methods.

If you are not laughing enough, keep a humor file of cartoons, pictures, and jokes; watch comedy movies; or spend time with people or pets who make you laugh (Box 11-4). Take a humor break during the most tense part of your day. Start thinking of something funny. If it does not seem that funny at first, stay with it.

If you truly want to start laughing, two groups are available for you to contact. The American Association for Therapeutic Humor can supply you with bibliographies on various aspects of humor as therapy and with a newsletter called *Laugh It Up*. The Humor Project provides workshops, courses, and seminars for people who wish to use humor as a positive force in their work. For a small fee, it also supplies an information packet on the positive power of humor as well as a magazine called *Laughing*

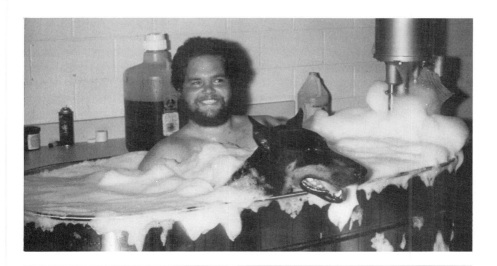

Figure 11-5 Light-hearted persons are a positive addition to any veterinary staff. They often help others through difficult times by providing comic relief at just the right moment.

BOX 11-4

Examples of Humorous Miscommunications

These examples of humorous miscommunications prove that some of the funniest are found in everyday life.

Sentences from actual letters sent to "welfare" offices in application for support:

- I am very much annoyed to find you have branded my son illiterate. This is a dirty lie, as I was married a week before he was born.
- You have changed my boy to a girl. Will this make any difference?
- Mrs. Jones has not had any clothes for a year and has been visited regularly by the clergy. She needs a lot of support.
- In accordance with your instructions, I am sending proof that I have given birth to twins in the enclosed envelope.
- I am forwarding my marriage certificate and six children. I had seven but one died which was baptized on a half sheet of paper.
- My husband got his project cut off two weeks ago and I haven't had any relief since.
- I want money as quick as I can get it. I have been in bed with the doctor for two weeks and he doesn't do me any good. If things don't improve, I will have to send for a new doctor.

And from church bulletins:

- This afternoon there will be a meeting in the south and north ends of the church. Children will be baptized at both ends.
- Tuesday at a 4 p.m. there will be an ice cream social. All ladies giving milk, come early.
- This being Easter Sunday, we will ask Mrs. Johnson to come forward and lay an egg on the altar.
- Thursday at 5 p.m. there will be a meeting of the Little Mothers Club. All those wishing to become little mothers please meet the pastor in his study.
- The ladies of the church have cast off clothing of every kind and they may be seen in the church basement on Friday afternoons.
- Tonight's sermon: "What is Hell?" Come early and listen to our choir practice.

From the Denver City Welfare Department, 1962, and John Jennings' column in The Tucson Citizen newspaper, Tucson, Arizona.

Matter. The addresses and telephone numbers for these organizations are listed in the Resource Appendix.

Humor should be used with caution, however. As pointed out earlier, some people are offended by the "warped" humor that comes from those who have been exposed to excessive stress. We remember a time when a stressed technician, a colleague of ours, had a terrible week with every animal that came into her service dying and "going home in a body bag." She told us she that was tempted to parrot the grocery store clerks and ask clients, "Which would you like for the body—paper or plastic?" Fortunately, she only shared this story with us. Obviously, the moral of this story is: There is a time and place for everything.

Health Care.   Two basic components of health care are nutrition and exercise. The psychologic and physical benefits of both are well-established. Proper diet and exercise not only make you feel better, they also prevent you from becoming ill in the future. Experts in nutrition have proven that deficiencies in certain vitamins, minerals, and proteins can significantly affect your energy levels, mood, and sleep patterns.[31]

Good eating habits go hand-in-hand with exercise. It does not take much to experience their benefits. In a review of more than 120 studies, Steven J. Petruzzello, PhD, of the University of Illinois at Urbana-Champaign found that doing as little as 6 minutes of aerobic exercise can reduce anxiety.[32] One of the most popular explanations for this effect is that exercise causes the body to release endorphins, which block pain and produce a sense of well-being. Another possibility is that the elevated body temperature induced by exercise may positively affect brain biochemistry, or, it may be that taking time out from normal activities gives relief.

If you feel that you do not have the time or resources to begin a complete exercise program, try walking. Of all the physical fitness activities, walking is the easiest, safest, and cheapest. To start, you need no equipment except comfortable shoes (Fig. 11-6). Choose an exercise program that you truly enjoy rather than one that feels like pure hard work and drudgery. You will be more likely to stay with it. Check with your physician before beginning any exercise program.

Time in Natural Settings.   Anyone who has taken a stroll on a deserted beach at sunrise, hiked into mountainous "back country," or simply sat on a park bench and watched the squirrels play, knows the healing power of nature. Anyone who has been mesmerized while watching the nature specials on the Discovery Channel or stared at the landscape photographs in National Geographic magazine has experienced its spell. You have personally experienced nature's positive effect on your well-being (Fig. 11-7).

Researchers are beginning to support what we intuitively know. In a 1991 study, Ulrich and colleagues[33] monitored the physiologic stress responses of university students as they watched an unpleasant film about work accidents. Immediately after the students viewed the film, they were shown a color-sound videotape of an environment; a nature scene or an attractive urban environment lacking nature. Findings showed that students recovered much faster and more completely from the stress of observing the accident film if they were then exposed to nature settings

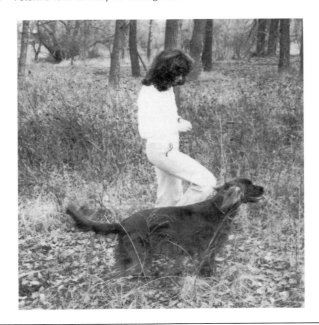

Figure 11-6 Walking is more enjoyable when companion animals go along.

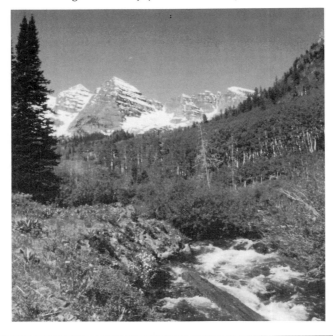

Figure 11-7 The best nature experience is "the real thing."
PHOTO COURTESY OF JENGER SMITH.

rather than to urban environments. Monitoring devices showed that the restoration benefit of nature took place within 3 to 4 minutes.

Another study by Ulrich[34] suggested that patients spend less time in the hospital, about three fourths of a day on average, if they have a nature view. In addition, patients who participated in that study needed fewer doses of strong pain killers and had fewer surgical complications. Ulrich also indicated that what people respond to as natural is not necessarily limited to wilderness. Agricultural fields, wooded parks in cities, and even golf courses were defined as "nature" by the survey participants.[35] Therefore, you do not have to go far to enjoy the benefits of nature.

Personal and Professional Development

As you learn how to communicate your concerns for clients during pet-loss-related crises, you will be more comfortable when intervening. The more comfortable you are when intervening, the lower your stress level will be. Thus, you will be repaid in full for any investment that you make to personal and professional development. Four ways exist in which to reduce stress through personal and professional development: develop communication skills, look for learning opportunities, use community educators, and seek therapy.

Develop Communication Skills. One way to raise your comfort level with a process is to get more information about ways to do it effectively. Evaluate your communication skills by surveying the significant persons around you. Find out what they think about your communication effectiveness. Ask for honest feedback and incorporate it. Look for good communication role models. Read books on effective communication; many are on the market.

Look for Learning Opportunities. Lifelong technical and nontechnical learning is a component of any bond-centered practice. This type of training should be an option for you and for every member of your staff. Technical training is available at the teaching hospitals nationwide. Nontechnical training can also be found in those institutions and in your local communities.

Three types of training will help you feel more comfortable in your role as helper. The first is general training on effective communication. Find a course that allows you to *practice* (through role-play) many of the basic skills presented in chapters 6 and 7. Most continuing education programs offer these courses. The second involves training in paraprofessional crisis intervention and is available through community crisis centers. The third is paraprofessional grief counseling, which is given by community hospice programs. Generally, in exchange for the training, you agree to give a predetermined number of volunteer hours to the training agency. Most people find the volunteer experience very helpful and extremely rewarding.

Technicians should not be left out of the training experience, given that they spend a relatively large amount of time with pet owners. Many times, pet owners will tell technicians things that they are unwilling to tell practitioners. Although generally a plus, it also puts additional pressure on the technical staff. Therefore, train technicians for success by adequately training them to intervene in pet loss.

Use Community Educators. If you are unable to participate in a comprehensive training program, arrange for a series of staff trainings from the local educational or mental health professionals in your area. Many provide workshops as a free community service or at a nominal fee. You can also establish a barter system with the trainer. He or she may agree to educational presentations at your clinic in exchange for veterinary care for companion animals.

Seek Therapy. If your stress level becomes too high, you may need to seek therapy from a trained mental health professional. Speaking to an objective person about the difficulties that you are experiencing can bring emotional relief and help you to see and solve problems in new and creative ways. The process of "venting" feelings has been found to be very beneficial. It may seem embarrassing to initiate contact with a therapist. You may feel that it indicates weakness on your part. Clinical experience shows, however, that the healthiest persons are the ones who know that they need help and who are able to reach out for it.

Time Management

Lack of time is a societal problem, and it is one of the most challenging aspects of veterinary medicine. In practice, you may be on call 24 hours a day and need to be available to handle your clients' medical and emotional emergencies at a moment's notice. In your "spare" time, you deal with client complaints, mediate staff disputes, and handle the financial aspects of your veterinary practice. Outside the demands of practice, you also strive to honor your obligations to family, friends, and community.

You already work hard to handle the challenges inherent in your profession. You may therefore be skeptical about implementing the techniques discussed throughout this book. You may think that the methods are financially unrealistic and too time-consuming. You may be saying, "What you are suggesting is impossible. I'm already so busy I can't keep up." It is possible to implement the bond-centered practice ideas, however, if they are paired with a commitment to time management. The four time management categories are: structured time, transition time, focused time, and clean time.

Structured Time. Most professionals spend most of their lives within a structured time framework. Structured time is time that is scheduled for specific activities, set to take place in agreed upon amounts of time. Structured time involves a schedule of appointments and meetings, all of which have beginning and ending points.

When structuring your time, start by establishing clinic hours that accommodate client needs *and* fit your personality. For example, if you are not a "morning" person, set your clinic hours from 10 a.m. to 6 p.m. On the other hand, if you tire by the end of the day and grow impatient with client demands, try to schedule most of your clients early and use the end of the day to complete patient records, read journals, or focus on other aspects of your practice.

When structuring your time, notice how often you change your schedule (for example, come in early, stay late, skip lunch) to accommodate client needs. If you do it "rarely" or "occasionally," you are probably in control of the way in which your time is structured. If, however, you do it "often" or "always," you are giving your control to others.

Transition Time.   Transition time relates to a period of time between activities. It is the time needed to pass from one thing to another; to "finish" what just occurred and to "focus" on what is about to occur. Transition time is used to recover your emotional composure and clarity of thinking. Transition time is generally brief. It is as simple as a 5-minute walk outdoors or sitting down at your desk to take a few deep breaths.

The key to regular use of transition time lies in knowing your schedule in advance and allowing time to take care of yourself during stressful periods. On a daily basis, for example, try not to schedule difficult clients or challenging patients back-to-back. Whenever possible, avoid scheduling more than one euthanasia in a day. On a weekly or monthly basis, plan ahead for increased stress due to staff absences, vacations, or off-site trainings. Allow extra time during holiday and tax seasons too. Do not expect to handle the same volume of clients when other time demands increase or when staff availability is decreased.

Focused Time.   Most people know it is difficult to do several things simultaneously and to do them well. Therefore, developing the ability to focus your mind and to fix your attention on one thing at a time is essential.

Prioritizing your interventions makes it is easier to maintain focus. Then, you recognize that you cannot and do not want to do everything, but you can commit yourself to the things that you define as important (for example, giving 5 minutes of grief education, performing client-present euthanasias, or hand-writing condolence cards). To help you to maintain your focus during euthanasias, for example, perform them during quieter times of the day, turn off your pager, and ensure that others are available to take care of emergencies for you. A commitment to an activity benefits your clients and you. When you give your full attention to something, it is more likely you that will feel good about it when it is completed.

Clean Time.   Clean time is exactly what it sounds like. It is time that is free of demands and responsibilities. It is time is not cluttered with the worries of work or home. Everyone needs clean time, yet, most say it is difficult to find. Some veterinarians tell us that it is impossible to get away from work. They say that business is too demanding or that they have no one to cover for them. We know some who have actually cancelled vacations with their families to care for sick patients.

Veterinarians must find clean time on a daily basis. It is essential. Force yourself to talk about something other than veterinary medicine. Read books or watch programs that stimulate discussion about other subjects. Avoid "shop talk" during breaks or when socializing with colleagues. Avoid taking paper work home because this habit contaminates clean time. Also, take time away from the clinic to pursue personal interests. Go fishing, take a dance class, volunteer, or travel. If you are unable to say "no" to the unexpected duties that inevitibly arise while you are away or cannot resist stopping in the office just to "check in," leave town.

Ensure that your employees get clean time too. Allow them to take a "mental health day" once or twice a year. With mental health days, staff members call in "well" rather than "sick" and spend the day doing something nice for themselves. Mental health days can be scheduled a bit ahead of time out of courtesy for others. This type of support for one another strengthens relationships in the clinic.

Two more points must be addressed in summarizing this segment on time management. First, delegate authority whenever possible. Most staff members blossom when given the opportunity to handle new tasks. It feels good to think creatively, to improve skills, and to be trusted with an important aspect of the practice. A technician, for example, can be responsible for stocking examination rooms with tissues, for researching card companies and ordering condolence cards, or for maintaining a small library of books about pet loss and grief. A receptionist may be able to write a brochure about the human-animal bond or about pet loss and grief.

Second, most CSU graduates now in practice tell us that they are actually busier in practice than they were in veterinary school. They work long hours are are often on emergency coverage. While in veterinary school, many of these students relied on negative coping habits to address high levels of stress. They told themselves that this high-stress period was time-limited and that they would take better care of themselves after graduation. The truth is that nothing magical happens to train you *how* to do that between graduation from veterinary school and the beginning of veterinary practice. You need to begin *now*.

Drawing Closure

Of all the stress management ideas discussed in this chapter, none is more important than this one. *Drawing closure* on an emotional level means that you bring your cases to an end. No nagging questions remain; no "what ifs" or "if onlys" invade your thoughts. You have let go of your cases, released them completely. When cases are fully closed, you realize that your best efforts were put forth, and you are able to turn your energies to new patients and clients.

Case closure occurs when you send condolence cards to clients or follow-up with them by phone. It takes place when you check out assumptions and seek answers to remaining questions about your clients' satisfaction with your services. It also occurs on a medical level as you track down necessary medical information to better understand your patients' illnesses or deaths. Closure can be drawn to cases in three ways: creating purposeful endings, debriefing, and consultation and supervision. Let us look at each.

Creating Purposeful Endings. Purposeful endings are ceremonies or rituals, intentionally created by you, that signal that a case, a life, a day, or a year has been brought to a close. Purposeful endings are vehicles for celebrating successes, honoring efforts, grieving losses, and saying thank you. They take form as thoughts, actions, or events.

Purposeful endings can be created in thousands of ways. You have probably already created some of your own. When you pet and say goodbye to the animals whom you euthanize, for example, or when you make a donation to an animal-oriented organization in memory of a special pet, you are participating in a purposeful ending. The only guidelines for creating a purposeful ending are that it be meaningful to you, respectful of the other coparticipants in the process, and realistic in terms of time and resources.

For example, at the end of the day, a purposeful ending helps you to let go of the concentration and focus that are necessary to do your work. It helps you shift your energy from work to your personal life. One veterinary professional told us that she spends a few minutes at the end of each day tidying-up her desk and returning materials to the filing cabinet. For her, the sound of the cabinet drawer closing with a "click" signifies the end of her work day and the transition into her personal life. Others use the time between leaving work and arriving home to detach from stress. Rather than reviewing the events of the day and planning the next one, they listen to soothing music or consciously observe the nature scenes around them. They have intentionally created a "decompression routine." Here are some examples of purposeful endings in terms of patient euthanasia:

- Say your own goodbye (simply or elaborately).
- Write a poem or verse to be said privately to and for the animals you euthanize.
- Perform an act of kindness for the animal before euthanasia (for example, students walk and feed treats to the junior surgery dogs the evening before surgery and euthanasia).

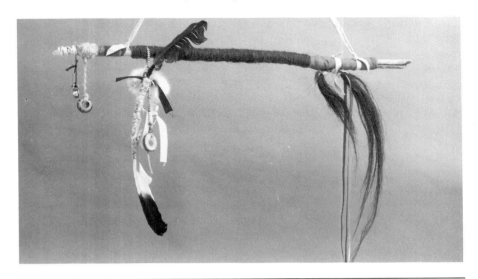

Figure 11-8 During staff debriefings, it is often helpful to use a prop to encourage people to speak. When the prop is passed to someone, that person is asked to speak. Anything can serve as debriefing prop; for example, beach balls or small bean bags work well. In CSU's junior elective on pet loss and client grief, a replica of a Native American talking stick serves as a debriefing prop. According to Indian legend, the person holding the talking stick has the floor and should not be interrupted when speaking. In class, then, the stick is passed from one class member to another as each student takes time to share his or her impressions and experiences from the week. This talking stick is dedicated to animals and is symbolically decorated with feathers, cat hair, dog fur, rabbit fur, and horse hair. It also contains pieces of coral to represent marine life and African beads to represent animals in the wild.

- Write about the events of the day in a journal.
- Meet with staff to discuss what you did well and what you should improve (Fig. 11-8).
- Plan a memorial ceremony for all the animals that died throughout the year, invite your clients.
- Sponsor a yearly "Blessing of the Animals" day with the support of religious leaders in the community (Fig. 11-9).

Because endings occur individually and in groups, involve your staff when brainstorming ideas for letting go. Everyone should have permission to draw closure in a way that is meaningful to them.

Debriefing. As discussed in Chapter 10, debriefing occurs when you talk openly with your staff about the emotional aspects of your cases. It involves discussing new or challenging events in your lives, sharing thoughts and feelings, and getting feedback and support for your actions. Debriefing takes place as successes and "failures" are shared in non-judgmental environments. In addition to the definition given in Chapter 10, debriefing can also be defined as *questioning or instructing an agent or employee at the end of a mission or period of service.* It is not a form of "deprogramming," and should not be used to force people to think in new ways.

Evaluating cases by debriefing allows you to acknowledge what was (and what was not) done well. It encourages your veterinary staff to discuss frustrations in not being able to cure or save particular animals. Debriefing can also be used to evaluate those demands which are self-imposed compared with those that are required and, thus, to modify behaviors in the future.

In a good debriefing session, whether one-on-one or in a group, the basic communication skills that are used with clients are used among staff members. Participants listen to and acknowledge the feelings of the speaker(s) without judgment. Open-ended questions are asked to help each staff member thoroughly understand the problem. Some examples are:

"How are you feeling?"

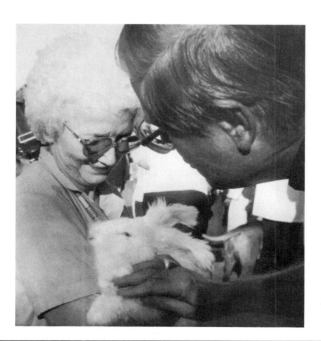

Figure 11-9 During a ceremony at the annual Delta Society Conference, ministers, priests, and rabbis bestow their blessings on the animals.
PHOTOGRAPH COURTESY OF THE DELTA SOCIETY.

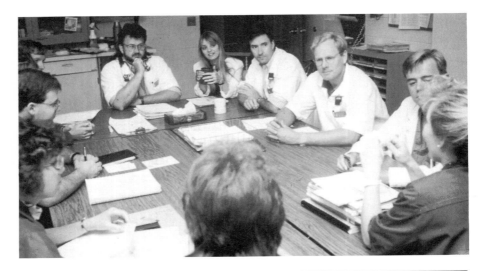

Figure 11-10 Routine staff debriefings that encourage discussion of emotions are extremely helpful. They combat feelings of sadness and frustration associated with patient and client care.

"Is there anything about the case that is bothering you?"

"What do you want to do about it?"

"How do other members of the staff handle that?"

"Is there anything more anyone would like to say?"

Other keys to debriefing are:

- Do not wait until the problem is overwhelming.
- Find a nonjudgmental listener.
- Meet in an environment that is conducive to the discussion of feelings.
- As the helpee, clarify your needs.
- As the helper, clarify what you can do to help.
- Set time limits for the discussion before starting.
- Have sessions as frequently as possible to prevent stress build-up.

As a veterinary professional, if you are to handle the stress associated with caregiving in a bond-centered practice, you need this time to process information, to share memories, and to express personal feelings about your patients' illnesses and deaths. Experts tell us that this is essential for avoiding burn-out. Soares says:

Veterinarians should meet deliberately to talk about having more satisfaction in their work. It's really important that veterinarians share with each other solutions they found and how they're feeling.[36] (p. 755) (Fig. 11-10)

Consultation or Supervision. At times, when dealing with particularly difficult cases, you may seek support or advice from other professionals outside your clinic. When you do, you are using consultation or supervision to bring closure to a case. Objective opinions are often needed if you have become negatively invested in cases. Discussions with other veterinarians or with members of the human service profession may normalize experiences and can help you to resolve conflicts about troubling cases. It may also help you set realistic limits in the future. When selecting someone with whom to consult or debrief, do so with care. A nonjudgmental listener will provide support, validate feelings, and do so without giving advice or raising questions about your competency.

CONCLUSION

Because we live in a society that rewards us for "overwork," it is difficult to create, and stick with, a stress management plan. If you make a commitment to establish a bond-centered practice, however, it is essential that you also commit to caring for yourself. It is also essential that you allow and encourage your staff to do the same. A rich and replenishing personal life will help you to keep this in perspective. We leave you with the words of renowned grief educator and psychiatrist Elisabeth Kubler-Ross: "After working with thousands of individuals who were dying, not one ever said, 'I wish I would have worked more.'"[37]

REFERENCES

1. Herzog, G., and Masback, C.: The 15 Minute Executive Stress-Relief Program. New York, Putnam Publishing, 1992.
2. Lazarus, R.S., and Folkman, S.: Stress, Appraisal, and Coping. New York, Springer Publishing Company, 1984.
3. Seyle, H.: Stress Without Distress. Philadelphia, J.B. Lippincott, 1974.
4. Edelwich, J.: Burn-out. New York, Human Services Press, 1980.
5. Elkins, A.D., and Elkins, J.R.: Professional burnout among U.S. veterinarians: How serious a problem? Vet. Med., *82*:1245–1250, 1987.
6. Graham, S.B.: When babies die: Death and the education of obstetrical residents. Med. Teacher., *13*:171–175, 1991.
7. Zuziak, P.: Stress and Burnout in the Profession, Part 1. J. Am. Vet. Med. Assoc., *198*:521–524, 1991.
8. Crowell-Davis, S.L., Crowe, D.S., and Levine, D.L.: Death and euthanasia: Attitudes of students and faculty at a veterinary teaching hospital. *In* Kay, W.J., Cohen, S.P., Fudin,

C.E., Kutscher, A.H., Nieburg, H.A., Grey, R.E., and Osman, M.M., eds.: Euthanasia of the Companion Animal: The Impact on Pet Owners, Veterinarians, and Society. Philadelphia, The Charles Press, 1988, pp. 199–207.

9. Hart, L.A., Hart, B.L., and Mader, B.: Humane euthanasia and companion animal death: Caring for the animal, the client, and the veterinarian. J. Am. Vet. Med. Assoc., *197*:1292–1299, 1990.

10. Swanson, T.R., and Swanson, M.J.: Acute uncertainty: The intensive care unit. *In* Pattison, E.M., ed.: The Experience of Dying. Englewood Cliffs, N.J., Prentice Hall, 1977, pp. 245–251.

11. Cook, A.S., and Oltjenbruns, K.: Dying and Grieving: Lifespan and Family Perspectives. New York, Holt, Rhinehart, and Winston, 1989.

12. Fulton, R.: Anticipatory grief, stress, and the surrogate griever. *In* Tache, J., Selye, H., and Day, S., eds.: Cancer, Stress, and Death. New York, Plenum Press, 1979, pp. 87–93.

13. Vachon, M.L.S.: Staff stress in the case of the terminally ill. Quality Rev. Bull., May:13–17, 1979.

14. Lazare, A.: Outpatient Psychiatry: Diagnosis and Treatment. Baltimore, Williams and Wilkins, 1979.

15. Wolfelt, A.D.: Exploring the topic of codependency in bereavement caregiving. Kirkland, Washington, Association of Death Education and Counseling, Forum Newsletter, *15*:7–8, 1991.

16. Cermack, T.: A Time to Heal. Los Angeles, St. Martin Press, 1988.

17. Whitfield, C. L.: Co-Dependence: Healing the Human Condition: The New Paradigm for Helping Professionals and People in Recovery. Deerfield Beach, Fl., Health Communications, 1991.

18. Wegscheider-Cruse, S.: The Miracle of Recovery. Deerfield Beach, Fl., Health Communications, 1989.

19. Soares, C., and Mader, B.: Home Away From Home: Emerging From Co-Dependency in the Caring Professions." Portland, Delta Society pre-conference workshop, October 9, 1991.

20. Bradshaw, J.: Homecoming. New York, Bantam Books, 1990.

21. Woititz, J.G.: Home Away from Home: The Art of Self Sabotage. Pompano Beach, Fl., Health Communications, 1987.

22. Beattie, M.: Co-dependent No More. New York, Harper-Hazeldon, 1987.

23. Cook, A.S., and Dworkin, D.S.: Helping the Bereaved: Therapeutic Interventions for Children, Adolescents, and Adults. New York, Basic Books, 1992.

24. Malenik,D., Hoyt, M.F., and Patterson, V.: Adults' reactions to the death of a parent: A preliminary study. Am. J. Psychiatry, *136*:1152–1156, 1979.

25. Benoliel, J.Q.: Loss and adaptation: Circumstances, contingencies, and consequences. Death Studies, *9*:217–233, 1985.

26. Lief, H.O., and Fox, D.C.: Training for detached concern in medical students. *In* Lief, H.I., Lief, V.I., and Lief, N.R., eds.: The Psychological Basis for Medical Practice. New York, Harper and Row, 1963, pp. 12–35.

27. Fry, W.F. Jr.: Humor, physiology, and the aging process. *In* Nahemow, L., McCluskey-Fawcett, K.A., and McGhee, P.E., eds.: Humor and Aging. New York, Academic Press, 1986, pp. 81–98.

28. Kushner, M.: The Light Touch. New York, Simon and Schuster, 1990.

29. Twidale, H.: Nowadays, being 'Old Sourpuss' is no joke. Working Woman, March 1986, p. 18.

30. San Jose Mercury News, July 30, 1986, p. 14E.

31. Davis, A.: Let's Eat Right to Keep Fit. New York, New American Library, 1970.

32. Working Mother, November 1992, p. 20.

33. Ulrich, R.S., Simons, R.F., Losito, B.D., Fiorito, E., Miles, M.A., and Zelson, M.: Stress

recovery during exposure to natural and urban environments. J. Environment. Psychol., *11*:201–230, 1991.

34. Ulrich, R.S.: View through a window may influence recovery from surgery. Science, *224*:420–421, 1984.

35. Ulrich, R.S.: Human responses to vegetation and landscapes. Landscape and Urban Planning, *13*:29–44, 1986.

36. Zuziak, P.: Stress and Burnout in the Profession, Part 2. J. Am. Vet. Med. Assoc., *198*:753–756, 1991.

37. Kubler-Ross, E.: Comment from the keynote address during Colorado State University's three-week symposium entitled Death: Another Stage of Growth. Fort Collins, Co., Fall, 1980.

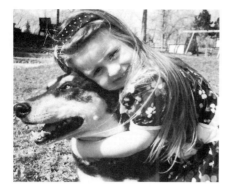

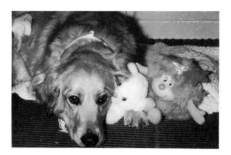

IV

Practice Issues

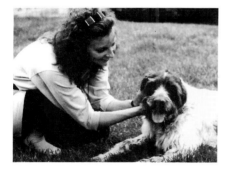

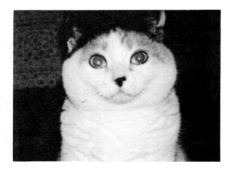

12

Helping a Variety of People

Pet owners represent a wide cross-section of people. They are male, female, young, old, and include those who are physically impaired or disabled. Pet owners come from all walks of life, all races, all cultures, and all socioeconomic groups. All pet owners have some needs in common; however, some have needs that are unique to their age, gender, or physical condition.

In a bond-centered practice, it is important to promote and acknowledge the human-animal bond with all of your clients. Five specific groups of pet owners are discussed in this chapter: men, women, older clients, clients who are disabled, and children. In this chapter, special emphasis is given to helping children because they are one of the most vulnerable populations you serve during pet loss.

MEN, WOMEN, AND GRIEF

You learned in Chapter 2 that grief is experienced differently by each person. Differences in grief experiences are often particularly pronounced between men and women. Many of these differences are societally and culturally based. Individual personalities and circumstances also affect people's grief responses.

The difference in the ways in which men and women grieve is called discrepant grieving (Fig. 12-1). Sometimes, the outward signs of discrepant grief seem to follow classic stereotypes. For example, it seems that women need closer relationships with significant others during grief and that men

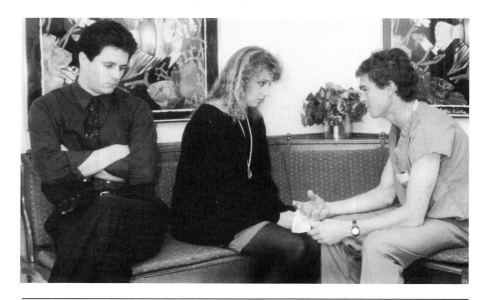

Figure 12-1 Men and women often exhibit different responses to loss.

prefer solitude. Continuing with the stereotypes, during grief, men seem to try to ignore their feelings by keeping busy and working long hours, whereas women often are unable to do anything *but* grieve. These differences can result in strained male-female relationships, especially when couples do not understand each others' needs or erroneously interpret their partners' behaviors. For example, men may view womens' needs for support and companionship as smothering, and women may view mens' needs to be alone or to stay busy as rejection.

Discrepant grieving may produce conflicts, hurt feelings, and differences in opinion regarding treatment options and choices surrounding euthanasia. You can be helpful in these situations by fulfilling the roles of educator and facilitator. When you recognize cases of discrepant grieving, you can make some simple statements that may ease tensions between your male and female clients. For example:

> Jane and Bob Smith's dog, Honey, has cancer, and it has become obvious that the time to euthanize Honey is near. She is not eating or interested in playing ball, which is her favorite thing in life. Jane has asked you about being with Honey when she dies, but Bob does not want to be there himself and thinks that Jane would be better off if she didn't witness Honey's death either. As he puts it, "It's time to get on with our

lives." They disagree on this issue and have asked for your advice.

You tell Jane and Bob that you respect each of their choices. You know that, because they both love Honey, each will have to grieve her death in his or her own way. Just as Bob is allowed to choose not to be present, Jane also needs to make her own choice. For Jane, that means being with Honey during euthanasia. You tell both Jane and Bob that, although they are making different choices, that does not mean that either choice is wrong. Although he does not want to be present during the procedure, you acknowledge that you know that Bob loves Honey too. You also gently remind him that it is okay to cry and to mourn someone we love, even when it feels uncomfortable to do so.

Remember that "taking sides" or supporting one way of grieving over another is not helpful. It is important to reassure both men and women that, although their reactions to loss may be different, neither is inappropriate. Your own biases, depending on your gender, may influence how comfortable you feel with the expression of grief. Make sure that you have created an atmosphere in which both men and women feel comfortable expressing their feelings.

To begin this discussion of men, women, and grief, we reiterate that these descriptions are generalities. Of course, some men express grief in ways that are more traditionally feminine and some women express grief in ways that are more traditionally masculine. Ultimately, regardless of the differences in men's and women's responses to loss, no current evidence suggests that overall adjustment to bereavement varies significantly based on gender.[1] Further research in this area is needed.

Men and Grief

Our culture's expectations of appropriate male behavior often conflict with the behaviors and feelings that are part of grief. For example, men are often expected and conditioned to be in control, to be rational, to be confident, and to be strong. Men are also expected to refrain from crying, from being afraid, from asking for help, and from being indecisive. These expectations provide the basis for the stereotypical male who, when faced with crisis or loss, is supposed to be unemotional, to know what to do, to be supportive and strong for the rest of his family, and to be in control of himself and of the situation.

Carol Staudacher, author of the book *Men and Grief*, has worked for years with grieving men and women.[2] She believes that societal expectations and conditioning have had a profound effect on the way in which men work through their losses. Although society is changing, and some men today are openly talking about and displaying various manifestations of grief, most still are not. Staudacher identifies five of the more common coping styles men use when they are not openly talking about and displaying their grief. They include:

1. Remaining silent.
2. Engaging in solitary mourning or "secret" grief.
3. Taking physical or legal action.
4. Becoming immersed in activities.
5. Exhibiting addictive behaviors.

Staudacher reports that many of the behaviors exhibited by grieving men stem from their desire to exert control. They want to control the expression of their emotions, and they want to control what is occurring around them. She says that when men use these types of behaviors to handle grief, it makes it more difficult for them to fully resolve their losses. Grief must be expressed and released to be resolved. Most of the time, grieving requires identifying and releasing emotions, talking and sharing thoughts, and accepting help and support from others.

How You Can Help Male Clients

You can help men who are experiencing grief by simply understanding the coping styles that they use and by acknowledging that these coping styles may have ramifications for you and your staff. For example, men who remain silent or engage in solitary or "secret mourning," may reject your offers of support or may abruptly cut off conversations that could elicit emotion. They may also become angry with you if they perceive that you have pushed them toward those very uncomfortable feelings. Mens' fears of showing emotion may also prompt them to act in ways that may seem out of character or inappropriate for the situation. For example, some may go out of town on business trips during crucial euthanasia decision-making times, or others may ask friends or family members to drop their pets off at your office for euthanasia. Both of these examples probably occur because, for some men, the fear of crying in public overrides their sense of compassion and responsibility for their pets. Men who feel awkward when addressing death may look to you for guidance when dealing with grief. For example, they may need your permission to clip fur from their dog's tail, to save a horseshoe, or to tell their pets goodbye. They may be too embarrassed to ask for these items and opportunities themselves. Self-disclosure about your own struggles with pet loss is one way to normalize your male clients' feelings.

Men who take physical or legal action to manage their grief may threaten to hurt or sue you. Most of the time, they are mad at their situations, not at you. Knowing that these actions are the only ways that they know to express their grief may help you to remain detached from their anger and may help you refrain from reacting defensively.

Some men cope with loss by becoming intoxicated. Alcohol or drugs are frequently used to numb the pain of loss for short periods. Being drunk or high gives men an excuse to become emotional. Intoxicated clients may show up at your practice for euthanasias or return after their pets' deaths have occurred. In such cases, you should inform clients that you are aware that they are under the influence of drugs or alcohol and that they will need to wait until they are sober or straight to proceed. If possible, call your clients' friends or family members so that they can offer support in this process. For safety and for legal reasons, try to discourage them from driving. If clients are in a belligerent state, call the police.

Finally, the key to helping men lies in avoiding assumptions about their lack of feelings. Send condolence cards, even if your male clients do not *appear* to be upset. Also, we have noticed that women typically get hugs from their veterinarians, whereas men get hand-shakes. Our clinical experience shows that even the most stoic men are responsive to hugs or to sensitive pats on their shoulders, especially during crises. Offer to comfort them in some appropriate way, even if they appear to be doing "just fine."

Women and Grief

Women generally define themselves within the context of responsible, caring relationships.[3] They are socialized to be empathic and maternal and to act as caretakers for others. They are typically nurturers, fulfilling this role at work and at home and attending to the basic needs of their loved ones. Womens' lives are often intertwined with the lives of their companion animals, given that women are routinely the principal caregivers for companion animals. Thus, when pets die, women feel not only the primary, immediate loss of their dear companions, but also the secondary losses of daily routines and rituals.

Societal expectations of women are often the exact opposite of those imposed on men. Women are expected to talk, to be emotional, and to depend on and need help from others. These expectations make it easier for women to express their grief and, by doing so, to partially resolve their losses. Thus, strong displays of grief such as shock, tearful outbursts, wailing, and even fainting are manifestations of grief more commonly exhibited by women than by men. Ironically, however, because of their expressiveness, women are often labeled as "too sentimental," "overly sensitive," "hysterical," or "out of it."

How You Can Help Female Clients

Regardless of the type of loss, most women appreciate the opportunity to sort out the details with a listener who is comfortable with the expression of strong emotions. Women often need to discuss their losses repeatedly, and the sooner the better. For this reason, most people who talk to therapists or attend support groups are women. To help women during times of loss, you can give them the names of several grief professionals with whom they can talk. You can also keep a list of pet owners who have experienced pet loss and who are willing and available to listen and to provide peer support.

Women are often faced with the fact that people want them to finish grieving and to "feel better" before they are able to do so. Well-meaning friends and family members may encourage them to "get on with life" by giving them new pets. You can help your female clients by reminding them that they may need more than a few weeks or months to get through grief and that, in fact, a year or more may be needed.

Some studies have shown that women are more likely than men to somaticize their grief.[4,5] Because most clients and most support staffs are women, it is even more essential for you to learn to understand, respond, and encourage the openly emotional grief styles of women.

Older Clients and Grief

A growing body of research documents the positive effects that companion animals can have on the physical and emotional well-being of older persons (Fig. 12-2).[6,7] One study showed, for example, that elderly owners who are strongly attached to their pets have better emotional health compared with elderly people who do not own pets.[8] In other studies, pet ownership has been shown to correlate positively with survival after discharge from a coronary unit[9] and with lower levels of accepted risk factors for cardiovascular disease.[10] Research into the relationships between pets and the elderly has been so persuasive that laws are beginning to change nationally to allow elderly pet owners to keep pets in retirement centers and nursing homes. It would seem logical that, if pets provide significant health benefits for older people, the deaths of their pets could also affect their health.

The longer people live, the more losses they experience. Loss is an inevitable part of life. Persons in their 60s, 70s, and older have probably experienced the deaths of many of the people who have been most important to them. For example, by this time, their parents and many close friends have probably died. Spouses may also be dead or be in failing health, and some may have even grieved the deaths of their children or siblings. These significant deaths can trigger realizations of one's own mortality.

For older pet owners, companion animals are often symbolically linked with deceased loved ones. Perhaps the dog who is now dying was an

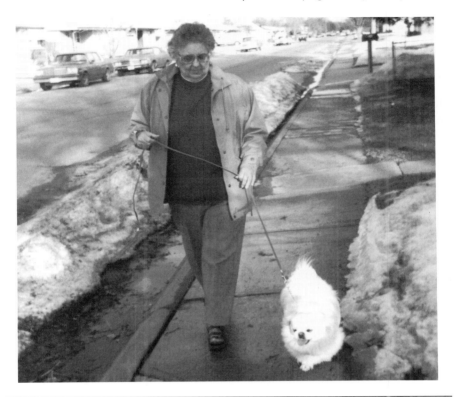

Figure 12-2 Older persons, particularly those who live alone, are often highly attached to their companion animals and share many daily activities with them.

anniversary present from a now deceased spouse, or the elderly cat may have originally belonged to a deceased sibling. It is likely that most people have not fully grieved all their losses. Thus, when older persons are faced with the deaths of companion animals, some unresolved grief will probably be triggered, along with possible fears and anxieties about their own deaths.

As people age, losses other than death also occur. For example, physical strength and stamina decline, making older people incapable of undertaking all the activities that they did when they were younger. Memory losses due to aging or Alzheimer's disease can also occur. Necessary medications may produce mental confusion and can reduce the ability to process information quickly. Retirement may bring a change in standard of living and a loss of daily routines. Therefore, older persons living on fixed incomes may not be able to afford complicated treatments for their pets and may be forced to make life and death decisions based on finances. Because of these factors, older persons may need extra support, care, and understanding when their pets are ill or dying.

How You Can Help Older Clients

Demographers project that, as the "baby boom" generation ages, 13 percent of the population will be over 65 years of age by the year 2000 and that 21 percent will be 65 or older by the year 2030.[11] You can expect an increasing number of your clients to be in this age group. Dealing with older people sometimes forces us to slow down too. It may be necessary to repeat information to someone who is hearing-impaired or who needs some extra time to comprehend what is being said. It may also be helpful for you to write down information or instructions because elderly people may not be able to remember detailed information after they leave your clinic. Older persons who live alone may want to call a sibling or child to help them make a decision about their pets' care.

Another concern about older people is that they may have lost most of their support network. To help them "fill in the gaps," you can keep a reference list of community resources available to senior citizens. Such resources could include transportation services or drug and pet stores that may offer senior discounts. You may also want to consider offering such discounts at your clinic.

If you do a great deal of work with older clients, you will find that it is common for them to reminisce about the past. They may tell you about other pets or family members who have died. These memories may be triggered by discussions about the pet who is now ill or dying. Discussions of death may also elicit comments about their own health or acknowledgment that their own lives are drawing to a close. Do not trivialize the importance of these feelings. Responses such as "Oh, Ruth, you'll live forever" are not helpful. Discussing the possibility of a pet's death may provide an older person with an important, but rare, opportunity to have an honest conversation with someone about how *they* feel about dying.

In conclusion, we provide a few final notes about working with elderly clients. First, because of generational differences, elderly pet owners may have more discomfort with the open expression of emotion than do younger clients. Second, elderly owners may have had, over the years, numerous experiences with pet death, euthanasia, and viewing bodies. Those situations may have been poorly handled, leaving elderly owners skeptical about grief support. In these cases, their current decisions may be based on outdated historical information that you may or may not be able to change with education. Third, many older pet owners function at levels that are more commonly associated with younger people. Remember to respect the years of learning that elderly people have. Each is an individual with his or her own level of education, life experience, and mental and physical competency. Do not assume that your older clients need special consideration until you have asked them directly or observed a decline in their functioning for yourself.

People with Disabilities and Grief

Treating companion animals who are also service animals for people who are visually or hearing-impaired and for those who are physically disabled involves some special considerations. Not only do service animals provide companionship, they are also relied on to provide their owners with a level of independence and functioning that would be difficult to achieve by other means (Fig. 12-3). Because of the work that these animals do, they may come to be viewed by their owners as true extensions of themselves. Thus, the death of a service animal may result in a loss of self-confidence and self-esteem for people who are impaired or disabled. In addition, if

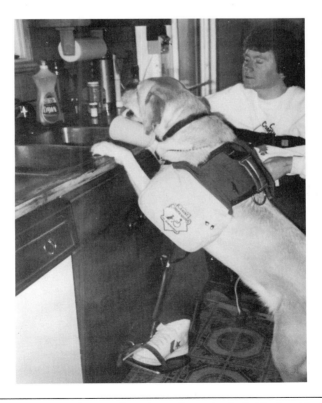

Figure 12-3 Service animals provide independence for individuals with disabilities.
PHOTOGRAPH COURTESY OF DALE COSKI.

service animals in failing health have to be retired before their deaths, owners may feel that they contributed to their animals' deaths by not allowing them to work.

When companion animals die, able-bodied owners can wait until they are emotionally ready before they adopt other pets. Owners of service animals may not have that option. To remain independent and undertake usual activities, they may have to obtain another animal immediately, thus possibly exacerbating the normal feelings of guilt and betrayal that accompany losing one companion animal and adopting another. Thus, owners may have difficult times immediately bonding with new animals. Such difficulties may, in turn, affect the degree to which the service animal and person are able to work as a team.

Children who are disabled are likely to form close bonds with their companion animals as a result of the loneliness imposed on them by restricted interactions with the rest of society. For children who are disabled, the role a service animal plays as friend and confidant may be greatly

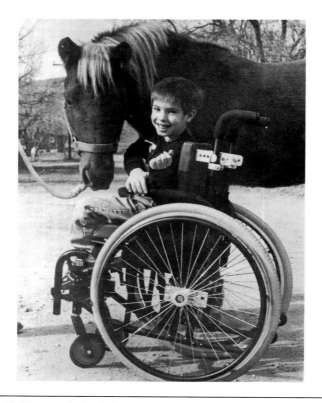

Figure 12-4 Children with disabilities appreciate the "unconditional acceptance" given by animals.

magnified (Fig. 12-4). For some, their service animal may be their *only* friend. If the animal has acted as a communication catalyst and has helped instigate conversations with others, the loss of the animal may make these children feel even more withdrawn, discouraged, or shy.

How You Can Help Clients Who Are Disabled

First, be sure that your veterinary facility is accessible to disabled persons. This accessibility should include the entrance to your clinic as well as the examination rooms, restrooms, and other client areas. Also, many people with disabilities live on limited incomes because they are unemployed or underemployed. Thus, you might consider instituting a reduced-fee policy for diagnostic tests, medications, and treatments on assistance animals.

When making treatment decisions about service animals, the way in which a particular drug, surgery, or other procedure will affect the animal's ability to work will need consideration. For instance, a service dog's condition may be treatable, but the treatment may not allow the dog to continue functioning as a service animal. Also, when treatment fails and euthanasia is imminent, people with disabilities may be sensitive to discussions involving quality-of-life issues. It is important to avoid giving the impression that lives with physical impairments are not worth living.

A few simple communication techniques will help you to feel more comfortable with and be more sensitive to the needs of service animal owners. These suggestions were made by staff members at the Kansas Specialty Dog Service:

- When talking to a person with a disability, speak directly to that person rather than to a helper or an interpreter.
- Do not assume that a person with a disability needs assistance in moving around. You can offer assistance, then give the person the opportunity to accept or decline the offer.
- If assistance is desired, either ask or wait to be instructed as to how you can help.
- Do not talk to people with disabilities as though they were children, and do not talk about them as though they were not in the room.
- Do not be embarrassed about using everyday language which inadvertently relates to a person's disability. Examples are "See you later," "Did you hear about . . . ," or "I've got to run."

Physically Disabled Clients

If you are not sure how to create the best environment when euthanizing service animals, ask their owners. We worked with a pet owner who was quadraplegic. She brought her German Shepherd's bean bag chair in for the euthanasia. The veterinarian lowered the examination table, and the client used the chair as a soft bridge between the table and the arm of her wheelchair. During the procedure, the dog and her owner were able to be close to one another without physical discomfort for either. Here are some other ideas:

- It is easier to establish communication on an equal basis if you place yourself at eye level with a person on crutches or in a wheelchair. To a person in a wheelchair, however, the chair is an extension of themselves. Therefore, it is inappropriate to lean or hang on it.
- People in wheelchairs will not be able to see what is happening to their dog on an examination table that is higher than they are. Lower the table if possible. A client-present euthanasia may best be conducted on the floor so that the owner can hold and comfort the animal.

Hearing-Impaired Clients

A good resource for pet owners who are hearing-impaired and grieving is the University of California, Davis' Pet Loss Support Hotline. Student volunteers not only help nondisabled pet owners, they also listen and give support to pet owners who are hearing-impaired through the use of a Telecommunications Device for the Deaf (TDD).[12] By dialing the phone and typing in messages on a keyboard, the person who is hearing- (or speech-) impaired can communicate with another TDD user directly or with a hearing person using a relay system. The device allows callers to have private, one-on-one conversations with helpers about the many feelings of loss that they are experiencing. For more information about the Pet Loss Support Hotline, see the Resource Appendix. Here are some other ideas:

- To get the attention of a person who is hearing-impaired, tap the person on the shoulder or wave your hand.
- When speaking, look directly at the person and speak clearly. Write down items of importance such as the diagnosis, treatment plan, cost estimate, and next appointment date. Then, you can be sure that you and your client have the same information.
- If a person who is hearing-impaired lip reads, keep your hands and other objects away from your face when speaking, and try to stand facing the light so that your face is more easily visible.
- When doing a client-present euthanasia, you might want to designate a touch on the arm or other signal to indicate

when you will begin injecting the drugs. This approach allows the person to look at and focus on the dog without having to watch you.

Visually Impaired Clients

When working with guide dogs belonging to people who are blind, remember that owners cannot know what you are doing to the dog unless you tell them. Describe your actions, and the dog's response, in detail. You might say, "I am going to lift your dog up on the table, which is located 2 feet to your right. I'm holding your dog now and he's licking my face." Here are other ideas:

- As you enter a room to see a client who is blind, be sure to identify yourself and anyone who is with you.
- When you talk to clients who are blind, use your normal speaking voice. Most people who are visually impaired are not hearing-impaired or mentally compromised.
- If clients need to give guide dogs injections at home, syringes can be notched to indicate the level of medication needed. If more than one medication is prescribed and if medications come in similar containers, rubber bands can be used to differentiate them.
- If you are conducting a client-present euthanasia, be sure to verbally describe each step (for example, when you are injecting the drug and how the animal has reacted).

As a final courtesy, be flexible when scheduling appointments for clients who are disabled. Many cannot drive and therefore rely on public transportation or rides from friends to get to a veterinary clinic. They may therefore not be able to meet a rigid time schedule.

CHILDREN AND COMPANION ANIMALS

Pet owners may also be children. In fact, research has shown that pet ownership is higher in families with children than in those without them.[13] Although children probably cannot be considered legal owners of animals, many have unique and significant relationships with their pets. Thus, when companion animals die, children—like pet owners of all ages—have individual needs and expectations of you. Some of those individual needs and expectations warrant specific discussion.

Veterinarians have told us that one of the more awkward situations they face in practice is deciding how children should be involved in the deaths of their pets. The wishes of practitioners and parents alike range from completely excluding children from death experiences (even to the point of lying to them about what has happened to their animals), to wanting them to be as involved in the process as possible, including being present during euthanasia. Both veterinarians and parents most often want to do what is best for children, although their own fears and anxieties sometimes interfere. However, unless all the adults involved understand the relationships between children, the human-animal bond, pet loss, and grief, none can do their best. In this chapter, therefore, we provide you with information that you can use when helping children and parents with pet loss.

The Relationships between Children and Companion Animals

A widely held belief in our society is that children and pets are made for each other (Fig. 12-5). Adults often say that they adopt pets for the kids. Within the last decade, researchers studying the human-animal bond have tried to understand more clearly the importance of and the problems related to children's relationships with their pets. First, it has been learned

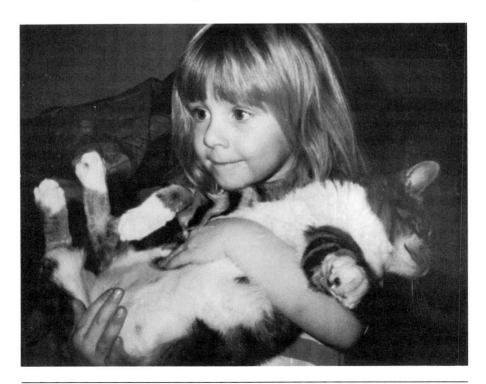

Figure 12-5 A child and her kitty.

that simply having pets in their homes does not guarantee that children will bond to them or that they will benefit from their presence.[14,15] Rather, the more important factors are the quality and intensity of children's attachments to their pets. Many variables affect the attachments that form between children and companion animals. These factors include the amount of time spent with pets, the knowledge that children have of their pets' characteristics and needs, and the roles that animals play in children's lives. Let us examine each of these variables more closely.

Time Spent with Pets

The desire to be close to or to maintain proximity with an attachment figure is a measure of attachment often used to measure the strength of the human-animal bond.[16] It is also used with animals and children.[17] Therefore, children who spend much of their leisure time with their animals may be more attached to them. For example, children who are often home alone before or after school or on weekends with only their pets for company may become more attached to their pets than do children who have other sources of emotional and social support (Fig. 12-6). Melson[18] found that the average amount of time spent with pets was positively correlated with children's reports of their emotional closeness to the animals.

Interest, Behaviors, and Emotions Directed toward Pets

Another measure of attachment is the degree to which the attachment figure can comfort and calm someone who is stressed.[19] For example, children who are home alone, ill, socially isolated, or in conflict with their parents or siblings or those whose families are in the midst of divorce, moving, or dealing with another family member's serious illness may not receive the support and attention that they need. Instead, they may turn to their pets as a source of comfort. Children who talk to their pets, and who consider them to be "special friends" with whom they can talk when they are upset, can be considered to be more attached to them than are children who do not engage in these behaviors.[20] Thus, children who often kiss, stroke, or caress their pets may be more attached to them than are those who hit them or push them away.

Understanding of Their Pet's Needs

As we said in Chapter 1, attachments to animals are more likely to develop when people know how to communicate with them. Thus, mutual communication between people and animals is more likely to occur when humans are knowledgeable about animals. Children who have primary responsibility for their companion animals and who become familiar with

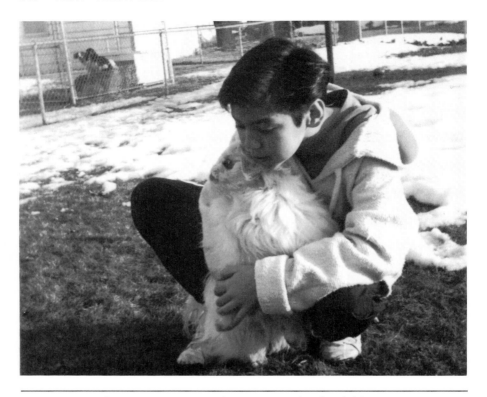

Figure 12-6 Pets provide companionship for children.

their animals' habits, behaviors, and care requirements usually become very attached to them. A good example of attachments formed in this way are the relationships that children who belong to 4-H clubs form with the animals whom they raise (Fig. 12-7). A significant number of clients and veterinarians have told us how painful it was for them or for children they know to sell or put up for slaughter the calves, lambs, or goats whom they had raised and for whom they had cared while participating in 4-H. Some reported that their feelings were either discouraged or ignored.

Recent evidence also indicates that certain types of relationships between pets and children can positively affect cognitive development,[21] perceived competence, empathy,[14] and social adjustment (Fig. 12-8).[22] The effects of such attachments are important because many children today grow up with working, divorced, or single parents and also live far away from extended families. Some children may therefore find it difficult to develop trusting friendships and may rely on their pets for emotional support. They may also receive consistent and unconditional love from

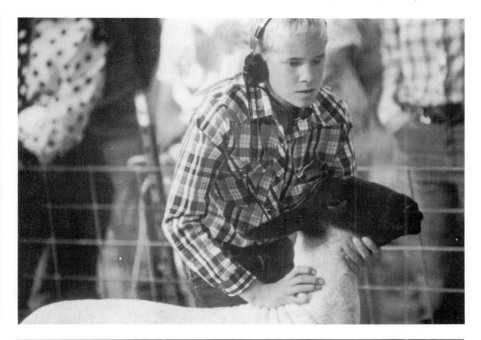

Figure 12-7 Youngsters invest a great deal of time and energy raising farm animals for 4-H competitions. This boy is visually impaired and is instructed by headset during the judging of his sheep.
PHOTOGRAPH COURTESY OF CSU COOPERATIVE EXTENSION.

their pets and be asked by busy parents to be responsible for much of their care. It is not surprising that the deaths of their companion animals are often significant losses for children.

The Impact of Pet Loss on Children

Myths about loss and grief exist in our culture, and we, as a society, abide by these myths. Some of the most damaging myths involve children. For example, many people believe that children are resilient during times of crisis and loss and that they do not grieve with the same intensity as adults. Because of this myth, people also believe that pets' deaths are fairly trivial losses for children.

Societal beliefs dictate societal behaviors. Thus, the experience of childhood pet loss rarely gets the attention that it deserves. No socially sanctioned rituals exist in which children can mourn their pets' deaths. Other people often expect and even demand that children recover rapidly from grief, and quick replacement of pets is usually encouraged and sometimes

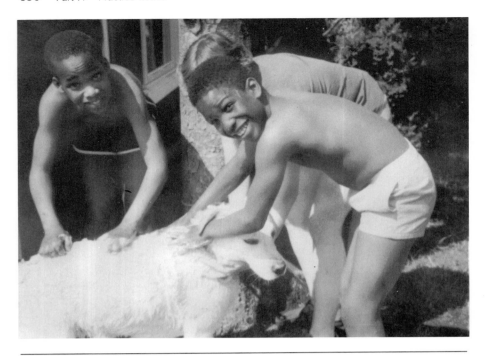

Figure 12-8 Children have success-oriented experiences when interacting with farm, domestic, and wild animals through programs like those offered at Green Chimneys Children's Services in Brewster, New York. Green Chimneys offers residential and nonresidential learning experiences in a rural setting and promotes care and concern for all living things.
PHOTO COURTESY OF GREEN CHIMNEYS.

even forced on them. In addition, children are commonly ignored during medical crises, left out of decision-making processes, and even lied to when the deaths of their pets occur. New information is dispelling these myths, however, and proving that, in reality, they could not be further from the truth.

During the last two decades, researchers have gathered much empiric and clinical evidence to support the idea that pet loss is very significant.[23] From research, experts have also gained a greater understanding of the true effect that pet loss has on children. They have found, for example, that children feel much the same way when pets are given away as they do when pets die because both experiences generate similar kinds of stress and feelings of grief.[24] Stewart's research[25] has shown that parents who do not give children the option of adopting new pets after the deaths of their former pets unwittingly create "unresolved bereavements" for their children. Her study suggests that, in time, another animal's presence may lessen feelings of grief for children.

Child development experts have long advised parents to prepare their children for loss by taking advantage of informal "teachable moments" involving death. At one time, suggested teachable moments included the discovery of lifeless birds or bugs in the yard, delivery of news regarding an elderly neighbor's heart attack, or the death of a family's pet. All these situations were deemed unemotional enough to allow opportunities to talk with children about death under nonthreatening circumstances. The underlying belief was that unemotional conversations about death would arm children with the basic knowledge necessary to help them cope when someone whom they really *did* love died.

Birds and bugs aside, the long-held belief that pet loss serves primarily as a "dress rehearsal" for the "real thing" has now fallen into disfavor. This change in beliefs constitutes a big step in the right direction. We now know that many children genuinely love their pets and that they are deeply affected by their deaths. Pet loss, then, does not present an opportunity for parents and children to have unemotional discussions about death and grief. Rather, it presents an opportunity for adults to ensure that children are informed, educated, included, comforted, and reassured about death so that they gain the confidence necessary to face loss and to recover from it.

Children, Pet Loss, and Parents

Many children are actively involved in their pets' daily health care. It is only fair to give them the option of also being involved in the circumstances surrounding their pets' deaths. (See the reading entitled "A Merciful Farewell" at the end of this chapter.) When companion animals die, however, it is instinctive for adults to want to protect children as much as possible. Thus, it is common for parents and veterinarians to make decisions about medical treatments without first discussing them with the children in the family. It is also common for adults to euthanize pets without creating opportunities for children to be present or at least to view their pets' bodies and to say goodbye.

Some parents lie to their children about what actually happened to their pets. They feel that it is kinder to tell children that their animals ran away or were given a new home rather than to say that their animals died or were euthanized. These tactics are not used maliciously by parents. In fact, quite the opposite is true. In times of crisis, many sensitive parents are simply inadequately prepared to discuss loss, death, and grief with their children. Thus, they deceive themselves into believing that they can spare their children pain by protecting them from painful experiences. This belief, however, is unfounded. It soon becomes evident that children who are shielded from one kind of pain must eventually deal with another. For example, a child who is told that her cat "ran away" must bear the pain of feeling rejected and abandoned by a pet whom she thought of as her best friend.

Even more upsetting than the pain of knowing about death is the pain of not knowing about death. Children are attuned to adults' nonverbal communication. They are experts at interpreting adults' voice tones, facial expressions, nervous gestures, body postures, and changes in eye contact. Even without words, most children know something is dreadfully wrong in a given situation; they just do not know what that "something" is. What they do know is that they are being deliberately excluded from something important.

When children are protected from experiences with death, they are denied opportunities to learn how to master their feelings of loss. When children are shielded from adults' expressions of grief, they are also denied the role models necessary to learn normal, healthy coping behaviors. One distressed parent who contacted us at The Changes Program called to find out "how she could quit crying before her son got home from school." During further questioning, we learned that the family's 13-year-old cat had been euthanized only an hour earlier. This mother was not insensitive. Rather, she was afraid that she would upset and frighten her son by reacting so strongly to her cat's death. The counselor reassured her that her emotional responses were normal and suggested that not reacting to the death of this beloved family member might seem more abnormal and confusing to her child.

During pet loss, parents often turn to veterinarians for information and guidance. They see you as the expert and assume you have much more experience and knowledge about coping with the deaths of pets than they do (Box 12-1). To you, this may feel like a delicate and personal situation that veterinarians should avoid. When it comes to children and pet loss, however, you have opportunities to either perpetuate unhealthy responses to pet loss or to influence positively the ways in which children handle grief in the future.

Children, Pet Loss, and Veterinarians

Some veterinarians regard the children who visit their practices as no more than distractions, interruptions, and potential chaos. Yet, children are important members of any veterinarian's clientele. In fact, some practitioners and veterinary management consultants believe that children actually increase the frequency of visits to veterinarians. A Charles, Charles, and Associates study[26] found that children often alerted parents to illnesses or problems with family pets and motivated parents to seek veterinary care. The findings also indicated that, in many instances, parents took sick or injured animals to veterinarians because they realized that seeing animals suffer had devastating effects on their children.

BOX 12-1

Suggested Resources for Veterinarians and Parents

It is helpful for veterinarians to have educational videotapes and handout materials available for both clients and staff to use. Here are some suggested resources.

The Affection Connection, *Will the Sadness Go Away?* Cooperative Extension Service, Kansas State University, 1991.
   This videotape is appropriate for use by veterinarians, parents, 4-H leaders, teachers, and others who deal with the issue of pet loss. It works in conjunction with the brochure entitled *Children and the Death of a Pet* (publication MF 956). Order copies of both from The Affection Connection, State 4-H Office, Umberger Hall, KSU, Manhattan, KS 66506-3404. The video and resource packet cost $50.00. One hundred copies of the brochure are $45.00.

Guideline Publications, *Death of a Pet: Answers to Questions for Children and Animal Lovers of All Ages.* P.O. Box 245, Stamford, NY 12167. Telephone: 1-800-552-1076.

The American Animal Hospital Association (AAHA). *The Loss of Your Pet, Counseling Clients, and Understanding Pet Loss.* AAHA Education Department, P.O. Box 150899, Denver, CO, 80215–0899.
   AAHA offers this videotape series on pet loss counseling designed for client use and for staff training. It can be ordered for $59.00 (members) and for $85.00 (nonmembers) from AAHA's national headquarters in Denver, Colorado. AAHA's Member Service Center can be reached by calling (800)-252-2242.

Boulden, J.: *Saying Good-bye Activity Book.* Jim Boulden Publications, Santa Rosa, CA, 1989.
   This coloring and activity book encourages children to explore their feelings about death. Copies can be ordered from Jim Boulden, P.O. Box 9358, Santa Rosa, CA 95405. Telephone: (707)-538-3797.

Sibbitt, S.: *Oh, Where Has My Pet Gone?* B. Libby Press, 1991.
   This pet loss memory book is appropriate for ages 3 through 103. This workbook combines the essential tasks of mourning into directed activities in order to provide a framework for healing. Order from B. Libby Press, 1426 Holdridge Circle, Wayzata, MN 55391. The price is $11.95 including shipping costs.

Veterinarians who want to work more effectively with young clients need to learn how to talk with children of different ages and how to assess individual situations (Box 12-2). If the first mistake that veterinarians make is to ignore children altogether, the second mistake is to assume that children are mini-adults, with the same level of cognitive and emotional development as their adult clients. The belief that children think, feel, and

BOX 12-2

Assessing Children's Needs during Pet Loss

Veterinarians can learn to assess which children may need extra support during their pets' deaths. The ways in which children handle pet loss depends on several key factors. These factors include:

- The child's age and level of cognitive and emotional maturity.
- The role that the pet played in the child's life.
- Other events currently taking place in the child's life (parental divorce, recent move, illness, and so forth).
- The role the child played (if any) in the death of the pet.
- The child's personal loss history.
- The child's ability to cope with crisis.
- The circumstances surrounding the pet's death.
- The parent(s)' confidence in assisting children with loss and grief.
- The quality and availability of other means of support.

If veterinarians determine that children are deficient, unskilled, or unsupported in several of these areas, they can assist parents by making appropriate referrals to human service professionals. Human service professionals might include teachers, school counselors, social workers, family therapists, members of the clergy, and counselors or support group facilitators who specialize in pet loss. It is wise to talk to human service professionals before referrals are made. Although human service professionals may be highly qualified and skilled at what they do, they may not be trained to address grief or issues of pet loss.

respond like adults has caused many parents and veterinarians to mishandle childrens' experiences of pet loss.

How Boys and Girls Grieve during Pet Loss

The following is a brief overview of child development, infancy through young adulthood, in terms of childrens' abilities to understand and cope with death and grief. The purpose of this guide is to show that children grieve as deeply as adults but that they express grief differently from adults due to their shorter attention spans and varying levels of cognitive development. These age and stage categories are somewhat arbitrary, and a great deal of overlap exists between them. Some 3-year-olds, for example, have the cognitive and physical abilities of 5-year-olds, whereas some teens are immature and think and behave more like 10-year-olds. Each child is unique, and the information presented in this overview should be used only as a guide.

Children respond to loss based on the knowledge and skills that are available to them at the time of loss. In general, children who have a broad knowledge base about life and death, many and varied copied skills, and strong emotional support from family and friends cope better with death and grief. Such children grieve in more age-appropriate ways. This guide, therefore, is intended to help parents create a foundation of knowledge, skill, and support for children so that each child will feel safe to grieve in his or her own way. You can use this information to educate and assist clients who are also parents.

Infants (Birth through 1 Year of Age)

When pets die, babies feel the escalated levels of stress that arise in families, but they are not aware of the cause of the tension. Infants respond to high stress levels by crying, whining, clinging, withdrawing, or regressing.

One can talk to babies about pet loss, but, obviously, they are not cognitively capable of comprehending death. Babies are best reassured by hugs, cuddling, and special time devoted to them. Family routines should be kept as normal as possible.

Toddlers and Preschoolers (2 through 4 Years of Age)

At this age, children still do not understand that death is permanent and universal. They miss their playmates and may ask many questions (Fig. 12-9). Toddlers and preschoolers are ready and willing to talk about death and are more relaxed and curious about it than any other age group. They have not yet been conditioned to think of death as taboo, nor to think of grief as shameful or embarrassing. Young children may or may not cry about their losses initially and their symptoms of grief will come and go with varying degrees of intensity.

Toddlers and preschoolers may express their confusion, fear, and sadness about death through play, open displays of emotion, or through their developing language skills. They may also express them by "acting out." Acting out is a way that children release feelings of pain, distress, and anxiety when they lack other, more positive vehicles for expression. Acting out behaviors might include hitting, kicking, throwing temper tantrums, or the intentional breaking of known and accepted rules. Toddlers and preschoolers may also display symptoms of separation anxiety, developing clinging behaviors or withdrawing from normal friends and activities. Psychosomatic complaints like stomach aches, sore throats, and chronic fatigue can also signal the presence of grief that has been suppressed. Changes in children's personalities, daily habits, social lives, and behaviors can be signs of grief that need more positive vehicles for expression.

Young children explore death through play. They might draw pictures, bury stuffed animals in their sandboxes, or plan funerals for their dolls.

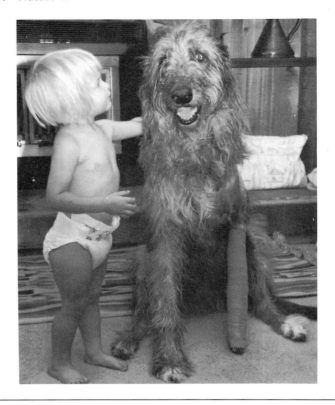

Figure 12-9 Toddlers learn about the human-animal bond through their own pets.

Although these activities may seem alarming and morbid to adults, they are normal, healthy responses for toddlers and preschoolers and should be encouraged. Children deal with new information and current issues through experimentation. Their activities do not, in most cases, require adult intervention.

Early School-Aged Children (5 through 8 Years of Age)

Early school-aged children are less willing to talk about death. They often personify death and think of it as The Grim Reaper, The Dark Angel, or as a monster-like form. Because they imagine death in concrete ways, they also think that they can hide from it or avoid it. This belief can cause early school-aged children to feel angry at someone who dies. They do not understand why their loved one did not just run away or hide when death came to get them.

Death also appears to be within their control because hero figures perform amazing feats to prevent it. Early school-aged children are in the "magical thinking" phase of cognitive development. In this phase, they believe that the world revolves around them and is, for the most part, under their control. They perceive this control as a huge responsibility and may feel that any death of which they become aware may have somehow been their fault. Their beliefs (along with the beliefs of younger children) are further confused by the television programs they watch. On TV, actors are "killed," only to reappear again next week on different programs. Cartoon characters are flattened, get up, and walk again. Death appears to be reversible.

As with younger children, early school-aged children may discuss death in morbid detail with their friends and may create elaborate stories to embellish the experience. For various reasons including peer pressure, busy schedules, and emotional inhibitions, grief may be delayed, with the manifestations and symptoms surfacing weeks and even months after a loss. Children may need to have the facts honestly restated and may need to be reassured that they are not responsible for what happened to their pets.

Generally, around the age of 8 years, early school-aged children realize that death is permanent and universal. This time can be troubling for them as they begin to ponder the mortality of those they love. It is important for these children to have opportunities to talk about their losses and to ask questions about death.

Late School-Aged Children (9 through 12 Years of Age)

Most older school-aged children know that death is irreversible and that it eventually happens to everyone. They are capable of sustaining intense periods of grief and can become preoccupied with a loss, particularly if they have had feelings of abandonment or rejection previously. For older school-age children, grief for a companion animal may be connected to another, equally disturbing death and can trigger memories of that loss.

Like younger children, older school-aged children may ask some shocking questions about death. For example, they may be curious about dismemberment during autopsies or deterioration of bodies after burials (Box 12-3). This is one way in which children cope with anxiety. It is most helpful for parents and veterinarians to give them honest answers and suggestions for active resolutions. Suggestions may include viewing their pets' bodies, helping to dig graves, visiting crematoriums, and participating in goodbye or memorial ceremonies. As with younger children, opportunities for heart-to-heart talks or question-and-answer times are usually appreciated.

BOX 12-3

Lab Coordinator Gives Kids a Friendly Look at Pathology

This story illustrates the "morbid" curiosity of late school-aged children (9–12 year olds). It also demonstrates how helpful it is to take children seriously by providing them with honest information and real-life experiences. (*Note:* The CSU Veterinary Teaching Hospital does not normally open its necropsy lab to the public because of health concerns, but in this case an exception was made.)

On December 10, 1991, we found a dead calico cat across the street from Andrew Colson's house. It was approximately 10 feet away from the street laying on its side. From the outside there was no blood or wounds. One of the eyes was somewhat sucked in, but there weren't any other marks on the cat. We decided to try to find out why the cat died.

Our hypothesis was that it either froze to death because it had been cold outside, or it could have been hit by a car. We brought it to Andrew's house, Mrs. Colson said we could not do any projects until we found the owner. First, we went from house to house asking, "Is this your cat" and we would hold it up. When we couldn't find the owner, Mrs. Colson told us to put up a sign at the entrance to the village. We made a sign that said, FOUND DEAD CAT, but she wouldn't let us put that up either. She said it was insensitive and you have to tell people in a nice way that their pet has died. Well, we never did find the owner so we buried the little cat in the snow by the garage because Mrs. Colson wouldn't put it in a freezer like we wanted.

Next, we started calling veterinarians. The vets said they would not do a necropsy on a dead cat because it would smell. We kept on calling and finally we called the Colorado State Veterinary Teaching Hospital and talked to Dennis Madden, coordinator of the necropsy lab. Mrs. Colson set up a time when we were able to come in.

On February 6, 1992, we got to get out of school and went to Fort Collins for the necropsy. When we get there we met Mr. Madden and went to the back of the school (which is actually an animal hospital were students learn to become veterinarians).

First, Mr. Madden, who was very funny and friendly (we thought he was going to be grouchy and mean) told us what it was like to be a pathologist. He showed us all the forms that he used to fill out. He explained that an autopsy is done on dead people and a necropsy on dead animals. He told us that they do about five to eight necropsies every day. Most were for people who wanted to know why their pet had died. While we were there, a farmer brought in two baby pigs that had died because all his baby pigs were dying. He wanted them to do a necropsy so he could find out what was killing them and give them medicine for it. Also, a ranger brought in a hoof from an elk and wanted to know if the elk had a disease because it would probably mean the whole herd had it.

Next, Mr. Madden prepared us to go in the room by giving us these plastic boots and a plastic apron and gloves to keep us from getting contamination on us and taking it home to our pets. When we walked inside, there were four different tables with a hose connected to clean each one off. We went to one of the four tables. When he started cutting the cat open, Andrew almost threw up, but we hadn't eaten any food all day just in case we might throw up, so nothing came out. He just threw up air. During the necropsy, Andrew had to sit by the trash can the whole time because he kept throwing up air.

Basically, he just went through all the different parts on the cat, but everything was the color of dark red inside the body because the cat was dead for such a long time. Also, the tissues and organs were soft and mushy instead of firm because they were so old.

First, he checked the cat for broken bones, then he skinned it, then he examined it and talked to us about all the different clues and marks he found. He took out all the organs one by one and talked to us about the different body parts. The results are written up in the necropsy report.

When he was finished, he threw all the parts away and rinsed off the table. Then he said, "Do you want to see what a fresh dead animal looks like?" We said, "Yeah!" He went back to a freezer and brought out a big dog and threw it on the table, politely though. Then he cut it open and showed us. All the organs and tissues were all different colors, the way they are supposed to be. You could even see the veins in the dog's heart. The inside organs were white or pink or grey or even blackish blue. In our cat everything had been red inside. Also all the things were firm. The dog had a really big heart because it was a race dog and an athlete. He even showed us the bladder and made the dog pee even though it was dead. We really enjoyed this project and learned a lot from it and are very grateful to Mr. Madden for helping us.

Andrew's Mother Expresses Her Thanks

Dear Dennis (Madden),

I want to thank you so very much for what you did for the boys. They are still talking about it now. It wasn't just walking them through the necropsy, but it was the respect you had for their curiosity, and the integrity with which you treated them like fellow peers in a communal project. Those two guys grew about two feet during their time with you (although the one probably lost a little weight throwing up in the trash can). I also realize how much time you took to really teach them. I know you were busy and yet you didn't let the boys see that. You gave them more than their share of time and all of your focus. You are a real leader, Dennis, and I wonder how many people's lives you have affected and may never even know.

As far as the science fair went, interestingly enough the teacher in charge of accepting projects told Andrew and Danny she thought it was inappropriate and indicated to me that I was raising a Jeffrey Dahmer and refused to accept the project (without having looked at the project). I talked to the boy's teacher who agreed that it was unfair and gave Andrew and Danny the chance to do an hour-long presentation to their own class. The results were fantastic. All the kids asked questions forever (especially about the dog peeing, how bad the cat's smell really was, and how many times Andrew threw up). They were spellbound. Their teacher gave them a "A" and told them it would have won the Science Fair and he wished he had gone to bat for them.

Box continued on following page

The boys still talk about the experience and I, as a mother, am most grateful. If there is ever anything I can do for you or your children I would love to return the favor. I teach children's theater and am a geriatric and child therapist and would be happy to bring those skills in return.

Thanks,
Heidi Colson

Andrew and Danny Say Thanks, Too. . .

Dear Mr. Madden,

I still have the smell of dead, rotten cat in my brain. Thanks so much for your time. We got an A+ for the report. . . . We couldn't have done it without you. Thanks for cutting the dog open.

Sincerally, (sic)
Andrew and Danny

Adolescents (13 through 17 Years of Age)

Adolescents are self-conscious and hyperemotional. Their feelings and thought processes are confusing and often contradictory. Adolescents will want to be treated like adults on one day and like younger children on the next. They will be devastated by their pets' deaths on one day and will say that it is "no big deal" on the next. Because most adolescents feel awkward about their bodies at this time, pets are often the only ones whom they allow to be physically close to them. Therefore, when pets die, many teenagers miss the tactile outlet that companion animals provide.

Parents and veterinarians must be cautious not to overburden teenagers during the experience of pet loss. Adolescents are sometimes asked to take responsibility for younger siblings during a family crisis and, when this responsibility is prolonged, their own grief processes are interrupted or postponed. Adults must also be careful not to engage teenagers' rebelliousness by insisting that they grieve in certain ways or within certain time frames. Basically, adolescents should be treated in the same ways as younger children, with adults offering them time to talk and to ask questions about their losses.

Young Adults (18 through 21 Years of Age)

When a young adult experiences pet loss, it is often due to the death of a childhood pet. When a childhood pet dies, an important part of a young adult's childhood also dies. Thus, the deaths of childhood pets often represent a rite of passage from childhood to adulthood because they sever the last link to a simpler, more innocent time. For young adults who had strong bonds with their pets, their pets' deaths truly represent the "end of an era."

Another common issue for young adults is the guilt that they may feel for "abandoning" their pets when they left home to attend college, to go to work, or to get married. Many feel guilty for not being present during their pets' deaths at a time when their pets may have needed them the most. Some also fear that their pets may have died feeling angry at them for being absent. Guilt is not easily erased, but young adults benefit from and appreciate words of comfort from sincere adults. Adults should verbally acknowledge the symbolic connections that exist between pets and young adults' childhoods. Like younger children, young adults should be reassured and provided with opportunities to discuss and resolve their feelings of grief and guilt.

How You Can Help Children

You can help parents and children prepare for and deal with pet loss in many ways. This guide includes suggestions for providing effective and well-informed guidance to children and parents who are your clients.

Build Personal Rapport with Young Clientele

One of the best ways you can help children is to continue to develop rapport with them each time you see them. Rapport-builders include allowing children to assist during their pets' examinations, involving them in their pets' treatments, and talking to them directly about their pets. For example, you can ask children questions like, "What do you think is wrong with Lucky?" and "Shall I give Skippy her shot on her right or left side?" or "Would you like to help me give Whitey her vaccination?"

While talking with children, it is helpful to use words that they understand and to draw pictures (use colored pens!) of what is happening to their pets. Talking with kids is more effective when you move to childrens' eye level; that is, squat or sit so you have direct eye contact with children. Establishing direct eye contact during medical updates and consultations lets children know that you are truly interested in their opinions, thoughts, and feelings.

Pets and children go together, so you will see hundreds of children over the course of a year. It is a good idea to write childrens' names in the patients' case files. It is also a good idea to provide waiting room or examination room play areas, treats (for both animals and kids!) and, when time allows, tours or special visits to private areas of the hospital. When children are familiar with you and with your veterinary facilities, it is easier to gain their trust and cooperation during times of crisis and pet loss. By the same token, when the rapport between you is strong, it is easier for them to convince you to meet their special needs.

For example, one 10-year-old child with whom we worked was allowed to go into the surgery suite to say goodbye to her horse. She told us:

I think Rex was afraid when he had to go into the surgery room without me. But, when I came into the room he knew I was there, even though he was unconscious, and he wasn't scared anymore. I didn't want him to die being afraid.

This child later asked her parents to bury her horse next to her swing set, which they did. Knowing Rex is nearby is a source of comfort for her, not a stressor.

Encourage Parents to be Honest with Children

You can help parents to talk honestly with their children about their pets' illnesses, injuries, treatments, and deaths. You can also make a com-

BOX 12-4

Suggested Reading List about Children and Grief

Reading to children about pet loss creates opportunities for discussions about death and grief. Here are some suggested resources.

Brown, M.: *The Dead Bird.* Harper Junior, 1958, (reprinted, 1990).
Buscaglia, L.: *The Fall of Freddie the Leaf: A Story for All Ages.* Slack Book Division, 1982.
Carrick, C.: *The Accident.* Clarion Books, 1981.
Cazet, D.: *A Fish in His Pocket.* Orchard Books, 1987.
Gipson, F.: *Old Yeller.* Harper & Row, 1956 (reprinted, 1989).
Grollman, E.: *Talking About Death: A Dialogue Between Parents and Children.* Putnam/Beacon Press, 1990.
Hamley, D.: *Tigger and Friends.* Lothrop, Lee & Shepard Books, 1989.
Heegaard, M.: *Coping With Death and Grief.* Lerner Publications Company, 1990.
Heegaard, M.: *When Someone Very Special Dies: Children Can Learn to Cope With Grief.* Woodland Press, 1988.
Hewett, J.: *Rosalie.* Lothrop, Lee, & Shepard Books, 1987.
Jewett, C.L.: *Helping Children Cope with Separation and Loss.* The Harvard Common Press, 1982.
Rogers, F.: *When a Pet Dies.* Putnam Publishing Group, 1988.
Sanford, D.: *It Must Hurt A Lot.* Multnomah Press, 1987.
Stein, S.B.: *About Dying: A Open Family Book for Parents and Children Together.* Walker & Company, 1984.
Varley, S.: *Badger's Parting Gifts.* Lothrop, Lee, & Shepard Books, 1984.
Viorst, J.: *The Tenth Good Thing About Barney.* Atheneum, 1971.
Warren, P. *Where Love Goes.* Me Books/Art After Five, 1992.
White, E.B.: *Charlotte's Web.* Harper Junior, 1952.
Wilhelm, H.: *I'll Always Love You.* Crown Publishing Group, 1985.
Wright, B.R.: *The Cat Next Door.* Holiday House Books, 1991.

mitment to be honest in your own interactions with children. It is important that you never agree to lie to children to protect them. In the long-run, lies create more problems because, when lies are exposed, childrens' abilities to trust, empathize, and grieve normally are damaged.

Most parents who ask you to lie to their children are really asking for help and support. Many of them are concerned that their own strong emotions may frighten or confuse their children. By asking you to collude with them in a lie, they are signaling a need for more information and guidance. You can have books, pamphlets, and videotapes about children and pet loss available for parents to check out. You can also suggest that parents and children read books about pet loss together. A suggested reading list is included in Box 12-4.

Encourage Parents to Include Children

Children of all ages can be included in decisions, euthanasias, and goodbye rituals and ceremonies. With adequate preparation, most children who are old enough to think and speak for themselves can choose whether to be present at euthanasia. They can also decide for themselves how to say goodbye to their pets, how to honor their pets' memories, and whether to see their pets' bodies. The key to exposing children to any of these potentially upsetting experiences is preparation. For example, if children want to be present at their pets' euthanasias, they need to be clearly told what will happen while they are in the room; what they will see; how their pets will look, feel, and behave; and what appropriate actions they can take after the pet is dead (for example, petting, hugging, crying, or spending time with their pets' bodies). In this case, preparation means that you and your young clients' parents structure the grief experience by giving children permission to think, feel, and behave in ways appropriate for them. This approach, of course, does not include allowing children to behave in ways that would cause harm to themselves or others.

After an animal's death, you can suggest that parents organize and participate in memorial ceremonies for their childrens' pets. Memorials are effective ways to say goodbye and to draw closure to relationships. Examples of memorial ceremonies and rituals include funerals (where children may read poems or stories that they have written about their pets), planting of trees or rosebushes as visual tributes to pets, creation of scrapbooks of photographs, and making donations to animal-related service organizations in memory of their pets.

Avoid Using Euphemisms

Children, like adults, respond well to straightforward explanations and concrete words. Using words and phrases like "died," "dead," and "helped to die" may seem harsh, but they help children clearly understand

and accept the reality of their pets' deaths. Remember, it is not *what* is said, but *how* it is said that has the greatest impact on children.

Thus, when working with young clients, you should avoid inaccurate terminology (euphemisms) like "put to sleep" and "went away." Because children are "put to sleep" every night, use of these words may cause them to fear that they may also die in their sleep. Children may also have negative responses to explanations like "Heidi got sick and died" or clichés like "Heidi is happy with the angels now." Because children get sick, the first phrase may mislead them to believe that all sicknesses end in death. Because children see people crying and acting depressed when a pet dies, the cliché about Heidi's happiness may confuse them about how they should feel. It may also make them resent and dislike angels!

You should also protect yourself from becoming a pet's executioner in children's eyes. Caution parents about using phrases like "The vet made Heidi die." Clarify that disease, injury, or euthanasia drugs caused the pet's death and that you helped to end the animal's suffering. Let children know that everyone (especially you) shares in their sadness.

Explain Body Care

When explaining body care to children, it is important to talk to them with sensitivity and with enough detail that they are able to understand what is happening to their pets' bodies. Keep childrens' cognitive abilities and developmental levels in mind as you select body care terminology. Remember to draw pictures and to use appropriate "props" (caskets, urns, cremains, and so forth) to explain what will occur.

Children are very imaginative and, often, what they can imagine is much worse than what actually occurs. Therefore, honesty is essential in this situation. When talking to children about disposing of animals' bodies after death, say something like:

> "When animals die, their bodies don't work anymore. They can't breathe, move about, eat, drink, or play. After a little while, they become stiff and cold and can even start to smell. This happens naturally to anyone who dies. Because we still love our animals, though, we must take care of their dead bodies. There are several ways to handle a pet's body after death. I can explain them if you and your parents want me to."

Think ahead about how you want to explain burial, cremation, disposal in a landfill, and rendering.

Burial.   To explain burial, say something like:

> "Burying means you dig a hole in the ground deep enough so other animals can't dig Bear's body up. Then you put Bear's

body in it. Some people like to put their pet's body in a blanket, cardboard box, or a casket before burying it. A casket is a box that is made especially for burying animals in the ground. We have some here at our clinic that I can show you if you like.

"You might want to put special toys or treats in the grave with Bear. Most people say another goodbye to their pets at the time of burial. I think this is a good idea.

"After Bear's body has been placed into the hole, it is covered with dirt. Then, this special place where you have buried Bear is called a grave. After the grave has been filled with dirt, you can place something special on top of it, like a big rock, some flowers, or a marker with Bear's name on it. Pets can be buried at home (check your city code), in pet cemeteries, or in other appropriate places. If the grave is close by, you can go and visit Bear's grave whenever you feel like talking to or remembering him. If you decide to bury Bear, it will be important to remember that pets don't feel anything when they are dead. They don't need to breathe and they don't need to eat. When they're dead, they cannot come back to life."

Cremation.   To explain cremation, say something like:

"When an animal's body is cremated, it is put into a large oven that gets very, very hot. It is larger and hotter than the ovens people have in their houses. It is an oven that is made especially for cremating animals. The temperature in the oven gets so hot that it causes the animal's body to burn and to crumble down into small pieces. The heat from the oven causes the fur, and all the other soft parts of the body to melt away or disappear. Then, all that remains are the bones. The bones are usually in very small pieces because the heat in the oven also causes them to crumble. These small bone pieces are called "cremains." The cremains usually look like a mixture of light colored sand and small pebbles or rocks.

"It might help you understand cremation if you think about a log in a fireplace. As the log gets hot in the fireplace, it gets smaller and smaller, leaving only ashes behind. You might also want to think about cremation as a form of recycling. During his life, Bear's body was in one form; but, now that he is dead, his body must go through a process that will change it into a different form. However you decide to think about cremation, the most important thing to remember is that animals don't feel anything after they're dead. Although we can feel a burn from things that are hot when we are alive, dead animals don't feel burns. They don't feel anything.

"After cremation, some people like to keep the cremains of their pets in a jar, a box, or an urn. Others scatter them in a special place. If people don't want their pet's cremains returned to them, we dispose of them. Would you like to see the cremains of another animal who died? Sometimes it helps to decide about cremation when you know beforehand how cremains really look."

Mass Burial in a Landfill.   To explain mass burial, say something like:

"When people decide not to bury their animals themselves or to cremate them, we often take care of their animals' bodies for them. We take the animals' bodies to a place where many different kinds of animals are buried together. This place is like a giant grave where animals and dirt are all mixed together. This place is called the landfill.

"The landfill is also used to bury people's trash. However, if you decide on mass burial for Bear's body, it will not be in with trash. It will only be buried with other animals. (Be sure to check with your local landfill to make certain this is true.) After Bear is buried with the other animals, you won't be able to visit his grave. But you can think about him whenever you like and remember the special times you shared together."

Rendering.   To explain rendering, say something like:

"When large animals die, it is very difficult to bury them and very expensive to cremate them. Because of these difficulties, most people send their horses, llamas, mules, cows, and so forth to rendering plants. These businesses use animals' bodies for other good purposes. Many animal foods, fertilizers, and even some kitty litter is partially made from the remains of dead animals. Because animals can't use their bodies after they are dead, rendering is one way to reuse or recycle them.

"Some people feel upset at the thought of having their animals rendered. Others believe that the spirit and personality of their pet was what made him or her special, not the body. Whatever you decide about rendering Bear's body, it's important to understand that, although rendering may be hard to think about, it is an effective way to take care of his remains."

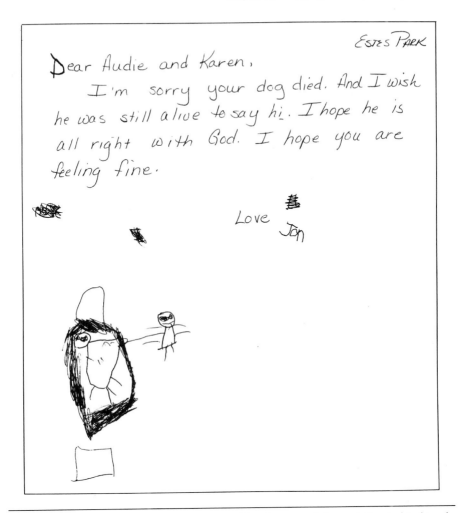

Figure 12-10 A mother helped her 4-year-old write a condolence letter to his friends after the death of their dog Gus.

Contact Significant Adults

After pets die, it is wise for parents to contact other adults who play significant roles in their childrens' lives. These adults may be teachers, care providers, and relatives. They should be asked to provide understanding and additional support to children during the grief process (Figs. 12-10 and 12-11). Grief is isolating and easier to bear when adults whom children

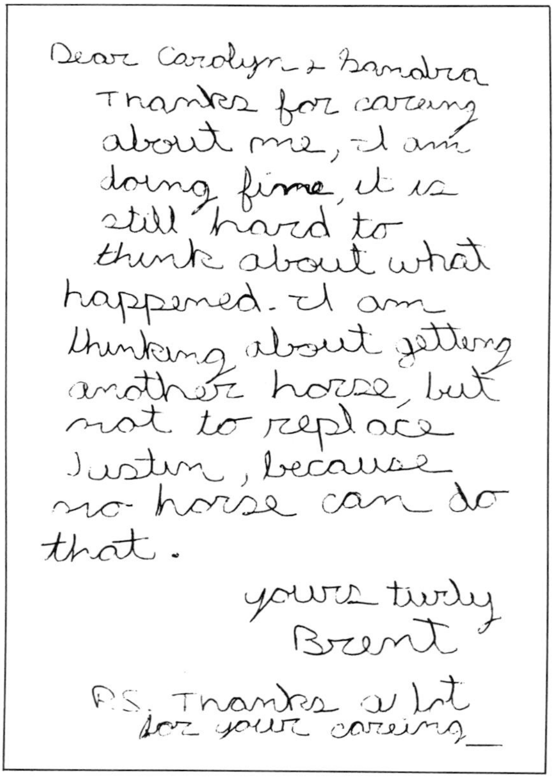

Dear Carolyn + Sandra
Thanks for caring
about me, I am
doing fine, it is
still hard to
think about what
happened. I am
thinking about getting
another horse, but
not to replace
Justin, because
no horse can do
that.
                    yours truly
                      Brent

P.S. Thanks a Lot
    for your caring

Figure 12-11 A young boy says thank you for caring.

respect talk to them about their own experiences with pet loss and grief. During conversations, adults should encourage a wide range of emotions, focusing on more than just sadness. Adults should also be prepared for children to express anger and blame and should not become defensive regarding childrens' comments.

Follow-up

One way in which you can follow-up with children after the deaths of their pets is by specifically naming them in the condolence cards you send. If time allows, you can also contact them directly to make sure that their grief is progressing normally. Children appreciate it when you contact them personally, and it helps you to avoid falling into the trap of getting your information about childrens' well-being from parents. Parents and children often have very different views of the same experience. Children may also talk more openly to you than to their parents. During your follow-up, be sure that both parents and children have plenty of reading material and the names and telephone numbers of local support services.

CONCLUSION

Along with the unique characteristics of the populations outlined in this chapter, special circumstances make the death of a pet particularly difficult to endure. The loss of a companion animal is emotionally painful under the best of circumstances. If other major disruptions are occurring in clients' lives simultaneously, the death may become overwhelming.

In today's rapid-paced society, it seems as if change is the rule rather than the exception. Most clients who walk through your door on a given day are probably either currently experiencing, or have experienced in the recent past, a major life crisis. These crises can include a divorce or separation, the birth of a child, the loss of a job or a job promotion including additional responsibilities, an illness or death in the family, a change in financial status, a move, and various other events. Under these circumstances, your clients may be short-tempered, frightened, anxious, and want any problems with their pets to be resolved quickly and with a positive outcome. People who are under a great deal of stress may need more time to make decisions or may get stuck in the decision-making process. They may also become angry more quickly or have unrealistic expectations. Helping clients who are dealing with a variety of these circumstances is the topic of the next chapter.

An example of how one family decided to euthanize their dog and to include their young child in the process follows.

A Merciful Farewell
Terry D'Erchia

Our 14-year-old Golden Retriever was dying. A routine blood screen revealed that she had kidney failure, which is irreversible but possibly controllable. We knew the end was near, but just how much good time we had left with our beautiful Sage was unknown.

Our first efforts to control the effects of the kidney disease were rewarding. After we put her on a specially-formulated diet and began giving her vitamins, as prescribed by our veterinarian, the blood test results improved dramatically and Sage's activity level was better than it had been in months. We cautiously hoped for a long reprieve for our beloved friend.

But it was not to be. First, Sage stopped eating the "magic food" which had stabilized her disease. We then tried a homemade recipe our veterinarian gave us and also began subcutaneous fluid injections. Once again, we gained a bit of good time, but Sage rapidly went downhill when she again refused to eat. We gave her medication to calm her stomach and increased the subcutaneous fluids. Nothing helped—and then Sage began trembling unaccountably and we realized that it was time to allow our valiant companion to die with dignity.

Although we were sure our decision was the only one we could accept for our suffering pet, it was excruciatingly difficult to actually carry it through. Our veterinarian was kind and compassionate and was willing to come to our home to perform the euthanasia. Still, though, we would be playing God; not a comfortable role to accept.

And what about our 7-year-old son? Would he understand or would he condemn us for "murdering" his dear friend? Initially, my husband wanted to shield our little boy from the pain. But after consulting with our veterinary hospital's grief counselor, we realized that our son deserved the opportunity to decide for himself whether or not he wanted to be present at Sage's euthanasia.

What a wise decision! Not only did our little boy then have the opportunity to spend Sage's last evening with us pampering her, feeding her forbidden treats, gently rolling a ball for her to catch (her greatest passion), but the discussion of Sage's suffering and the responsibility we felt to end her pain opened up invaluable lines of communication within our family. His disturbing questions regarding human suffering and terminal illness revealed his maturing sense of morality. Although there were no wholly satisfactory answers to such questions, they were important for us to discuss.

When the overdose of anesthesia was given, he was the one who comforted Mom. He held the flashlight at the grave site and scattered wild flowers over Sage's body. But, after all, he had helped her in life—aiding with the injections and the preparation of special food, making sure our big Collie puppy didn't knock her down—and so it was fitting that he should be allowed to say goodbye.

In the end, Sage left us painlessly and peacefully. We all cried and shared our grief at our great loss. But we know our noble friend was given a precious gift—a dignified end with no suffering. She will always be alive in our hearts and can never be replaced. Our 11-month-old puppy is an important part of our family circle, but, as an individual, very, very different from our old friend. He is not a substitute for Sage, but his presence does soften the edge of the pain which will remain for awhile. And I know that some day we will truly lay our wise and generous friend to rest in our hearts, and will be able to smile when we remember all the joy she selflessly gave us.

REFERENCES

1. Cook, A. and Oltjenbruns, K.: Dying and Grieving: Lifespan and Family Perspectives. New York, Holt, Rinehart and Winston, 1989.

2. Staudacher, C.: Men and Grief: A Guide for Men Surviving the Death of a Loved One, A Resource for Caregivers and Mental Health Professionals. Oakland, Calif., New Harbinger Publications, 1991.
3. Gilligan, C.: In a Different Voice. Cambridge, Mass., Harvard University Press, 1982.
4. Parkes, C.M., and Brown, R.J.: Health after bereavement: A controlled study of young Boston widows and widowers. Psychosom. Med., 34:449–461, 1972.
5. Sanders, C.M.: A comparison of adult bereavement in the death of a spouse, child, and parent. Omega, 10:303–322, 1979.
6. Lago, D., Connell, C.M., and Knight, B.: A companion animal program. In Smyer, M.A., and Gatz, M., eds.: Mental Health and Aging. Beverly Hills, Calif., Sage Publishing, 1983, pp. 165–185.
7. Ory, M.G., and Goldberg, E.L.: Pet possession and life satisfaction in elderly women. In Katcher, A.H., and Beck, A.M., eds.: New Perspectives on Our Lives with Companion Animals. Philadelphia, University of Pennsylvania Press, 1983, pp. 303–317.
8. Stallones, L.: Companion animals and health of the elderly: Part 3. People, Animals, Environment, 4:18–19, 1990.
9. Friedmann, E., Katcher A.H., Lynch, J.J., and Thomas, S.A.: Animal companions and one year survival of patients after discharge from a coronary care unit. California Vet., 8:45–50, 1982.
10. Anderson, W.P., Reid, C.M., and Jennings, G.L.: Pet ownership and risk factors for cardiovascular disease. Med. J. Aust., 157:298–301, 1992.
11. Spencer, G.: Projections of the population of the United States, by age, sex, and race: 1983–2080. Current Population Reports: Population Estimates and Projections, Series P-25, No. 952, Washington, D.C., U.S. Government Printing Office, 1984.
12. Miller, J.A., and Sharp, E.V.: The deaf can hear and the speechless can speak. Animal Imprints, Center for Animals in Society Newsletter, Number 10. Davis, Calif., University of California, 1992/1993.
13. Messant P: Correlates and effects of pet ownership. In Anderson, R.K., Hart, B.L., and Hart, L.A., eds.: The Pet Connection, University of Minnesota, Minneapolis, CENSHARE, 1984, pp. 331–340.
14. Melson, G.F., Sparks, C., and Peet, S.: Children's ideas about pets and their care. Paper presented at the annual meeting of the Delta Society, November 10–12, Parsipanny, N.J., 1989.
15. Poresky, R., Hendrix, C., Mosier, J., and Samuelson, M.L.: The companion animal bonding scale: Internal reliability and construct validity. Psychol. Rep., 60:743–746, 1987.
16. Cairns, R.B.: Attachment behavior in mammals. Psychol. Rev., 73:409–429, 1966.
17. Bowlby, J.: Attachment and loss. New York, Basic Books, 1969.
18. Melson, G.F.: Availability of and involvement with pets by children: Determinants and correlates. Anthrozoos, 2:45–52, 1988.
19. Ainsworth, M.D.S.: Attachment as related to mother-infant interaction. In Rosenblatt, J., Hinde, R., Beer, C., and Busnel, M.C., eds.: Advances in the Study of Behavior. New York, Academic Press, 1979, pp. 2–51.
20. Bryant, B.: Characterizing the family life and social-emotional development of children who are highly involved with pets. Paper presented at the annual meeting of the Delta Society, Vancouver, Canada, October 4–6, 1987.
21. Kidd, A.H., and Kidd, R.M.: Childrens' attitudes towards their pets. Psychol. Rep., 57:15–31, 1985.
22. Melson, G.F., and Taylor, S.: Pet ownership and attachment in young children: Relations to behavior problems and social competence. Paper presented at the annual meeting of the Delta Society, Houston, Texas, October 11–13, 1990.
23. Gage, G., and Holcomb, R.: Couples' perceptions of the stressfulness of the death of the family pet. Family Relations, 40:103–105, 1991.
24. Bryant, B.: The richness of the child-pet relationship: A consideration of both benefits and costs of pets to children. Anthrozoos, 3:253–261, 1990.

25. Stewart, M.: Loss of a pet-loss or a person: A comparison study of bereavement. *In* Katcher, A. and, Beck, A., eds.: New Perspectives on Our Lives with Companion Animals. Philadelphia, University of Pennsylvania Press, 1983, pp. 390–404.
26. Troutman, C.M.: The Veterinary Services Market for Companion Animals. Overland Park, Kan., Charles, Charles Research Group and the American Veterinary Medical Association, 1988.

13

Helping in a Variety of Situations

Not all interactions with emotional clients concern companion animal death or euthanasia. Veterinarians handle many kinds of emotional situations everyday. These situations often include medical emergencies, delivering "bad" news, and responding to client anger.

In these situations, however, the underlying threat of loss and the presence of grief can complicate veterinarian-client interactions. Symptoms of grief can manifest in feelings of anxiety, irritability, anger, blame, confusion, and, occasionally, even in thoughts of suicide. When not recognized, understood, and addressed, grief manifestations can escalate and create greater tension. Sometimes the manifestations of client grief can become so hard to manage that the veterinarian-client relationship comes to an impasse, especially when disagreement exists about what should happen next.

If you are truly committed to honing your communication skills and to helping clients during grief, these situations can be viewed as opportunities and challenges. However, they require you to harness the full strength of your helping abilities and to be very clear about your own capabilities and predetermined helping roles.

As we stated previously, your goal when intervening in any loss or grief-related situation is to facilitate your clients' experiences so that they can attain the most positive grief outcomes possible. Again, it is vital for you to remember that each client's grief outcome will be different. Some clients will be ready and able to accept your help, and others will not. Some clients will make full use of the positive coping skills and social support systems available to them, and others will not. You will only be able to help to the extent that your clients will allow you to help.

In Chapter 3, we profiled the average veterinary client. This chapter brings us back for a second, closer look at another portion of your clientele. As we said in Chapter 3, your clients are pet owners, but they are first human beings. Some humans are mentally and emotionally well-adjusted, and some are not. Some humans are honest and straightforward, and others are devious and manipulative. We are the first to admit that the clients who exhibit emotional, albeit normal, responses to pet loss or even to the threat of pet loss are often the most difficult to handle. Some make offensive comments or display annoying behaviors. Others linger after business hours or make unreasonable demands.

In this chapter, we discuss ideas and strategies for dealing with some of the more complicated and challenging grief-related situations that you will encounter. No right and wrong answers exist in terms of handling these situations—only ways of helping that have proven to be more effective than others. The topics discussed in this chapter represent the dozen situations about which veterinarians most often ask us during case consultations. In all of these situations, the TEAM model and the verbal and nonverbal communication techniques discussed previously form the foundations of the suggested helping interventions.

Any of the situations discussed in this chapter could "blow up" in your face and become fodder for grievances or lawsuits filed against you. For this reason, we strongly urge you to keep copious case notes in your client files regarding any and all pertinent veterinarian-client conversations and interactions. We also encourage you to document any attempts you make to resolve the problem. When you are in a helping role, you want to believe and expect the best from clients, but it is naive not to take steps to protect yourself.

SITUATION ONE: "In Medical Emergencies, I Know How to Help My Patients, but How Can I Best Help Clients During Their Accompanying Emotional Crises?"

> Frank Coleman rushes his dog, Rusty, to your veterinary clinic on a Friday afternoon at 4:45 p.m. It seems that Frank walked across the street to visit a neighbor after arriving home from work. Rusty was hit by a car as she ran from the yard to follow him. Her injuries are severe, and her life is in danger. You know that the time you have to try to save Rusty is short. You need to diagnose and treat your client's pet, but Frank is clutching Rusty to his chest and has launched into a monologue describing his reactions to the accident. He will not give you the dog.

"She's always been a good dog," Frank is saying as he cradles Rusty in his arms. "She's my son's dog, really. My wife and I are divorced and she's the first thing he looks for when he comes to my house to visit. Sometimes I don't know what to say to my son, but we can always talk about Rusty. We go on walks together, we take her in the car. . ."

Suddenly, Frank shoves Rusty into your arms, sits down in a chair in your waiting room, and holds his head in his hands. "My son's coming tomorrow for a week-long visit. You have to fix Rusty!" he shouts. "If she's not there, I don't know what my son will do! In fact, if he finds out that I let her get hit by a car, he'll probably never want to come see me again. If that happens, I don't know what I'll do!"

By this time, Frank is crying and his voice has taken on an edge of desperation. He gets up and begins to pace across the room. With a sudden burst of anger, he shouts, "Go fix her, Doc! Don't just stand there, go fix her!"

Frank Coleman is in crisis. Crises are defined as the changes in people's lives that cause them to drop to lower levels of functioning.[1] An operational definition of crisis can be partially based on its observable characteristics. Some common characteristics include: feeling out of control, panicked, confused, experiencing distortions in time (for example, when events seem to move very quickly or when time feels frozen), having tunnel vision (for example, the inability to consider more than one solution to a problem), and having difficulty recalling information. When people are in crisis, they show symptoms of shock and anxiety. Many are also unable to think clearly or to follow the course of normal conversations. Some people in the acute stage of crisis display intense emotion or erratic and irrational behavior. When people are in crisis, the knowledge and skills that they normally use to cope with life either no longer work or are forgotten. Crises are caused by people's responses to stress. Usually, stress itself does not cause emotional crisis. Instead, crises occur when people feel helpless to respond to stress effectively.

The body and mind can only sustain the stress of crisis for so long. After a period of time (unique to each individual and each crisis, but generally estimated at about 72 hours), people either resolve crises in healthy ways (for example, by identifying alternatives and seeking help) or handle them in negative ways (for example, by using denial, self-destructive behaviors, or directing their attentions toward other distractions, often another crisis). The aim of crisis intervention is to direct people toward healthy and positive resolutions for their problems.

In general, crisis intervention has two main goals:

1. To assist clients in finding their own solutions to their problems.

2. To stabilize the situation and assist clients in returning to their original levels of functioning. Effective crisis intervention does not aim to bring people to higher levels of functioning. That is the realm of psychotherapy.

When intervening in crisis, it is important to help clients deal with what is going on *now*, while assessing which of their needs will require attention later. Situational crises such as medical emergencies demand a "first things first" approach to helping (for example, saving pets' lives or deciding about treatment options), but they also require that clients in crisis receive both emotional relief and linkage to the resources that can continue to assist them in the days and weeks ahead. Let us return to the case study that began this section and examine what might be done to stabilize Frank Coleman's crisis situation.

Clients in crisis are helped by structure. The first step in providing structure for Mr. Coleman might be to gently, yet firmly guide him into an office or examination room. Doing so accomplishes two things: It restores some control over the situation and provides Mr. Coleman with privacy and fewer distractions. He may then be able to maintain a tighter focus on the situation at hand. It also spares other clients, who may be waiting for their own appointments, from feeling they should somehow deal with Mr. Coleman's pain. Sometimes, during a crisis, bystanders attempt to help and inadvertently exacerbate the situation. By removing a client in crisis from the public eye, you prevent such problems from happening. In addition, handling crises with skill and compassion lets other pet owners know that, should they ever be in a similar position with their pets, they can count on you and your staff to handle their crises with sensitivity. This approach deepens your clients' loyalty and commitment to you and to your practice.

After structure has been brought to a crisis situation, you can maintain it by keeping clients well-informed about their pets' medical status. If possible, a technician or receptionist can wait with Mr. Coleman while you examine his dog, or, at the very least, they can periodically return to the room to provide him with frequent updates on his pet's medical status. When you return to the room with your findings, you can continue to structure the situation by giving Mr. Coleman concise directions regarding the steps that will occur next. Statements like:

"Please have a seat,"

"Follow me over here to the view box. I want to be sure you understand the x-rays,"

and

"I'm going to give you some time to think about this and review what we've talked about while I go back to attend to

Rusty. I'll be back to answer your questions in about 10 minutes."

are examples of gentle, directive statements that provide appropriate structure during crisis.

As medical information begins to overwhelm pet owners, some also become overwhelmed by emotions. Some clients work hard to suppress and hide the emotions that are overtaking them. When they lose the struggle and openly display their sadness, confusion, or grief, your overall control of the situation is in jeopardy. This is because, if emotions are ignored, many clients feel that they are not receiving proper care or attention; yet, if emotions are overemphasized, clients often feel embarrassed. In a crisis, it is therefore imperative to address, without being overly solicitous, whatever emotion is present. Acknowledging emotion brings it from a covert to an overt level. This acknowledgment is important because, when clients are preoccupied with either the expression or suppression of emotion, they have neither the ability nor the inclination to listen attentively to what you are telling them. All of their energy is being distributed toward whatever they are experiencing emotionally.

There are many nurturing ways to address clients' emotions. Many of these make use of nonverbal communication. For example, a nurturing and non-nurturing way exists in which to hand tissues to clients who are crying. The non-nurturing way is to avoid eye contact, pick up the tissue box, and wave it in the clients' general direction as they struggle to gain composure. The nurturing way is to pull one or two tissues from the box, make direct eye contact with the clients, and hand them the tissues. In the previous case scenario, handing Mr. Coleman a tissue while saying something like:

"I see how much you love Rusty. I would expect you to cry in this situation."

would reassure Mr. Coleman and give him permission to respond (for example, cry harder or regain his composure) in whatever way feels right to him.

You could also use touch and a soothing voice to express your concern to Mr. Coleman. In addition, self-disclosing about a similar personal experience could normalize his feelings and let him know that you also often respond emotionally to crises. Clinical experience suggests that, during a crisis, it is important to pay attention to what clients *say* they want and need, in addition to what you might *assume* they want and need. Without client acceptance, your helping efforts during crisis can be fruitless, but, when clients feel that their concerns are validated, they relax and are better able to listen to important medical information. At this point, they can be told about treatment procedures, staff roles, and clinic policies and philosophies.

Sometimes, animals are brought to your clinic by people other than their owners. These animals may have been injured without their owners' knowledge. If animals have no identifying information, it is a good idea to photograph them so that, if they die, they might later be identified by the owner. We had one such incident at CSU. A dog was brought in on emergency, died, and was cremated before the owners could be located. Because the dog had no identifying information, the attending veterinarian had no way of knowing how to reach the owners. A few days later, a young couple arrived at the Veterinary Teaching Hospital, inquiring whether or not we had treated a small dog. The critical care unit staff recalled the "John Doe Dog" and agreed to talk with the couple. After hearing their description, the doctor told them that he was quite certain that the dog he had treated was theirs. They wanted to make sure, however, so the grief counselor encouraged them to bring in a photograph of their dog so the clinician could make a positive identification. This was done, and the clients, although saddened to positively learn of the death of their dog, were relieved to know what had happened to her.

Another point regarding veterinary medical emergencies involves client visitation privileges. Research from human medicine has indicated that most families want and need contact with loved ones who are in intensive care;[2] yet, in veterinary medicine, many veterinarians persist in either severely restricting visiting hours with companion animals or in forbidding client visits altogether. Clinical experience shows that depriving clients of contact with their ill or injured companion animals usually just heightens their anxiety. Therefore, everyone's needs seem to be better served when clients are invited and even encouraged to visit their pets while they are hospitalized (Boxes 13-1 and 13-2.) Such visits are especially important if patients are expected to die.

If you are worried about how clients might respond to seeing their pets hooked up to emergency equipment and monitors, take time beforehand to prepare them for what they will see. For most highly attached pet owners, the opportunity to visit their pets and to perhaps say goodbye to them one last time far outweighs any discomfort that they may have about seeing their pets in critical condition.

One final point about dealing with emergencies involves ensuring that your clients are calmed and stable enough to drive home afterward. It is a good idea to remind clients that it is hard to function normally during crisis and that even "second-nature" activities like driving can feel complex and overwhelming for some people. Therefore, you can ask clients to call a friend or family member who can drive them home or, at least, offer clients a cup of tea and a quiet place to sit until they feel recovered enough to drive themselves. One of our students told us about a unique service offered by

BOX 13-1

The Critical Care Unit Client Information

Clients should be informed in advance about rules governing their behavior in critical care areas. A client information handout such as the one below facilitates the process.

Guidelines for Visitors

- Visiting hours are by appointment only. See your pet's primary clinician (veterinarian) for details.
- Each visitation period will be limited to 30 minutes.
- Children *are* permitted but must be under direct adult supervision.
- Questions regarding your pet's condition should be directed to your pet's primary clinician.
- Visitors must limit their interactions to their own pet.
- Do not try to remove your pet from its cage or from the critical care unit without permission from your pet's primary clinician.
- Do not feed your pet unless authorized by the primary clinician.
- Unescorted visitors are *not* permitted in the critical care unit. Your pet's primary clinician must accompany visitors.
- Under certain circumstances, visitors may be asked to leave before their visiting period is over. Visitors are *required* to obey any instructions from critical care unit staff or faculty. This policy is in the best interest of all of our patients in critical care.

This handout was developed by the Colorado State University Veterinary Teaching Hospital's critical care faculty and staff, 1993.

the emergency practice in which he worked. The veterinarians at this practice made an arrangement with one of their local taxi services so that cabs were available, even late at night, to take distraught owners home and to bring them back the following day to retrieve their cars.

SITUATION TWO: "Medical Emergencies Often Go from Bad to Worse. What's the Best Way to Deliver Bad News to Clients?"

Many times, veterinarians must deliver "bad" news to clients. News that can be considered "bad" is usually loss- and grief-related: diagnosing a chronic or terminal illness, informing clients about their pet's sudden or unexpected death, or relating information about disease recurrence or treatment failure. Breaking bad news may confirm pre-existing suspicions for frightened or worried clients; therefore, both delivering and receiving

BOX 13-2

The Critical Care Unit Visitation Protocol

Visitation programs run more smoothly when all participants understand the established guidelines. To this end, protocols such as the following should be posted for staff and client review.

- Client visits must be scheduled in advance with the critical care unit (CCU) faculty, resident, or staff on duty.
- Client visitors are *not* permitted during CCU case rounds (8:30 to 9:30 a.m., 4:30 to 5:30 p.m., 9:30 to 10:30 p.m.).
- Client visits are to be avoided during three- and four-times daily treatment periods (7:00 to 8:00 a.m., 1:00 to 2:00 p.m., 3:00 to 4:00 p.m., 7:00 to 8:00 p.m.)
- Client visits will *not* be allowed after 10:00 p.m., unless personally escorted by the primary clinician *and* approval has been obtained from the CCU personnel on duty.
- Client visits will be limited to 30 minutes, unless approved by CCU personnel.
- Only one group of visitors will be permitted in the CCU at any given time.
- Children are permitted but must be accompanied by an adult and remain under adult supervision.
- The primary clinician must accompany all visitors to the CCU.
- Visitors may not be left unattended in the CCU. The primary clinician or primary student must be in attendance to answer questions.
- The primary clinician is responsible for explaining the visitation protocol to clients. It is the primary clinician's responsibility to ensure proper conduct on the part of visitors to the CCU.
- The primary clinician should introduce visitors to the CCU faculty, residents, staff, and students working with their pet.
- Specific questions regarding patient status should be directed to the primary clinician.
- General questions regarding CCU operation and equipment may be answered by CCU personnel *as time permits*.
- Patients should remain in their cages during visits unless approved by the primary clinician *and* CCU personnel.
- Visitors should be made as comfortable as possible during their visit to the CCU. This provision includes appropriate seating, adequate accessibility to their pet, and professional conduct by personnel present in the CCU.
- The CCU faculty, residents, or staff have the right (and responsibility) to eject unruly visitors from the CCU. The primary clinician is required to respect the opinions of CCU personnel on this matter. Students with concerns about visitor behavior should address their concerns to CCU personnel on duty.
- Temporary removal of a patient from the CCU to an examination room for visitation is still permitted provided the primary clinician approves.

These guidelines were developed by the Colorado State University Veterinary Teaching Hospital's critical care faculty and staff, 1993.

bad news can trigger feelings of guilt and anxiety and can be unsettling both for pet owners and veterinarians.

Sufficient data exist to prove that problems with communication between doctors and human patients are extremely common and that these problems adversely affect case management.[3] More specifically, evidence from human medicine suggests that communication about "bad" news is handled badly,[4] possibly because doctors fear being blamed, fear the unknown, fear the expression of emotion, and fear that they do not know all the answers.[5] Also, evidence suggests that large clinical workloads may impair communication skills.[6] We can assume that, under busy, stressful conditions, doctors perceive they have no time for the tactful delivery of bad news. Logically, these research findings can be applied to veterinary medicine, with the same factors affecting the communication that occurs between veterinarians and clients.

If veterinary professionals fail to win client trust during the delivery of bad news, effective case management is jeopardized; therefore, time invested in educating and reassuring clients during this crucial time pays off later. Clinical experience has shown that most angry, time-consuming interactions that occur later between clients and their veterinarian are traceable to previous episodes of poor communication during the delivery of bad news.[7] Your goals when delivering emotionally upsetting news to clients are to provide medical information while establishing trust and rapport with your clients. Both goals are accomplished by patiently and consistently addressing client concerns.

Three methods of approach[8] can be used when delivering bad news: (1) the blunt and unfeeling way; (2) the kind and sad way; and (3) the understanding and positive way. The last is probably the preferred way. To convey bad news with an understanding and positive attitude, communication concerning it should be delivered in stages because it takes time for clients to fully realize the magnitude of what they have been told. In fact, clients will remember little about the first conversation and will have many questions to ask during the next. Veterinarians who rely on one consultation to cover all the bad news details will probably find that their communication has failed.

Sometimes, bad news must be delivered by telephone. The helping literature gives conflicting suggestions about use of the telephone during this situation. For example, one expert suggests that, when telephoning clients with the news that a pet has died, you should first state that the pet is seriously ill,[9] rather than dead, and ask them to come to your clinic as soon as possible. This expert feels that doing so helps keep clients from panicking and may prevent them from having an accident on the way to your clinic. A Gallup Poll survey of the public supports this approach, with 64 percent in favor prolonging the truth until it can be given face-to-face and 26 percent against it.[10]

We understand the attractiveness of this approach to delivering bad news but disagree with it for one main reason. It is dishonest. When the client arrives at your office, you are forced to either reveal that you lied to them on the phone and that, in reality, their pet was already dead, or you must lie to them again and tell them that their pet died while they were en route. It seems to us that the first scenario could easily cause your clients to doubt and mistrust what you say to them from that point forward. It could also be seen as condescending and insulting to them because you obviously withheld important information from them, thinking that it would be too hard for them to handle. Besides being even more dishonest, the second scenario could cause clients to feel guilty that they did not make it to your clinic in time to be with their pets and to say good-bye before they died. Needless to say, feelings of guilt often complicate the grief process.

We believe that telephone tact can be taught and that, if you present information in a helpful way, the telephone can be an effective way to deliver bad news to clients. One way to achieve this goal is to simply change the context in which information is given. Using the telephone to deliver bad news can be viewed as cold and impersonal; however, effective use of verbal communication techniques can create a context of sensitivity and compassion. Crisis intervention expert Karl Slaikeu says that the goal when creating this context is not to deny what happened or to soften the blow, but instead to arrange the realities so people can begin to assimilate them and take the first steps toward working through grief.[11] During phone calls, the sensitive "arrangement of realities" is perhaps best accomplished when veterinarians prepare clients emotionally for what is to come, predict the ways in which clients may feel or respond when the news is given, and then proceed to offer clients information in brief, step-by-step conversations. For example, when using the telephone to deliver bad news about a pet's sudden death, you might first say:

> "Mrs. Brown, I have some bad news that may be upsetting
> for you to hear." (Preparing client emotionally, predicting
> how client might feel or respond.)

You might follow this statement by offering Mrs. Brown a choice regarding the way in which she wants to hear the news to which you have referred. In other words, you might ask:

> "Would you like me to tell you now, or do you want to come
> down to my office?"

With a lead in like this, nine times out of ten, clients will say that they want the news now, over the telephone. Then you can continue with:

> "We tried everything we knew how to do, but FiFi died dur-
> ing surgery. I want you to know that she was anesthetized

and felt no pain. I also want you to know that all of us here were with her when she died." (Brief explanation of situation.)

After saying this much, you should stop because, at this point, some sort of emotional reaction will usually come from the client. This reaction might be sobbing, cries of disbelief, anger, or complete silence. It is important then to ask what the client needs next. Some logical choices to offer might include providing her with more detailed medical information now, providing it to her in an hour or so by calling her again, or setting an appointment to see her later in the day so you can discuss the details face-to-face in your office. Regardless of her choice concerning further discussions with you, you also should offer her the option of viewing FiFi's body.

Keep several things in mind when using the telephone as a means of delivering bad news. First, because you have no nonverbal cues such as facial gestures and eye contact, the main vehicle for establishing trust and rapport and for conveying understanding and concern is your voice. Thus, the tone, pacing, and pitch of your voice are extremely important. To be calming and reassuring, your voice must be quiet, slow-paced, and empathetic. Instead of becoming caught up in your clients' panic (often reflected in their voices by high pitch and rapid rate of speech), you must counter with attentive, calm, and controlled speech.

You must also be aware of ways to use silence effectively. Without nonverbal cues as guides, telephone silence is much more ambiguous. It is sometimes difficult to know whether clients are crying, are collecting their thoughts, are unsure about what to say next or how to answer your questions, or if you have offended them somehow. You can acknowledge their silences and your clients' stress by making comments like:

"I'm right here for you. Take your time."

"I can imagine how hard this is for you to talk about. Cry if you need to . . . I would cry, too, if I were facing this situation."

"All of this is pretty overwhelming."

"You've been very quiet for a while now. Do you want to continue talking with me at this time?"

Sometimes, clients use the telephone to deliver bad news to you. They may call during a medical emergency or to let you know they are discouraged with treatment and ready to euthanize their pet. Face-to-face interactions with clients generally occur on your "turf," with the length of the contact also predetermined and structured by you. When they use the telephone, however, clients increase their control over conversations with you. For example, by using the telephone to contact you, clients not only begin interactions when they want to, they are also more in charge of what is discussed and when and how conversations end, thus creating potential problems for you. For example, sometimes you cannot talk when a client calls you. When this happens, as with any helping interaction, you can assess your client's needs and respond to them accordingly. Here are some examples of the kinds of emotional telephone interactions with which you may be presented and suggestions about ways in which to respond to them. Keep in mind that, because most of the calls that come in to clinics are initially handled by receptionists, many of these comments are most appropriately made by them:

- *Responding to immediate, but not life-threatening crisis:*

"I can hear in your voice that you need help with this right now, Diane. I need your phone number and the person best able to help you will call you back within 5 minutes."

- *Responding to present, but not urgent emotion:*

"Diane, I can hear the concern in your voice, and this sounds like something we need more time to sort through. Because I (or 'the doctor' if your receptionist is talking) am in the midst of a case with another pet owner, I'd like to set up an appointment with you so we can talk further about this. Would you like to come in or shall we make arrangements to talk again on the phone?"

- *Responding to a call back or request for information:*

"I'll be happy to talk with you about this, Diane, but, due to my appointment schedule, this just isn't a good time. Can we arrange a time when we can talk longer and more easily?"

- *Responding when you have just a few minutes and need to get to the main reason for the call:*

"Diane, I have just a few minutes before my next appointment, and I want to help you if I can. What is the main reason for your call today?"

To conclude this section, we point out several common courtesies to keep in mind when using the telephone to deliver bad news:

- Do not leave messages regarding emotional topics like death, relapse, or body care arrangements on answering machines. Simply leave your name and telephone number and ask your clients to return your call.
- Be aware that clients you contact at work may be unable to talk freely with you about emotional issues. Before you be-

gin, ask them if this is a convenient time to talk or if they would prefer to arrange a telephone appointment when they can speak more freely from a more private area.

- Maintain your clients' confidentiality. If you reach family members or coworkers with whom you have not met or spoken, do not give them details about your patients' conditions. Simply leave a message with your name and number or call back at another time.
- Prepare yourself for potentially emotional calls by finding a quiet, controlled environment where you will not be distracted or interrupted. Also, if possible, turn off pagers and other phones.
- Give clients choices regarding how much detail and the kind of information you share with them. For example, you might say, "I would be happy to explain the details of Mickey's surgery to you. Would you like to have that information?" Each caller's needs for information will vary, so it is best not to make assumptions.

Veterinary medicine has four general categories of bad news: unexpected death, diagnosis, treatment ups and downs, and telling clients that is it time to decide about euthanasia. Each has some unique aspects in terms of effective communication. Situations Three through Seven examine each of these individually.

SITUATION THREE: "How Do I Break Bad News about a Patient's Sudden or Unexpected Death?"

The following example illustrates one way in which the delivery of bad news can be grossly mishandled:

A family of four returned from a week-long vacation and stopped at the boarding kennel to pick up their dog. The kennel was associated with a local veterinary practice. When the father gave his name to the receptionist, she seemed flustered and asked them to wait while she got the veterinarian. Mr. and Mrs. Booth and their two young sons took seats in the waiting room. Soon the veterinarian appeared and asked them to join him in a nearby examination room. Mr. Booth was the last to enter and, when he had closed the door behind him, the veterinarian picked up a large object wrapped in a black plastic bag and handed it to him.

"He died the first day you were gone," the veterinarian said by way of explanation. At first, the Booths were speechless. Then, the boys began to cry.

"Are you serious?" Mrs. Booth asked in disbelief. "Are you sure this is our dog?"

The veterinarian nodded his head and checked his records. Male black lab named Fred, right?" he asked. No one said anything, but Mrs. Booth opened the bag and peeked inside. She began to cry, too.

"Why didn't you call us and notify us?" Mr. Booth asked. "We left you the number where we could be reached."

"I don't have time to track pet owners all over the country." The veterinarian replied. "Besides, I thought you'd take the news better in person."

The Booths took their dog home and buried him. The next day, they contacted the state veterinary board and filed a grievance against the veterinarian. Later, they contacted a lawyer and brought a lawsuit against him.

Long after the family recovered from Fred's death, they dwelt on the insensitive way they were given the news. In their own ways, each of them reviewed the experience over and over and found it hard to let go of the antagonism that they felt for the veterinarian. In fact, even today, the experience continues to have a very negative influence on the way that they feel about veterinary medicine, in general.

No strategies or methods exist to allow veterinarians to break bad news painlessly. No matter how carefully veterinarians handle their clients' feelings, awkward moments and manifestations of grief will arise. Veterinarians who deliver bad news should prepare themselves to deal with shock, disbelief, anger, sadness, and even hysteria because the way in which clients react to bad news is largely unpredictable. Sometimes clients react with rage, confusion, or aimless pacing. Suspicious accusations may also be directed at the veterinarian, or clients may direct overwhelming feelings of guilt at themselves. In contrast, numbness and shock may cause some clients to appear calm, stoic, and in control. In the wake of bad news, this control can seem eerie, confusing, and grossly inappropriate.

Just as you want to sensitively "arrange reality" when you are delivering bad news by telephone, you also want to create an understanding and positive context for the face-to-face delivery of bad news. For example, in the case scenario about the Booths, the veterinarian might have begun by saying,

> "Mr. and Mrs. Booth, Danny, and Mike, I have some news
> that I'm sure will be difficult for you to hear."

He might then have gone on to describe what happened to Fred, how they
tried to save him, and how he actually died. If appropriate, he may have
also told them how and where Fred's body was held while waiting for the
family to return. Based on our experience, the Booths would focus better
on the veterinarian's words if Fred's body was not in the room at the time.
Then, afterward, if the Booths requested it, he could be brought into the
room. If Fred's body was soiled due to urination, defecation, treatment, or
surgery, the veterinarian or technician could have washed, dried, and
brushed it before presenting it to the owners to see. In addition, he could
have placed the body in a more aesthetically pleasing container and positioned it so it would be more conducive to viewing. Also, all catheters and
tape could have been removed.

Research has attempted to determine whether preparation (information
about what is about to happen and the effect it will have) facilitates subsequent physical and psychologic healing.[12] Most studies regarding preparation have been done on people who are facing surgery. These studies show
that whether or not preparatory information is helpful depends on the
person's typical mode of handling stress. In other words, people who tend
to deny or avoid stressful situations do not benefit from information about
surgery, but those with a history of attacking or facing problems head-on
do. This research underlines the need to consider individual differences in
coping styles when delivering bad news. One way to assess your clients'
coping styles is simply to ask them what they want. For example, in the
Booths' case, you might say:

> "I have more detailed information about how Fred died.
> Would you like me to give you that or have you heard all that
> you want to hear?"

Probably the best course of action when telling clients about their pets'
unexpected deaths is to provide them with the basic facts and then stand
by, prepared to listen and absorb their various emotional responses without becoming defensive, guilty, hurried, overly responsive, and without
offering intellectual explanations. When the Booths expressed their dissatisfaction with how Fred's death was handled (for example, anger that the
veterinarian did not contact them immediately instead of waiting for them
to return), the veterinarian could have listened to their concerns and then
simply apologized. He might have said:

> "I made my decision based on what I thought would be best
> for you, and I'm truly sorry if it caused you even more un-
> happiness."

SITUATION FOUR: "How Do I Sensitively Deliver Diagnoses That Have Potentially Terminal Outcomes?"

When veterinarians are uncomfortable delivering "bad" diagnoses to clients, they often relay information in booming "lecture" voices or in unemotional monotones that are void of empathy. They also tend to "protect" themselves from pet owners' potentially strong emotional reactions by placing physical and emotional barriers between themselves and their clients. Examination tables, chairs, and clipboards are all examples of protective barriers. Putting the entire expanse of the examination room between clients and themselves works for many veterinarians when nothing else is available.

The delivery of a diagnosis works better when you explain test results, radiographs, and prognoses in a soft voice with your words spoken a bit more slowly than usual. As we have said previously, it is also enhanced when discussions with clients take place in relaxed, yet structured environments in which the arrangement of furniture allows you and your clients to sit down and to have direct eye contact. The removal of physical barriers such as examination tables, desks, and clipboards also allows you to touch clients, should additional support be required.

Structuring the environment means planning ahead for potentially emotional conversations by taking control of the physical parts of the interaction. Preparations may include arranging chairs for face-to-face conversation, gathering educational props and materials, or stocking the room with facial tissues. You can even set up videotape equipment so that pet owners are able to view educational programs that are specific to their pet's disease or treatment.

People are also part of structured environments. Animal health technicians or other staff members can be helpful to clients who receive disturbing diagnoses when they take notes or draw pictures of complicated medical information as you talk. Sometimes, they can even arrange or facilitate supportive or informational meetings with other clients whose pets have similar conditions.

Some veterinarians tape-record their diagnosis deliveries and descriptions of treatment options. They give these tapes to clients so that they can literally take information home with them. Tape-recording the diagnosis allows clients to listen to the information again when they are in a more relaxed, familiar environment and also allows them to share the information with other family members. In a survey of 41 human patients whose physicians used tape recordings, 77 percent of patients wrote extremely positive comments about the technique, and no negative statements were made.[13] When delivering diagnoses, great value can be found in making written information available for patients to read.

Well-planned diagnostic presentations greatly increase clients' understanding of disease and its treatment. They also go a long way to calm clients' fears and to ease their feelings of anxiety. It cannot be overemphasized that the diagnostic encounters that occur between you and your clients set the groundwork for all other interactions that follow.

When clients have had a chance to assimilate the diagnostic news that you have told them, they may have questions like:

> "How long does my pet have?"

> "Is my pet in pain?"

and

> "How am I going to get through this?"

You can reassure them by giving them honest, concrete information and by saying something like:

> "My staff and I will help you in every way we can. We also work with a person in town who understands the love of animals and does a wonderful job helping pet owners make difficult decisions. We will give you her name."

In addition, you can help clients to mobilize their personal support systems by suggesting that they call a sympathetic friend or family member. You can assess your clients' coping skills by asking them how they usually handle crises, how they take care of themselves, and on whom they rely for support in their personal lives. If they have no one, you can help them to make connections with the counseling resources that are available through your office, your area veterinary medical society, or the community in general.

If clients exhibit extreme displays of emotion, such as panic attacks or sobbing, help them work through their waves of emotion. Never leave the room because you assume that your clients want to be alone. The act of leaving the room may communicate embarrassment and disapproval. Clients' extreme emotions may alert you to the possibility that a diagnosis is tied to another experience they have had with a similar illness, injury, or death. As long as you show genuine concern, it is okay to ask your clients:

> "What is your personal experience with this disease? Has someone close to you dealt with or died from this?"

It goes without saying that, if you are unable to spend any time with clients, you should not ask this kind of question. If you can spend some, but not great amounts of time, with upset clients, try to find another staff member or a human service professional who can, or, alternatively, have the client contact a friend or family member by phone. While they are talking, you can check in with them often.

It is not helpful to clients to discuss bad news in ambiguous, evasive ways. False promises and euphemisms do not help pet owners. In fact, such evasions can destroy the trust that clients have placed in you when they prove to be unfounded or misleading. A sympathetic, yet honest, discussion of the problem is far more beneficial because it strikes a balance between unrealistic hope and unrelenting honesty.

SITUATION FIVE: "Long-Term Treatment Takes Its Toll on Clients. How Can I Best Support Them Through the Ups and Downs?"

Most clients appreciate having the choice of several treatment options including whatever reasonable and humane alternatives exist between palliation and cure. Depending on the situation, clients can also be offered the option of taking their pet "home to die" with no further intervention. Depending on the medical status of the animal, a fourth option that can be offered is euthanasia. Two other ideas that are much appreciated by pet owners are permission to seek second opinions from other veterinarians and referrals to veterinary medical specialists.

Many believe that directing clients to specialists causes them to abandon their referring veterinarians. To the contrary, clinical experience indicates that clients appreciate their referring veterinarians much more when they realize the degree to which referrals to specialists can affect their pets' quality of life and survival. Timely referrals usually deepen pet owners' loyalty to and trust in their veterinarians.

Your two main goals during treatment are to prolong the quantity and quality of pets' lives and to successfully guide pet owners through the emotional ups and downs of treatment. Treating pets is often expensive and emotionally exhausting; therefore, any discussion of treatment options should be accompanied by a discussion of estimated costs and the value that veterinary medicine places on animals' quality of life. Quantity of life is meaningless without quality of life; however, quality of life means different things to different people. For some, it is manifested in their pets' abilities to chase balls or to greet them in the evenings. For others, it is in simply knowing that their pets are eating and sleeping through peaceful, painless days.

The quality-of-life issue that seems to hold the most significance for owners is pain. Most responsible owners are hesitant about treatment when they feel that their pets may suffer long-term or chronic pain. Most are also prepared to stop treatment when the spread of disease or extensive injuries causes their companion animals undue discomfort. When a cure is not possible, palliative procedures can improve the patient's quality of life but do not necessarily improve the odds of survival. It is within your role as a helper to help clients stay clear on the difference between quantity and quality of life.

Several predictable crisis points can occur during treatment: recurrence of disease, unexpected complications from surgery, unexpected death, and the decision to stop treatment or to euthanize. As treatment progresses, veterinarians should strike a balance between sustaining client hope and providing honest, realistic assessments about the animal's chance for recovery. Despite all of the scientific knowledge that you have at your disposal, the hard fact is that medicine at large entails a degree of uncertainty. Because you can rarely, if ever, offer clients guarantees, it is important to emphasize that, although you may advocate for certain treatments, you should never push clients to treat or not to treat. Pet owners must be comfortable with each step taken and must be assured that treatment is in their pets' best interests.

Pet owners respond to their pets' treatments in many ways. Two of the most extreme responses are fierce dedication or deep doubt. It is predictable that clients showing either of these responses are more anxious about facing the imminent deaths of their pets.

Clients who are fiercely dedicated to their pets sometimes give up huge portions of their personal lives to care for their companion animals. In extreme cases, some even spend several months sleeping on floors beside their pets or quit their jobs to be 100 percent available to them. Clients with deep doubts about treatment often second-guess each decision and begin every day with anxiety. The question, "Is today the day that Pepper will die?" is never far from their thoughts.

With advances in veterinary medicine, so many conventional and experimental treatments are available that it is easy for owners to settle into a false sense of security about never-ending treatment options. When all treatment methods fail, however, feelings of helplessness and hopelessness similar to the ones that overcame clients at the initial diagnosis resurface.

During this phase, it is your responsibility to continue to relay honest information about the amount of discomfort that the companion animal is experiencing and to gently remind clients about the low probability for quality life in the future. False hope at this time encourages denial and is ultimately unfair both to your clients and patients.

Sometimes, pet owners themselves find hope in the form of unconventional treatments. They may ask you about acupuncture, rice diets, or herbal remedies. If you are not an advocate of unconventional treatment, it is important for you to clearly state your beliefs and to let clients know that, in your opinion, they may even compromise their pets' chances for survival. If clients persist, however, you should refrain from skeptical or cynical comments about any unorthodox treatments that clients may suggest. These options may seem to you like naive attempts at treatment, but some veterinarians have seen them work! More importantly, unconventional treatments often allow pet owners to feel that they are providing their companion animals with every chance for recovery and that they are continuing to participate actively in their pets' treatment.

As you continue to monitor the progression of your patients' illnesses or injuries, you can discuss with owners what signals to watch for as death draws near. As we said in Chapter 8, you can encourage owners to establish personal "bottom lines" for their pets' levels of deterioration. For some, the bottom line is their pet's lack of interest in eating or in going for walks. For others, it is the agony of watching their pet struggle to breathe or to "get comfortable." For many clients, it is either their pet's inability to respond to them or their pet's struggle to muster even a small response that aids their final decision to euthanize. Clinical experience shows that most pet owners "know" instinctively when their pets' fight to stay alive is over and that their decision to euthanize is supported by treatment team members most of the time (Fig. 13-1).

Although agreement may exist about timing, the euthanasia of a companion animal after intense treatment is an emotionally draining experience for everyone involved in the case. Results from studies in human medicine show that deaths after long, lingering illnesses are among the hardest losses that people face.[14] Survivors often feel exhausted after they have cared for loved ones who have lingered and who have needed considerable physical care during and after treatment. These findings are equally relevant to pet loss. Like human caregivers, pet owners and veterinary professionals who provide extensive nursing care for pets frequently struggle with conflicting feelings of grief and relief after their pets die.

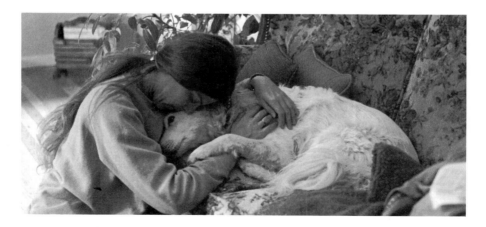

Figure 13-1 Spending time with companion animals is one of the best ways to make decisions regarding their medical needs.   PHOTO COURTESY OF BARBARA MILLMAN.

SITUATION SIX: "How Can I Help Clients Who Can't Make the Decision to Euthanize Their Pets?"

One of the most difficult times for pet owners, and for you, comes when euthanasia decisions are needed, but when pet owners are unwilling or unable to say their final goodbyes. In Chapter 8, we discussed some basic ways to support clients in the decision-making process that precedes euthanasia. We suggested what you could say and do to help clients to clarify their wishes regarding their animals' deaths, thus minimizing regrets later. At times, however, clients who struggle with the decision to euthanize get "stuck" in the process and need additional guidance from you. Several strategies are helpful during these times.

First, when helping owners make euthanasia decisions, be sure that they know that you fully understand the difficulty of the decision-making process. You can do so by validating how difficult it is to know when the exact time to end a life has come. You can also acknowledge your clients' relationships with their animals, their shared histories, and the immediate circumstances that make euthanasia especially difficult. Also, early in your conversation, you can ask clients about their philosophic positions regarding the subject of euthanasia. Some people, particularly those in the medical professions, are uncomfortable with euthanasia. Others may be opposed to it for religious or ethical reasons (for example, activists who promote animal rights). Also, as discussed in Chapters 8 and 9, you should review the euthanasia procedure to ensure that it is clearly understood. It is impossible for clients to see euthanasia as a helpful option if they do not truly understand it.

This aim is facilitated, in part, by giving clients accurate and detailed information about their animals' condition, the medical procedures necessary to sustain life, and the actual euthanasia procedure. These detailed descriptions are essential when helping clients gain clarity about choices to prolong or stop life. Also, be sure that clients clearly understand their animals' suffering. If possible, relate suffering to a human illness so pet owners are able to empathize with their pets. Say, for example:

> "Right now, Moose is probably feeling like we do when we have a really vicious flu. It hurts just to move and it is impossible for him to get comfortable. His temperature is extremely high and he is having a hard time breathing. He is frequently crying out and I believe he is experiencing quite a bit of pain. Unfortunately, there is no longer anything I can do to relieve his symptoms and, from now on, the odds are high that he will only get worse."

It is also helpful to share your perspective and observations with clients. For example, you can say:

> "You see Shadow every day, but I only see her once a week. Since I don't see her decline gradually, the deterioration caused by her disease seems more dramatic to me. For instance, I can tell you that, since I saw her last, she has changed considerably. She has lost weight and muscle tone and she is far less responsive than she was last week."

If animals are hospitalized, allowing owners to visit them may also help them to understand the gravity of their pets' situations. Whenever possible, you should arrange for owners to take their animals home for several hours, or even overnight so that they can experience first-hand the amount of care that their animals require as well as the amount of pain that their animals are experiencing. In most cases, when pet owners are forced to interact with their suffering pets, their denial is broken, and a decision to euthanize is reached.

Second, because euthanasia is a threatening topic, pet owners are better able to explore the possibility of euthanizing their pets if they are given opportunities to incrementally incorporate information about it. In other words, most clients cannot change directions as quickly as veterinarians and make the leap from trying to save their animals to helping them die. You can help clients bridge this gap between "trying" and "dying" by first introducing the idea that the time to think about saying goodbye has arrived. Your hope is to help them turn their focus from continuing to strive to provide their pets with an ever-diminishing quality of life to providing them with a quality death.

Bridging the gap between "trying" and "dying" is also facilitated by helping clients to explore their feelings (often subconscious) and concerns about letting go of their pets. Some questions that may help clients during this time are:

> "What would a quality death look like?"

> "How will you say goodbye?"

> "When you look back on CP's death, what kinds of things will be important to you about how he died?"

> "What is the worse thing that could happen regarding Sandy's death?"

Most pet owners respond to these questions by saying that they want the chance to say goodbye to their pets and that they do not want their pets to suffer or die without them. This occasion provides an opportunity for you to talk about the possible consequences of waiting to euthanize, because clients are unlikely to get what they want if euthanasia is delayed. During this time, for example, you might say:

"Although there is nothing more we can do for Angie medically, there is a lot we can do for her—and for you—emotionally. Let's turn our attention to finding ways to make the last hours or days that you have with Angie emotionally satisfying and meaningful."

Then help clients find special ways to say goodbye and to make decisions about body care, memorials, and timing of euthanasia.

If the above questions do not help your clients move toward euthanasia, additional questions may be helpful. The purpose of this new line of questioning is to ensure that pet owners' actions are based in reality. To paraphrase decision-making expert Spencer Johnson, poor decisions are based on illusions that we believe at the time, and better decisions are based on realities we recognize in time.[15] These questions are designed to help clients recognize the realities of their pets' situations in time to spare clients and patients further emotional and physical pain. They must be asked sensitively, without any sense of judgment in your voice, and prefaced with a comment like:

"I am going to ask you something that may be difficult for you to hear."

Then ask, for example:

"If you prolong Derby's life, is it for you or for her?"

"Are you hoping that Griffin will die on his own so you can avoid making the decision to help him die?"

"Are you telling yourself that the euthanasia will be easier tomorrow or several days or weeks from now?"

If the client answers "yes" to this last question, you need to explore the reasons why this might be true. For example, the client's spouse may be currently out of town, but will be home in a few days. On the other hand, no concrete reasons may exist to warrant a delay in the procedure, and the client may be operating under the illusion that time will ease the emotional pain. If so, you can extend your discussion to include statements like the following:

"I want to assure you that it will not be any easier emotionally to euthanize Griffin later on. The reality is that you will never be completely ready to say goodbye to this wonderful friend. It is going to hurt no matter when his death occurs."

Caring for hopelessly ill animals is also difficult for veterinary professionals. We recall one case in which the decision-making process became so prolonged and intense that, after the procedure was completed, the relieved veterinarian gently said to the client, "On behalf of Rocky and all sick or hurt animals everywhere, thank you for letting him go." As this example shows, these cases take their toll, so we strongly recommend that you also find support for handling your own stress.

In a small number of cases (probably less than 1 percent of your clientele), you will need to tell clients that you can no longer ethically treat their animals. These statements about stopping treatment should only be made after all other avenues for facilitating clients' decision-making have been exhausted. Clients should not be forced to euthanize but should be given the option of seeking treatment from another veterinarian.

On the other side of the coin, when pets are critically ill or injured, very little time is available to plan and to make decisions. However, the need to do so does not change. Putting aside, for now, decision-making regarding treatment options, if pets are not going to survive their injuries or illnesses, owners still need to make decisions about presence at euthanasia and body care options. They may, however, have only 5 minutes to decide instead of 5 weeks or 5 months. When decisions must be made quickly, you will need to give owners very clear information about their choices and as much time as possible to make decisions (without compromising the animal's well-being). You can tell owners, for example, that they will need to tell you within the next 10 minutes whether they want to be present. You should then provide any information that they may need to make their decisions as well as private time (perhaps with other family members) to discuss the matter.

If necessary, body care decisions can be made after euthanasias occur; however, owners may not be prepared to make that decision quickly. Owners may want to talk with other family members who may not be present or may need time to think about their options. Other family members may also want to view the body. Under these circumstances, you can offer to hold the body for a reasonable period until a decision can be made.

If clients choose to view their pets' bodies after euthanasia, they should be well-prepared for the experience. They should be told exactly what to expect (for example, the pet's eyes will be open, the body may be stiff or cold, depending on how recently death occurred). If the pet suffered a traumatic accident or died during surgery, you should also tell the client what injuries or incisions they will see. If the body is quite disfigured, it can be wrapped in a towel or blanket, allowing the client to see only the head. Clients also benefit from being told what they can do while viewing their pets. Thus, it is helpful when veterinarians tell clients that they can touch, hold, or even groom their pets' bodies.

SITUATION SEVEN: "Many Clients Feel Responsible for Their Pets' Deaths. How Can I Help Clients Deal with Guilt?"

Guilt is the critic, the inner voice that judges thoughts, actions, behaviors, decisions, and feelings. If clients have tendencies toward feeling responsibility or fault for any and all events that happen, they probably have an overall orientation toward guilt. This tendency probably comes from childhood experiences and the messages received from parents and teachers as well as from societal expectations.

Sometimes guilt is justified, and other times it is not. For example, some clients do something to cause or precipitate their pets' deaths. They may be negligent or abusive in the way they treat their companion animals or they may knowingly take part in potentially dangerous situations such as walking their pets off-leash along busy, urban streets. In these cases, feelings of guilt are probably justified.

Justified or not, however, guilt is common, even when clients could have done nothing to prevent whatever happened to their pets. For example, many clients feel guilty when their pets are diagnosed with terminal illnesses such as cancer or congestive heart failure because they feel that they should have noticed their pets' symptoms sooner. In addition, many clients feel guilty after electing to stop treatment or after euthanizing their pets, even if their decisions were clearly in their animals' best interests. In these cases, guilt probably stems from the owners' beliefs that they have breached the "contracts" that they made with their pets—contracts that focused on keeping their pets alive, safe, and healthy. The help that you offer clients who feel guilty varies according to whether or not their guilt is justified.

When guilt *is* justified, you cannot make the guilty feelings disappear. Even if you say, "Don't feel so bad," or "It wasn't your fault," clients know that you are not telling the truth. They know it really *was* their fault, and their guilty feelings usually remain. As a helper, it is important for you to remember that you cannot change or "fix" another person's guilty feelings. What you can do is acknowledge their guilt and create opportunities for them to work through them. For example, if a client let his dog walk off-leash and the dog was hit by a car and killed, you might say something like:

> "I can see how guilty you feel about this, Mark, and I know you would do anything to turn back the clock and do this day over."

You might follow this statement by asking your client what he might want to say to his dog, in terms of saying goodbye or even apologizing for the

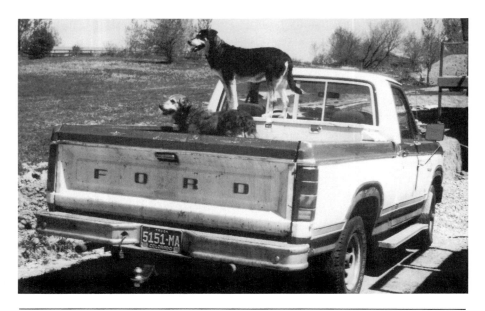

Figure 13-2 Many potential health risks exist for animals. When pets are accidently injured or killed, most owners feel guilty.

accident. Some clients even like the idea of writing a letter to their pet or of compensating for their negligence by donating to or volunteering with an animal-related organization.

Client guilt is also present, and somewhat justified, even when accidents are unforeseen or unpreventable. Such accidents might include chemical or antifreeze poisoning, deaths that occur while animals are being boarded or transported, or deaths that occur from improper care or feeding of animals (Fig. 13-2). Ways to help clients deal with this kind of guilt are to (1) gently ask them to stop judging themselves and (2) to help them learn from their experiences. When people stop judging themselves, they begin to understand that they did the best they could at the time, given the information that was available to them. Many realize that, logically, they could not have prevented their pets' deaths because they did not know that the danger existed. After they have gained this perspective, many clients have the ability to learn a positive lesson from an otherwise negative experience.

Quite often, clients who have learned a lesson from pet loss want to share their newfound knowledge with others. In general, they attempt to educate and enlighten other pet owners so other animals will not meet the same fate, thus reassuring them that their own pets did not die in vain. We have had many clients who turned their experiences with pet loss into valuable community services. For example, one client, whose small dog died of acute antifreezing poisoning, learned after her pet's death that resort owners often winterize the toilets in their mountain cabins by pouring antifreeze in them. She and her family had spent the weekend in one of these cabins and her dog had probably developed kidney failure because she had, on several occasions, drunk water from the toilet. Although this client had no knowledge of this winterizing practice before her pet's death, she felt guilty because, ultimately, her dog's death could have been prevented. To assuage her guilt, she created a handout for resort patrons, educating and warning them of this practice. She distributed the flyers among all of the mountain resorts in the area. She also wrote a letter to the editor of the local newspaper and spread the word about antifreeze poisoning in whatever way she could. Later, her guilt felt lessened because, in her heart, she believed that she prevented the deaths of many other companion animals.

Most clients who feel guilty also feel embarrassed that they placed their pets in danger by making inappropriate decisions or by engaging in questionable activities. Thus, on some level, they are also wondering how this event has affected your opinion of them. If you can separate the person from the behavior, you can probably honestly say something like:

> "Jack, I can see that this mistake is making you feel terribly guilty. However, I believe you are a responsible and conscientious pet owner who never intended to bring any harm to Scrooge."

This statement won't do much to alleviate your client's guilt, but it will reassure him that you still support him and don't wish to see him "punish" himself over the accident.

When guilt is *not* justified, it is equally difficult to "make the guilty feelings go away." Some clients, no matter what you say, will remain convinced that the little, seemingly insignificant things they did or did not do caused their companion animals' deaths. We had one client, for example, who believed that his dog's lung cancer was caused by sleeping next to the toilet and another who believed that her horse died prematurely because she failed to ride him every day. Clients hold these beliefs for a multitude of reasons, none of which are within the scope of your abilities (or responsibilities!) to resolve. The best you can do to help chronically guilty clients is to review the medical facts and acknowledge the guilt that they are feeling.

Guilt is also *not* justified when clients decide to euthanize a very sick or injured pet, although, to some extent, it is almost always present. Again, the feelings of guilt that arise after euthanasia can't be completely taken away, but they can be minimized. As a helper, you can gently tell clients that people often use guilt to distract themselves from the pain, sadness, and loneliness that accompany grief. You can also remind clients that you consider euthanasia to be a privilege and a gift. You can also say something like:

> "Medically, you did everything you could possibly do for
> Pistol and, in the end, you gave him a peaceful death. If you
> could do this all over again, would you do anything differ-
> ent?"

After reviewing their decisions, clients *usually* respond to this question by saying "no" and by feeling reassured that they acted in their pets' best interests each step of the way.

Occasionally, you will see clients who deserve to feel guilty. Perhaps they have been grossly negligent or even abusive to their pets. In these cases, your goal is not to alleviate your clients' guilt, but to act as an advocate for the animal. In most instances, these are not the kinds of clients you want to cultivate. Rather, they are the ones you want to report to the authorities and hopefully prevent from owning other animals in the future.

SITUATION EIGHT: "Some Clients Mention Suicide and I Don't Know if They Mean It or Not. What Do I Do?"

There are no clear-cut socioeconomic patterns that predict suicidal intent, but age and gender differences do seem to exist.[16] At present, elderly people have the highest suicide rates, and suicide is the third most common cause of death among adolescents 15 to 19 years of age and the second leading cause of death for college students and young adults between the ages of 20 to 24. Also, men comprise three fourths of all suicides each year. Occasionally, you may encounter clients who make comments like:

> "If Lady dies, I don't think I can go on."

> "I can't imagine my life without Duke."

> "When this cat dies, I just might go with her!"

Remarks such as these are probably normal reactions to impending loss. It is difficult for many pet owners to imagine what their daily routines will be like without their pets. Thus, losing such significant relationships can feel overwhelming.

On rare occasions, however, clients may be seriously considering sui- cide if their animal dies. Therefore, you need to know how to determine

BOX 13-3

Suicide Facts and Myths

There are many myths about suicide. The following represents a partial list.

- Myth: People who talk about suicide do not commit suicide.
  Fact: Of any ten persons who kill themselves, eight have given definite warnings of their suicidal intentions.

- Myth: Suicide happens without warning.
  Fact: Studies reveal that people who are suicidal give many clues and warnings regarding their suicidal intentions.

- Myth: Suicidal people are fully intent on dying.
  Fact: Most suicidal people are undecided about living or dying and "gamble with death," leaving it to others to save them. Most attempt to let others know how they are feeling.

- Myth: Once people are suicidal, they are suicidal forever.
  Fact: People who wish to kill themselves are suicidal for a limited period of time.

- Myth: Improvement following a suicidal crisis means the suicidal risk is over.
  Fact: Most suicides occur within about three months following the beginning of "improvement," when people have the energy to put their suicidal plans into effect.

- Myth: Suicide strikes much more often among the rich or, conversely, it occurs most exclusively among the poor.
  Fact: Suicide is neither the rich man's disease nor the poor man's curse. Suicide is very "democratic" and is represented proportionately among all levels of society.

This list is adapted from one originally formulated by E. Schneidman in 1952 and later published by Schneidman, E., and Mandelkorn, P.: How to prevent suicide. In Schneidman, E., Farberow, N., and Litman, R. (eds.): The Psychology of Suicide. New York, Science House, 1970.

the difference between a normal grief reaction and a potential suicide. You also need to know the limits of your responsibility in the latter situation.

Many myths exist about suicide (Box 13-3). One common myth is that, if you ask people directly about their suicidal intentions, you will somehow condone the act, thus encouraging them to kill themselves. Actually the opposite is true. Asking someone directly if they are planning to kill themselves can lower their anxiety level and make the event less likely to occur. Even so, when confronted with a suicide threat, people often respond with something like:

> "You don't want to do that. Think how much you have to be grateful for."

A comment like this not only shuts down the conversation, it makes people who are already feeling guilty about having suicidal thoughts feel even more guilty. It also serves to drive them further into feelings of isolation because they become convinced that no one else understands how they feel. A better way to handle clients' suicidal statements is to deal directly with reality. To do so, you should ask specific questions about how your clients feel and why they would want to die. Also, you should not use euphemisms about death. Euphemisms connote anxiety with the subject matter at hand. If you, as a helper, are too anxious to talk about suicide, you will not be able to help your clients deal realistically with feelings.

When talking to clients about your concerns regarding suicide, your own embarrassment about possibly misreading their comments or intruding on their private thoughts is secondary to ensuring that their lives are not in jeopardy. Think about how you would feel if you did not ask about suicide and your worst fears were realized. A few direct questions can provide you with the information you need to assess the situation. However, too many questions can sound like an interrogation. Simply ask your client:

"Are you thinking of killing yourself if Lady dies?"

Most often the client's answer to your question will be something like:

"No, of course not. I'm just so upset—I don't want to lose her."

In this case, you can calm down and be fairly sure that your client's comments represent a normal grief reaction. However, if the answer is something other than that, something like:

"Yes, I've thought about it from time to time. She's all I have."

you should take steps to first, assess the lethality of your clients' situation; second, support your clients through their immediate crisis; and third, either refer your clients to an appropriate human service agency or professional or contact the appropriate resources yourself.

How do you accomplish these tasks? First, all suicidal comments and threats should be taken seriously. Suicidal people usually are not mentally ill but have become so distressed and distraught that they have evolved a very narrowed range of options and, ultimately, are unable to see any other solution to their problems. Most persons who attempt suicide, however, are ambivalent about the act. That is, they do not truly want to kill themselves, they simply want to find an end to their overwhelming feelings of emotional pain. Due to this ambivalence, most people who commit suicide have given some previous indication of their intentions.

In studies of traits that often lead to suicide, three words crop up repeatedly. They are loss, loneliness, and hopelessness. Everyone experiences these feelings once in awhile, but those who are suicidal are overwhelmed by them. People who are suicidal generally believe that they cannot be helped because their problems seem too huge to surmount. Clients who are suicidal may have recently suffered other losses such as divorce or the death of a family member. They may have confided a history of sexual or physical abuse, or you may have noticed symptoms of drug or alcohol abuse. People who are suicidal have often interacted with various helping agencies and counselors, yet feel that they have received little or no help and, consequently, are going to continue to suffer for the rest of their lives. Thus, they see no reason to continue living.

Your degree of aggressiveness in ensuring that potentially suicidal clients receive help depends partially on what is called the "lethality" of their situations. To assess lethality, you need to determine whether your clients have specific plans for killing themselves and how quickly they could put their plans into action. For example, has your client collected medication and determined the dosage that would be fatal? Does your client now have the bottle of pills in hand, or would the client have to first obtain a prescription and then go to the drugstore to pick them up? You also need to assess if the method your client has chosen has a high probability of quick success (for example, slashing wrists compared with using a handgun). You also need to ascertain whether your client is isolated and alone or in close proximity to someone who can help.

If suicidal clients are not in immediate danger, encourage them to call a crisis or suicide hotline, a friend or relative, their family physician, a member of the clergy, or a therapist if they have one. You may also choose to call one of these persons yourself on their behalf. If you decide that you *must* notify someone, always tell clients of your intentions. Explain that, if they are unwilling to make the call themselves, you will make the call for them. Try to say this in a firm, supportive way rather than in a scolding or threatening manner. At this point, most clients will agree to call someone.

Some helpers attempt to make contracts with suicidal clients, insisting they agree to call them before they carry through with a plan. In general, this approach is not a good idea for veterinarians. If clients call you during a time when the lethality of the situation is high, you may quickly be in "over your head" in terms of your training and capabilities as a helper. If veterinarians receive calls from suicidal clients, they may also be tempted to directly intervene to try to prevent a death. You should never go to a client's house or attempt to rescue them, no matter where they may be. Suicidal clients do have the potential to turn homicidal, and your own life could be in danger if you attempt any kind of direct intervention.

Just because you have established helping relationships with your clients does not mean that you personally play a significant role in preventing their potential suicides. In fact, your main role is probably to stall for time until the professionals that you or your clients have contacted reach them. If, by questioning clients, you determine that they are in a position to complete a suicide, the lethality can be considered high and you should take steps to support them through their immediate crises *and* to contact someone who is trained to intervene in suicide.

In your position as a paraprofessional helper, the overriding strategy for suicide intervention is to halt any self-destructive behavior during that dark, crisis time when your client feels total despair. In most cases, people are only suicidal for a short time. Soon after, they gain control, restructure their lives, and go on. Therefore, the best intervention that you can use is to get help. In most communities, help is not difficult to find. For example, suicide or crisis intervention centers all across the country are staffed with qualified people whom you can call for advice or debriefing. In addition, many mental health agencies have a professional on staff who is authorized to hospitalize people (on a short-term basis) for observation and for their own protection. Many hospitals also offer this service. Finally, the most effective and immediate action that you can take is to call the police. The rule of thumb in determining whether to contact law enforcement authorities is to do so whenever someone makes a serious threat to do "harm to self or others." This code is used by police officers as a guide for intervening in potentially dangerous situations. After notification of your concerns about suicide, the police can do what is called a "welfare check." That is, they can locate your client and either intervene to prevent a suicide that is occurring or make sure that the danger of suicide is not imminent.

Surprisingly, people often commit suicide when their symptoms of depression seem to be improving. During this time, they become more communicative and resume many of their former activities. Seeing this behavior, their family and friends relax, believing the suicide crisis has passed. All too often, however, when those around them least expect it, suicidal people take their own lives. Two possible reasons explain this occurrence.

First, depression saps people of their energy and sense of purpose, and they need these resources to find the motivation to take action. In other words, in depressed states, people may want to kill themselves, but simply cannot find the energy to plan and carry through with it. As the most severe symptoms of depression lift, however, the ability to think more clearly and to act more forcefully returns, and suicide often becomes a reality.

The second reason is that, when deeply depressed persons actually make the decision to take their own lives, their resolve to carry out their plans may offer them profound relief. They may release all of the tension, anxiety, and worry that has gone into their decision-making process and feel that their spirits have been lifted and that their attitude and outlook on life has been greatly improved. People who are suicidal may actually enjoy their final days, making plans and looking forward to the end of their troubles.

Although the death of a pet may precipitate a suicide reaction, it has also been reported that clients preparing for suicide may bring their pets in for euthanasia so that they will not be left without care. One veterinarian told us about the following case:

> "In my first year of practice, an elderly client of mine brought in each of her three dogs over a span of several months for euthanasia. Since I knew that she really loved these dogs I was concerned about her decision to euthanize. When I questioned her about it she said that they got under her feet and she was afraid she would fall and hurt herself. Although I wasn't satisfied with the answer, I felt that I shouldn't pursue the matter. I had heard that some older folks prepared for suicide by euthanizing their pets but I didn't know how to bring it up. I didn't think I should. Two days after I euthanized the last of her three dogs, she killed herself. After twenty years of practice, it still bothers me."

Although thoughts of and even comments about suicide are quite common, truly suicidal clients are uncommon. Chances are that you will never encounter one. If you do, you should talk with a trained human service professional who can advise you as to what actions to take and about who can also support you. Being involved in someone's attempted or completed suicide can be devastating. If it happens, you will need to talk to someone about it. Above all, no one can assume responsibility for someone else's life, and you will need to be reassured that you were not responsible, either directly or indirectly, for your client's decision.

SITUATION NINE: "How Can I Diffuse a Client's Anger?"

Practitioners cannot completely avoid belligerent, angry clients. Although such persons represent only about 5 percent of a typical practice, they can cause 95 percent of its human relations problems.[17] When clients are angry, it is worth your while to find out why, because, to paraphrase veterinarian and practice management consultant Dennis McCurnin, if the problem is not resolved, you can lose a client, receive bad word of mouth publicity about your practice, and never know what you can do to prevent future problems.[17]

Our clinical experience shows that most client anger stems from minor, correctable issues like billing errors, appointment delays, and hurt feelings. McCurnin adds that, in general, most client dissatisfaction stems from misunderstandings concerning fees, performance of unauthorized services, and undesirable results of treatment or services. No matter what the cause, most angry clients want to be taken seriously, heard, and offered apologies, if appropriate.

If you are like most people, listening and apologizing may seem out of the question when you are confronted with anger. Being the target of anger probably makes you feel scared, vulnerable, and insecure. It might also make you worry that you will be blamed for something that you did not do *or* punished for something that you did! Anger may also make you feel concerned that your client may turn destructive and that you might be threatened or even hurt.

As we said about guilt, you learned how to react to anger during your childhood. If you have had no reason to consciously learn to respond to anger in a different, more adult way, you probably still revert to childlike behaviors when someone becomes angry at you. Chances are that, as a child, you reacted to anger by either feeling victimized, learning to cower and take anger into yourself, or by feeling defensive, learning to yell, fight back, and become angry yourself. Adult tantrums are probably manifestations of tactics learned during childhood. These tactics arise when people feel powerless and vulnerable, and they help them cope with fear, frustration, and helplessness. As a child, you learned these tactics worked because it got you what you wanted.

As Lorrainne Bilodeau writes in her book *The Anger Workbook*:

> Emotions were never meant to be destructive or harmful. In fact, the opposite is true. An emotion is a physiological sensation, the same as hunger. Like hunger, which signals the need for nourishment, each feeling functions to satisfy or warn of a human need. For this reason, feelings cannot be classified as 'good' or 'bad,' 'positive' or 'negative.' They are merely utilitarian. It is therefore counterproductive to curb or control emotions, release them, resolve them, or ventilate them. Instead, it is necessary to recognize each feeling, understand its function, and then choose a behavior that responds to that function. . .
>
> Anger is no exception. . . . It is not the emotion that is destructive, but the way a person expresses it.[18] (p. 95)

What does this quote have to teach us about coping with client anger? It suggests that you should not focus so much on the emotion of anger itself, but on the way in which it is being expressed. In short, you probably should not try to fix, change, or eliminate your client's angry feelings. However, it might be effective if you address and attempt to modify the way in which clients express anger (Box 13-4).

BOX 13-4

How to Deal with Anger

Many clients use anger to cope with feelings of fear, frustration, and helplessness. Since excuses and defensive comments usually increase these feelings, they are ineffective when dealing with anger. There are many more positive actions that can be used.

- *Keep your cool.* Responding in like fashion to any tirades usually escalates conflict. In most cases, arguments become polarized into "I'm right" and "You're wrong" power struggles, leaving little or no room for compromise. The best approach is to stay calm and help clients regain control.
- *Conduct discussion in private.* An audience often adds "fuel to the fire." Thus, discussions involving anger should take place in private. Ask irate clients to join you in a private area. This allows you to gain some control over the situation. It also interrupts their angry outbursts, helping the client to "cool down."
- *Let clients vent.* Angry clients usually feel better after "letting off steam." More times than not, they don't mean to attack you personally. Rather, you are most likely the handiest target. Don't take angry attacks and abusive language personally, but do let clients know when your own limits have been reached *before* you get angry yourself.
- *Get clients to sit down with you.* Sitting is a less aggressive posture. It also allows you to make better use of nonverbal communication techniques such as direct eye contact, open body posture, and touching.
- *Use clients' names.* Calling clients by name gets their attention and helps establish rapport.
- *Listen and demonstrate empathy for client concerns.* Determine what your clients' problems are and restate their problems using paraphrase and remarks such as, "Yes, I understand." Also, find some basis for agreement and compromise. Demonstrate your flexibility with comments like, "You have a point there." Avoid the word "but" as it tends to negate everything that was said prior to its use. Once clients know you are not hostile and have their interests at heart, you are much better positioned to resolve their problems.

Adapted from McCurnin, D. M.: The vocal minority: Difficult clients and how to deal with them. Topics in Veterinary Medicine, Summer 1990, pp. 5–12.

The best way to accomplish this task is to not become defensive. Everyone has the right to feel angry, but they do not have the right to use that anger to hurt others. The key to dealing with anger, therefore, is to not take it personally. In other words, the key is to *respond* to anger rather than *react* to it. A difference exists between reacting and responding. One definition for the word "react" is to reply with revulsion or to behave in a reverse or contrary way.[19] This definition implies the need to balance or to counter anothers' words or actions. When you react, for example, you dig in your heels and insist that you are right whenever clients accuse you of being wrong (even if you know deep inside that your clients have some valid points). In the process of balancing or countering your clients' points of view, you succeed only in polarizing the argument between you. When angry arguments get polarized, the relationship reaches an impasse, and usually no room remains for compromise or for resolution.

In contrast, one of the definitions for the word "respond" is to show sensitivity to behavior or change.[19] To respond, therefore, means to recognize and acknowledge what the behaviors of others mean in regard to their needs and feelings. When you respond, you "keep your cool" rather than rush in with your anger or defensive excuses to balance the argument. In short, you "see the big picture" and go with the argument rather than fight against it. Responding keeps the sides of an argument from becoming polarized. In summary, if you are reacting to anger, you are taking someone else's words and behaviors personally, and if you are responding, you are not.

Occasions arise, however, in which people make you a target for their anger and express their feelings in the form of verbal attack. In these situations, Ms. Bilodeau[18] suggests that you use a calm, but firm voice and say something like:

> "I'm willing to listen to you as long as you stop attacking me."

> "I want to hear what you're angry about and I can't while you continue to put me down."

If your client refuses to calm down and discuss the problem rationally, you need to be assertive and excuse yourself and leave. Alternatively, you can ask your client to leave.

When clients calm down enough to discuss the issue at hand, you must use your active listening skills to truly hear what they are saying. You can paraphrase what they are telling you to be sure that you understand the information correctly. If you discover a discrepancy between what you are hearing and what your client is saying, you can ask for further clarification. You can let clients know that you are trying to understand their positions and their side of the story. Also, you can ask for specific details and substantiation about the accusations.

After listening to the details of your clients' arguments, your response should be honest. If your clients are right, and you did make a mistake or overlook their feelings, tell them the truth and then ask if, together, you can find a way to work to develop a plan for resolving the conflict. Honesty and compromise may seem difficult, but it is the way mature, responsible professionals respond to anger. It is important for the sake of your own ethics and integrity to take responsibility for your actions.

If, on the other hand, you did not make a mistake or intentionally hurt your clients' feelings, present the facts as *you* see them. When you genuinely believe in yourself and in the facts of a situation, you do not have to defend your actions. Your sincerity will be naturally communicated through your eye contact, facial expressions, postures, and body language. Your case will stand on its own.

You must remember an important point when dealing with client anger. Simply because you are attempting to respond to anger in a calm, adult way, does not mean that your client will respond to your efforts. Thus, after trying to help and to resolve the situation, you can do nothing if clients will not accept your attempts to negotiate. They may want to continue with their tantrums, and they may want to hang on to their anger because anger may have an extremely useful purpose in their lives. It may act to cover up and defend against the real emotions they are feeling, which are deep sadness and hurt.

When clients are grieving, it is often preferable for them to continue to blame and to feel angry with you than to go beyond their emotional defenses and experience the genuine hurt and pain of loss, particularly among men. As we said in Chapter 12, during grief, men are more likely than women to react with anger. This anger often translates into physical or legal action. Sometimes, after you have sincerely and actively listened to your clients' complaints, it helps to gently point this out to them. For example, you might say something like:

> "You know, Bob, I can hear that you're feeling angry, yet I can also see that, underneath your anger is the sadness, loneliness, and grief you feel over losing Midnight."

A statement like this can be risky because, although it might "break the ice" and allow you to really help clients deal with grief, it might also make them feel more vulnerable and exposed, thus, in turn, making them feel even angrier. If anger is the route that clients choose, they will have to decide for themselves when and whether to believe or forgive you. They will also have to decide for themselves when and whether they are ready to grieve. In the meantime, you can be assured that you have done your part and that the rest is up to them.

SITUATION TEN: "How Do I Handle Threats or Homicidal Clients?"

As with clients who are suicidal, clients who are homicidal are extremely rare; however, you should never rely on this statistic. If you suspect that a person's anger may be expressed violently, get away! Your responsibility as a helper never extends to remaining in a place or near a person where you may be in imminent danger. Get away from the source of potential harm and seek professional intervention from the police. When confronted by a person who is homicidal, it is important to remember three facts:

- You did not cause the violent behavior.
- The behavior will not stop automatically.
- You have every right to seek help.

Police officers are trained to assist people who are in potentially violent situations. Never worry that contacting the authorities may be an over-reaction to a homicidal threat. As the old saying goes, you are better off safe than sorry—or dead!

In her seminars and staff trainings, Susan Cohen, Director of Counseling at New York's Animal Medical Center, makes the following recommendations (personal communication) about dealing with clients who may be threatening or homicidal.

1. If your client appears to be emotionally disturbed, but not threatening:
   - Relax.
   - Treat the client with ordinary respect.
   - Go along with the client's delusion (for example, "Okay, Miss Frank, let's see if Snowball has fireants in her ears").
   - Stay on the subject and stay in the present. Don't get sidetracked (for example, "That's very interesting, Mr. Martin, but let's try to help Blackie with his tooth problem").
2. If your client threatens you in general:
   - Try to prevent the situation from becoming worse by:
     a) Staying calm (for example, breathing deeply).
     b) Avoiding arguments.
   - Try to keep a clear route to an unlocked door.
   - Do not crowd the client or box him in.
3. If your client threatens you, but has no weapon:
   - Try to get help by signalling someone.
   - If necessary, run.
   - Yell for help. Don't be afraid to embarrass yourself.
   - Do not use force if you can avoid it.
4. If the client has a weapon:
   - Speak softly.
   - Speak as little as possible.
   - Do not look the client in the eye, because this appears challenging.
   - Defer in actions and words. Say, "You're in control here, Mr. Dunne. Tell me what you want me to do."
   - Make no sudden or unexplained moves. Say, "Lucky's file is in the top drawer of my cabinet. Do you want me to get it?"

- Do not challenge the client or try to counsel him or her. Do not say, "Now Mr. Dunne, put down that gun. You know you don't really want to do this."

Beyond these ideas, whether you are able to get out of potentially dangerous situations depends, in great part, on the condition of homicidal clients and on what they choose to do. For example, a 1986 survey of prisoners who were convicted of violent crimes showed that 53.5 percent admitted to being under the influence of alcohol, drugs, or a combination of both when they committed the acts for which they were imprisoned.[18] When alcohol or other drugs are involved, it is almost impossible to change people's anger or patterns of aggression until the substance abuse stops. Alcohol and drugs cloud people's thought processes, distort reality, and impair judgment. Thus, when you are dealing with a substance-abusing person, the danger obviously increases.

Perhaps the best way to deal with potentially dangerous or homicidal situations is to take steps to prevent them altogether. If you work in an unsafe area, do not work alone or late at night. If you are forced to work alone, do not agree to see unfamiliar clients or those who are known to be emotionally unstable. If you work in an emergency clinic where evening and late night hours are part of your job, have an emergency plan in place. For example, train your staff to handle potentially violent situations by contacting the proper authorities. You can also be sure that both you and your staff have adequate access to an emergency alarm system and that you have code words or signals that alert one another to your need for immediate help. In extreme cases, it may even be worthwhile to hire a security guard or to install a security door. The bottom line is that you need to take whatever precautions are necessary to protect your own life and the lives of your coworkers. Do not ever minimize the threat of danger and, if you find yourself in danger, do not attempt to be a hero. Get help however and wherever you can.

SITUATION ELEVEN: "How Can I Handle Clients Who Can't Afford or Don't Want to Pay a Fair Price for Veterinary Services?"

Almost every veterinarian has heard comments similar to the following:

"You mean you'd let him die because I can't pay for that expensive surgery? Isn't his life worth anything to you? Why can't you do it for free? You're a veterinarian, you're supposed to love animals!"

When an animal's life is hanging in the balance, most veterinarians find it very difficult to react in rational ways to impassioned pleas such as that shown above. This is because a wide range of emotions, often including anger, resentment, guilt, and fear, are triggered immediately by the client's implied accusation of professional insensitivity. Perhaps you get triggered because a part of you agrees with the client, and you find yourself wondering,

> "I don't want this animal to die, so why can't I do this for free?"

At the same time, you may feel resentful and angry that an attempt has been made to make you responsible for the pet's probable death because the client cannot (or will not) pay for the treatment. No "right" response exists in this and other financial dilemmas, but we hope that the following discussion will help you arrive at some effective methods for handling them.

Perhaps the first consideration is to step back a moment and think about what prompts clients to make such unfair statements. First, financial conflicts are usually highly charged with emotions and anticipatory grief. Thus, if clients are facing the possible loss of their pets, they may feel frightened and out of control. Second, if they are not regular consumers of veterinary services, their expectations of the costs involved with veterinary care are probably unrealistic. Third, they are undoubtedly feeling guilty and sad that their inability (or unwillingness) to pay may ultimately result in their pets' death. Consciously or unconsciously, they may be attempting to shift these emotional burdens to you. In the midst of emotional turmoil, the client has made you a target for all of these feelings. However, because you *are* a person, you *do* have feelings, it is very difficult to let your client's comments slide by without taking them personally.

However, depersonalizing your client's comments is exactly what you need to do. Depersonalizing means understanding that your client's comments are not necessarily directed at you, but more at the general situation. To accomplish this task, you may want to implement some of the many communication and helping skills discussed elsewhere in this book. For example, attending to and verbalizing the emotionally charged nature of the situation may help to decrease the tension so that a more productive discussion of options can follow. Saying something like:

> "It must be frightening to realize how much effort it's going to take to treat Scruffy. I know Scruffy's illness has been a real shock to you."

A statement such as this could then be followed by a detailed description of all the steps in treatment and their costs.

Understanding your own emotional reactions to the situation may also be helpful. Part of the problem you face is societal. Companion animals are undervalued in our society, as is suggested by the pet overpopulation problem and the way in which society trivializes the death of a pet. If the inherent worth of animals is sometimes ignored or devalued, then the medical services that you provide for animals are also undervalued.

Sometimes, veterinarians underestimate the value of their services and do not fully believe that the care they are providing is worth every penny (and often more) of the fees that they are charging.[20] If you do not believe that what you are offering is valuable and worth the price, it will probably be difficult for you to help your clients to believe it. Thus, it may be helpful to you to work on changing your attitude regarding the value of your work.

Another part of the problem you face is personal. Remember the discussion of codependency in Chapter 11? Most of us, women more than men, are socialized with a desire to please others and to have people like and accept us. For example, many veterinarians tell us that it is important to them to have their clients also be their friends. Other veterinarians have said that, although giving clients a break on their fees can cost them several thousand dollars each year, it is worth it to avoid being yelled at about charges. It takes some personal work to accept the old adage that "you can't please all of the people all of the time," and to not feel like a "bad" person when you cannot.

This idea applies not only to medical services, both basic and "high-tech," but especially to the extended services involved in establishing a bond-centered practice. When you take a half-hour to consult with a client about making a euthanasia decision, do a home euthanasia, facilitate a client-present euthanasia, or take time to explain the nature of a pet loss support group, you are providing services that are just as valuable and useful as are vaccinations, teeth cleanings, or physical examinations. Although you may decide to subsidize part of these costs as a way of retaining clients, you are justified in charging for your time and expertise. Even for the time you spend with clients for which you choose not to charge, practice management consultant Tom Catanzaro recommends documenting the value of these services on the bill followed by a "N/C" (no charge) notation so that clients are aware of the monetary value of the time that you spend with them.[21]

On a slightly different financial tangent, what can you do or say when faced with caring, highly-attached pet owners who honestly cannot afford the treatments required to save their animals' lives? What words can you use to inform people that you cannot provide veterinary medical care for free? A couple of ideas may be to say something like:

> "I know how much you love Scruffy. I care about Scruffy too. However, just as your financial constraints do not reflect the depth of your love for Scruffy, my commitment to my patients cannot be judged by my own financial limitations. I'd

like to work with you to see if we can come up with some options that will allow both of us to do the best we can for Scruffy within the practical financial limitations we have to live with."

"This is the worst part of my job. I became a veterinarian because I want to help animals and I feel sad and frustrated when I can't."

You also need to decide what other acceptable alternatives you can offer your clients. Usually, more than the two choices of treating an animal if they *can* pay and not treating the animal if they *cannot* pay exist. Various possibilities used by practicing veterinarians are:

- Offering clients a payment plan. The appropriateness of this alternative probably needs to be assessed on a case-by-case basis, depending on how well you know each client.
- Being willing to barter or trade with clients for other services. Perhaps your client owns a lawn care service and your lawn at home or your practice grounds need a substantial amount of yard work done. Would both you and the client be willing to have the costs of veterinary care traded for an equal value of lawn care?
- Establishing an "owner assistance" program. You may want to establish a separate fund to which any client can contribute. This fund would be used solely to care for animals whose owners cannot afford to pay. Compassionate pet owners often look for ways to help animals, and this option may appeal to your more financially solvent clients because they would have the advantage of knowing exactly how their contributions were being used.
- You may decide to donate services equal to a certain percentage (for example, 1 percent) of your gross or net income for the year to a client subsidy fund. The money in this fund would be used to subsidize patients' care when their owners could not afford to pay. Many veterinarians who establish this sort of fund "divide" the money equally among the members of their staff. For instance, if the fund contains $1,000.00 and four staff members work in the practice, each member has access to $250.00. Throughout each fiscal year, each staff member has the freedom to decide which cases and which services they will personally "charge" against this account. For example, if a young child and his mother bring in a puppy who has been hit by a car and they truly cannot afford treatment, a staff member may

elect to use his or her share of the subsidy fund to help the family pay. When services equal to an individual's share of the account are depleted, however, the option to subsidize clients is not available to them again until the next year. As with any charitable policy, it is important to devise some written rules and regulations to govern this fund. For example, you may establish a rule that the money cannot be used to help family members or personal friends. You may also want to develop some kind of client screening process so that you can ensure that only the people who truly need assistance have access to the money.

- Making owners aware of and actively promoting pet health insurance. This approach may ease the burden of expensive treatment in some cases. (More information about companies offering pet health insurance can be obtained from the Resource Appendix.)

Be aware that, regardless of these or any other options you choose, you are setting a precedent for what clients can expect from you. If you offer a financial alternative to one client, you may be asked to do the same for someone else. Word of your generosity (and flexibility) is bound to get out, particularly if you live in a small town or tight-knit rural community. Although you may not want to make *all* options available to *all* clients (for example, payment plans) you need to be clear regarding what criteria you will use in each case.

SITUATION TWELVE: "How Do I Keep My Sanity When Working with Clients Who Are Emotionally Unstable?"

Occasionally, you may encounter clients whose bonds with their animals could be considered abnormal or even pathologic. These pet owners may have no human friends or family members on whom they can rely. Thus, they invest all of their emotions in their pets. Pet owners who have abnormal or pathologic attachments to their pets often anthropomorphize them to the extent that they truly believe that their animals are the only ones who can understand and care for them. These clients usually isolate themselves from human society to such a degree that, without their companion animals, they feel that they have no support or reason to live.

Any client can be demanding and "needy" some of the time. You learned in Chapter 4 that grievers often display behaviors that could result in them being labeled as "difficult" clients. A difference, exists, however, between these "difficult" clients and those who might be termed manipu-

BOX 13-5

Working with Chronic Clients

For some people visits to the veterinarians fulfill long-term needs for human contact. They may also be used by clients to gain sympathy for their own situations, even if they have no intentions of taking action to address their problems. In the helping professions, these people are often called chronic clients.

Although it can be difficult to identify chronic clients, it gets easier with experience. You can assess whether or not clients might be termed chronic by monitoring your own responses to them. For example, if you find yourself feeling frustrated, ineffectual, and drained after each contact with certain clients, it may be because you are investing great amounts of time and energy in helping them resolve their problems, only to find that they are consistently unwilling to help themselves. Chronic clients can leave helpers feeling angry and incompetent. Therefore, it is important for helpers to remember that successful clients visits are measured by the quality of services provided, not by the actions clients are willing or able to take.

Chronic Clients often Exhibit Any or All of the Following Characteristics:

- Unwillingness to take action to deal with personal problems
- Unwillingness to follow through on referrals or to seek professional help
- Generally stating the same concerns and/or telling the same stories over and over again on each subsequent visit
- Being manipulative or hard to direct during visits
- Out of touch with reality
- Under the influence of alcohol and/or illegal or prescription drugs
- Evasive, making it difficult to ascertain the point of the visit
- Demanding and abusive to you if you do not do what they want

From The Crisis and Information Helpline of Larimer County, Crisis Intervention Training Manual, Fort Collins, Colo., 1986.

lative. One of the ways that you can recognize truly difficult or manipulative clients is by their consistent confrontational style, even when a crisis or loss is not occurring.

You *will* encounter these clients, and they *will* test your interpersonal skills. Regardless of how supportive, understanding, and empathic you are, some clients will demand more than you can or want to give. In the human services field, these persons are often referred to as "chronic clients" (Box 13-5). One hallmark characteristic of chronic clients is that they often show an unwillingness to act on any suggestions or help that you offer them. This unwillingness may or may not be conscious and may be shown by their persistence in repeating the same information or explaining the problem over and over. Talking to chronic clients can be very frustrating because they may ramble and give you a great deal of irrelevant information. You may have a difficult time getting them to stick to the subject. It may not always be easy to tell exactly what they want or expect from you. However, if they do ask something of you and you do not do what they ask, they may become demanding and verbally abusive.

As we discussed in Chapter 3, you are not a psychologist, social worker, member of the clergy, or a suicide prevention counselor. The first step in dealing with chronic clients is to clearly set your limits and boundaries in terms of what you can (and cannot) do for them. For example, if clients develop patterns of prolonged office visits or drawn-out telephone conversations, you may need to clearly state the amount of time that you have available to spend. You may need to say:

> "My next appointment is at 4 p.m., so I'll only be able to talk with you about this for 10 minutes."

Directly asking clients about the reasons for their calls or visits may also help to shorten your interactions with them.

> "I'm still unclear as to why you called today. Tell me exactly what you need."

You will also need to clearly define what services you can (and cannot) provide.

> "I'll make arrangements for the cremation service to pick up your pet's body, but I can't take the body there myself."

It is very helpful to think through your professional limits and boundaries before you encounter chronic clients. Then, you are prepared to respond to their requests when they occur. It is also important that you remain committed to your limits because chronic clients will often reword their questions and requests several times until they get the response that they seek from you.

Some clients go beyond the bounds of normal grief and exhibit truly obnoxious behavior. In these cases, we support your right, as a veterinarian, to "fire" them. We have "fired" a few clients ourselves over the years, although we have not made these decisions lightly. In every case where we have asked clients to no longer use our services, the clients have, in one way or another, abused our overtures of support. Their needs and demands have exceeded the limits and boundaries of what we were prepared and willing to offer them. Thus, after telling them very clearly what we could do for them and having them repeatedly refuse to cooperate with us, we have asked them not to return.

CONCLUSION

As we said in the beginning of this chapter, your attempts to help in any of these situations can go awry. Your overtures can be misunderstood, misinterpreted, or even unappreciated. Yet, although these risks exist, we still believe that, as the provider of a valuable human service and a professional who encounters people during vulnerable and emotionally fragile times, it is your ethical responsibility to respond to clients when they are in need.

Adhering to ethical responsibilities can, however, create ethical dilemmas. A few of the common ethical dilemmas associated with helping during times of pet loss and client grief are explored in the next chapter.

R E F E R E N C E S

1. The Crisis and Information Helpline of Larimer County: Crisis Intervention Training Manual. Fort Collins, Colo., 1986.
2. Alspach, G: Visions of healthcare: A view from the other side. Crit. Care Nurse, *12*:13–17, 1992.
3. Simpson, M., Buckman, R., Stewart, M., et al.: Doctor-patient communication: The Toronto consensus statement. Br. Med. J. *303*:1385–1387, 1991.
4. Platt, F.W.: Clinical hypocompetence: The interview. Ann. Intern. Med. *91*:898–902, 1979.
5. Buckman, R.: Breaking bad news: Why is it still so difficult? Br. Med. J., *288*:1597–1599, 1984.
6. Graham, S.B.: When babies die: Death and the education of obstetrical residents. Med. Teacher, *13*:171–175, 1991.
7. Butler, C., Lagoni, L., Dickinson, K., and Withrow, S.J.: Cancer. *In* Cohen, S.P., and Fudin, C.E., eds.: Problems in Veterinary Medicine: Animal Illness and Human Emotion, *3*:21–37, 1991.
8. Brewin, T.R.: Three ways of giving bad news. Lancet *337*:1207–1209, 1991.
9. Bacon, A.K.: Death on the table: Some thoughts on how to handle an anaesthetic-related death. Anaesthesia, *44*:245–248, 1989.
10. Viswanathan, R., Clark, J.J., and Viswanathan, K.: Physicians' and the public's attitudes on communication about death. Arch. Intern. Med. *146*:2029–2033, October 1986.
11. Slaikeu, K.A: Crisis Intervention: A Handbook for Practice and Research. Newton, Mass., Allyn and Bacon, 1984.
12. Cohen, S., and Lazarus, R.S.: Active coping processes, coping dispositions, and recovery from surgery. Psychosom. Med. *35*:375–389, 1973.
13. Hogbin, B.: Getting it taped: The "bad news" consultation with cancer patients. Br. J. Hosp. Med., *41*:330–332, 1989.
14. Sanders, C.M.: Effects of sudden illness versus chronic illness death on bereavement outcomes. Omega, *13*:227–241, 1982.
15. Johnson, S.: "Yes," or "No:" The Guide to Better Decisions. New York, HarperCollins, 1992.
16. Flanders, S.A.: Library in a Book: Suicide, New York, Facts on File, 1991.
17. McCurnin, D.M.: The vocal minority: Difficult clients and how to deal with them. Topics Vet. Med., Summer 1990, pp. 5–12.
18. Bilodeau, L.: The Anger Workbook. Minneapolis, CompCare Publishers, 1992.

19. Thompson, D., ed.: The Pocket Oxford Dictionary of Current English, 8th ed. New York, Oxford University Press, 1992.
20. Kay, W.J., Burk, R.L., Kerrigan, E.P., and Rodriquez, C.: Fee setting and collection. *In* McCurnin, D.M., ed.: Veterinary Practice Management, Philadelphia, J.B. Lippincott Company, 1988, pp. 189–216.
21. Lofflin, J. Raising your fees with confidence. Vet. Econom. *32*:26–45, 1991.

14

The Ethics of Helping

In Chapter 5, we presented the basic tenets of helping relationships (Box 5-1) and discussed the importance of setting limits and boundaries on assuming responsibility for others. Within this context, some of the ethical considerations of helping others were mentioned. You are undoubtedly aware, not only from the information presented in this book but also from your personal experiences in veterinary medicine, that the process of helping others often creates moral and ethical dilemmas for the helper.

Ethics are rules of professional conduct that are based on moral principles.[1] Veterinary medicine has been described as "inherently a moral enterprise."[2] The word "moral" implies judgment that is made between right and wrong. Ethical behavior, therefore is action based on the "right thing to do." Despite the fact that courses in ethics have been taught for years at some veterinary schools, widespread interest in veterinary ethics has only recently developed, and the field is growing rapidly.

Ethical questions in veterinary medicine may be even more difficult to answer than those belonging to other professions, including human medicine, because veterinarians must contend with the dilemmas, not only of their animal patients, but also of their human clients.[2] Sometimes, what is best for the patient may not be best for the client (and vice versa).

High standards and adherence to a code of ethics are basic tenets of veterinary medicine. The Principles of Veterinary Ethics and The Veterinarian's Oath both act as standards by which an individual may determine the propriety of conduct in relationships with clients, colleagues, and the public. Traditionally, veterinary ethics has focused primarily on blatant or readily agreed upon wrongdoings such as "quack" treatments, overcharging clients, or conducting unnecessary diagnostic treatments or medical procedures. Ethical standards for professional interactions, including such issues as advertising, fee splitting, and "client stealing" from referrals, have also been established. Today, veterinary ethics is a rapidly changing area. It is difficult to keep up with technologic advances in veterinary medicine and the parallel increase in questions that "high-tech" medicine creates regarding the status of animals in our society. The Principles of Veterinary Ethics and the Veterinarian's Oath, for example, do not offer specific guidelines for veterinarians who find themselves in the midst of difficult ethical or emotional situations particular to the human-animal bond. They also do not adequately reflect the growing interest veterinarians seem to have in helping clients during pet loss. As Bernard Rollin pointed out, the 1973 edition of the *Principles of Veterinary Medical Ethics* contained 30 entries discussing advertising, and none concerning the ethics of euthanasia.[3]

Professional curricula for many fields, including veterinary medicine, may either consciously or unconsciously be designed to perpetuate the existing standards, rules, and regulations of the profession and may actively or passively discourage conflicting viewpoints or questions regarding standard procedures. Thus, practitioners may not perceive ethical questions in the policies or procedures that are widely accepted in their field. In the past, for example, the use of succinylcholine without anesthetic as a method of restraint for horse castrations was an accepted procedure. For many years, the use of multiple recovery surgeries on dogs and cats was accepted as a method of teaching surgery skills to junior veterinary students (Fig. 14-1). Postsurgical pain medication for animals was generally deemed unnecessary. Discouraging client presence during euthanasia was standard practice. Performing euthanasias at the request of clients, regardless of their reasons, was viewed as the veterinarian's obligation. All of these examples contain ethical or moral dilemmas that were not recognized, or were ignored, during the time at which they were widely accepted procedures.

Today, the ethical dilemmas that veterinarians encounter almost daily (for example, animal welfare issues, "convenience" euthanasias, and pet overpopulation) are the result of their relationships with peers, clients, patients, and society at large. For example, many ethical questions arise when veterinary professionals work with dying patients and their patients' human families. Many of these situations did not exist as ethical dilemmas 20 years ago. We asked some of our colleagues to relate their thoughts about the challenges presented by pet loss-related ethical dilemmas. Examples of their comments include:

> "Deciding how to handle the demand for high-tech medicine. Is it right to encourage pet owners to spend great amounts of money on animals when many people can't afford basic

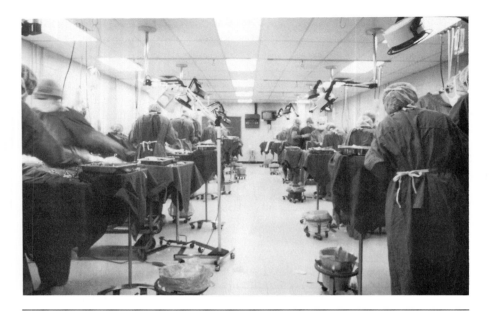

Figure 14-1 These veterinary students are developing their surgery skills without having to face the ethical dilemma of multiple-recovery surgeries.

health care? On the other hand, is it unethical to not offer or not have available "high-tech" treatments and diagnostic equipment if clients want it and can afford it? Must I, as a responsible business person, invest in this equipment?"

"Wondering how to confront colleagues who cheat their clients financially. Telling them that I think it is wrong to charge dedicated, committed pet owners more than usual or charge them for unnecessary procedures just because they know they can get away with it."

"Wondering if we are elevating animals to the status of human beings by making such a fuss over their deaths and over their owners' grief. If we are, is there anything intrinsically wrong with that? Are animals worthy of intense grief? Is it right for us to encourage strong grief reactions?"

"Wondering whether or not to allow children to be present at their pets' euthanasias or to visit the dead bodies of their pets. Is this really good for young children? Is it really helpful? For that matter, is it really good for adults to witness death, particularly when the death is that of a large animal?"

"Struggling with how I feel about veterinarians who use peoples' misfortune and times of grief to build their practices. For example, veterinarians who advertise their practices with a sort of 'animal funeral home' approach, offering everything from home euthanasias to on-site cremation and urn selection. I think taking it this far is morbid and I don't think that's right."

"Deciding how much 'pro bono' medical care I can give to clients who truly love their pets, but can't afford the treatment. How far can I go without becoming a sucker for people who know how to manipulate the human services system?"

"Deciding where I stand on animal rights and animal welfare issues. Whether or not animals should be used in research."

"Making a decision regarding my personal position on the euthanasia of healthy animals. I don't believe in convenience euthanasias, yet it's not really a black or white issue."

"Deciding whose best interests are my first priority. Is my priority the pet (medical concerns) or the pet owner (emotional and practice management concerns)?"

ETHICAL DECISION-MAKING

The process of solving ethical dilemmas can be viewed as having four components. The first is the recognition or interpretation of a problem as an ethical dilemma. The second is making a judgment about the appropriate course of action. Third is placing a priority on ethical values, and fourth is deciding to implement the course of action.[4] The way in which an ethical or moral dilemma is resolved depends first on the way it is perceived or described. This perception, in turn, depends on the moral orientation of the individual.[5]

Justice or Care

Perhaps the most well-known cognitive moral development theory is that of Kohlberg. His model is a six-stage, hierarchical sequence of moral reasoning that culminates with justice.[6] People move from stage to stage based on the degree to which they approximate justice or use the principle of justice in resolving moral conflicts. Kohlberg's theory regards justice as the moral ideal. His theory has gained wide attention and been validated by hundreds of studies substantiating his claims.

In response to Kohlberg's theory, Gilligan emphasized the concept of moral orientation or moral voice. Moral orientation refers to the framework in which a moral dilemma is perceived and described.[7] A person who takes a justice approach in resolving ethical questions considers what is fair for all and views relationships in terms of equality and inequality. A justice orientation is concerned with issues of individual rights and adherence to standards and principles. A person with a care orientation views relationships in terms of attachment and detachment. A care orientation is concerned with the complexities of sustained attachments, compassion, forgiveness, and close personal relationships. From a care perspective, morality requires not hurting others, condemning all violence and exploitation, and nurturing relationships between people. In short, making ethical choices from a justice orientation ensures that everyone is treated fairly, whereas making decisions from a care orientation prevents others from feeling deserted, isolated, or abandoned.

The moral orientations of 20 new veterinary medical graduates were studied before their entry into private practice.[5] The results are summarized in Table 14-1. Most of the new graduates recognized the presence of justice concepts in moral dilemmas, but substantially fewer recognized a care orientation. Less than half relied primarily on one or the other orientation when describing ethical dilemmas, and only 10 percent relied on both. Barely a third used one of these concepts for resolution of ethical conflicts. Although the sample in this study was small, it raises questions about the framework that veterinarians use to resolve ethical dilemmas.

Table 14-1
Moral Orientation of Veterinary Students

	Justice (%)	Care (%)	Both (%)
Presence	90	65	55
Predominance	45	45	10
Alignment	35	30	30

Presence refers to the recognition of the concept when describing the ethical dilemma. Predominance refers to whether or not one of the concepts is used exclusively or substantially more than the other when describing the ethical dilemma. Alignment refers to whether or not one of the concepts is accepted or used more as the preferred basis for resolving ethical conflicts.

Summarized from Self, D.J., Jecher, N.S., Baldwin, D.C., et al.: Moral orientations of justice and care among veterinarians entering veterinary practice. J. Am. Vet. Med. Assoc., 199:569–573, 1991.

The Influences of Women, Urban Lifestyles, and Veterinary Medical Education

Gilligan's research supports the claim that men, as a group, exhibit justice orientation predominantly and that women exhibit care orientation predominantly. In the survey by Self and colleagues,[5] slight differences in moral reasoning were shown between male and female veterinarians. A justice orientation was used 67 percent of the time by men but only 33 percent of the time by women. Conversely, 44 percent of men used a care orientation compared with 56 percent of women.

A glance at the practice of modern veterinary medicine shows that it is no longer a profession practiced predominantly by men. In fact, today a trend can be seen toward "feminization" of the field. Women now constitute more than half of the veterinary student population in the United States (Fig. 14-2), and most veterinary technicians, support staff, and clients are women and are from urban backgrounds.[8]

The move from rural agricultural settings to predominantly urban backgrounds has also influenced the veterinary field. As Dean Loew of Tufts University says:

> Our population is changing. Ninety percent of the people in this
> country live in urban areas, 98 percent are not farmers. The root of
> the animal rights conflict is shaped by a new urban view of animals,
> which is that of the pet owner who sees animal issues through the

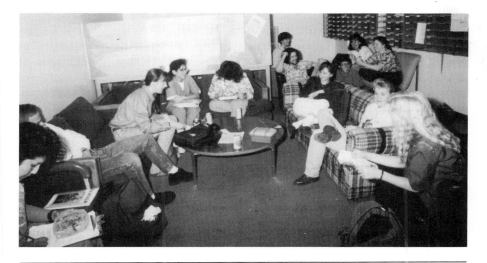

Figure 14-2 This candid shot of a student lounge illustrates that female students now outnumber male students at most veterinary schools.

prism of an individual animal. This perception is in opposition to the view of scientists, researchers, and farmers who see animals in terms of species that have a utilitarian role.[8] (p. 1354)

More than ever before, the attitudes, values, and needs of urban women are affecting the daily practice of veterinary medicine. This change is also having an effect on veterinary ethics.

Some evidence indicates that veterinary medical education may also influence the moral development of its students. In fact, veterinary education might inhibit it.[2] A recent study of 20 veterinary students measured moral reasoning ability at the beginning and at the end of their veterinary medical education. Two important findings emerged: First, the students' scores reported when they entered veterinary school did not differ significantly from those reported when they finished. Previous use of the test with young adults of the same age as average veterinary students has shown that scores would normally be expected to reflect growth and development in moral reasoning as the students matured over a 4-year period. Second, the variance of the scores decreased over the 4 years, meaning the students became increasingly similar in the level of their moral development. These preliminary results could indicate that veterinary students are not receiving sufficient training to assist them in identifying ethical dilemmas or in providing them with a framework from which to make their own, independent decisions.

Given the above information about veterinary ethics and ethical decision-making, the purpose of this chapter is twofold. First, we want to attempt to increase your awareness of the presence of ethical questions in helping relationships, particularly those involving animal death or euthanasia. You may not have thought about the practice dilemmas presented in this chapter because they may not correspond to the traditional view of ethical issues. Second, we want to emphasize the bond-centered veterinary practice perspective, which we believe encompasses the moral orientations of both justice and care.

Six common pet loss-related dilemmas are presented in this chapter. It is *not* our goal to make decisions or to arrive at a course of action for each of the examples discussed. Instead, we wish to help you to consider new information and new ways of thinking during ethical decision-making.

CASE EXAMPLES

The examples discussed in the following pages are all adapted from clinical situations that we have encountered. The names and details have been changed to protect the confidentiality of our clients and colleagues. In each case, you are assumed to be the veterinarian. You may discover whether you favor a justice or care orientation to ethical decision-making by examining your responses to each of these situations.

Case 1: Client Consent

> Chester, a 12-year-old cat belonging to the Mann family, became ill the night before the family left town for a 2-week vacation. They left Chester with you on their way out of town. They are very concerned about Chester and promise to call you frequently to see how he is doing.
>
> While you are still trying to determine what's wrong with Chester, he dies. Although you haven't heard from the Manns, you feel certain that they would want to know why Chester died. You want to know as well, so that you can be personally reassured, as well as reassure them, that his death was not due to any negligence on your part. The ethical question is, should you go ahead and perform a necropsy without your client's consent? You know if you wait too long, a necropsy will not be as useful due to deterioration of the body. Because you have no storage capability, it is standard practice for your clinic to have a pet's body cremated after death unless instructed otherwise. The Manns have not informed you of any other preferences for body care. Should you go ahead and send Chester's body to be cremated after the necropsy?

Both legal and emotional issues exist in this situation. Because animals are legally viewed as property, it is clear that the pet owner is the only person who has the right to determine what should be done with an animal's body.[9] Death does not change the right of ownership. (The only exception to this rule is if the animal died of a zoonotic disease.) Thus, technically, you cannot do a necropsy or make decisions about body care without the owner's consent. It remains unclear, however, to what lengths veterinarians must go to contact owners or to store bodies.[9] Also, unexpected deaths are often very difficult for pet owners. You know that the Manns will probably want to say goodbye to Chester and will need to know how and why he died.

Various factors would probably influence your course of action. For example, how long has the family been out of contact with you? What are the most likely causes of Chester's death? Would it be reasonable to wait a day or even 2 for the Manns to contact you before making any decisions? Would you handle the situation differently if the Manns had been clients for years or if this was only their first or second visit to your clinic? What impression did both you and the Manns have regarding Chester's prognosis when they left? Would an immediate necropsy be more or less important if you were concerned about the appropriateness of your treatment or diagnostic procedures? With regard to storing the body or cremating it, would it make a difference if, instead of being a 10-pound cat, Chester was a 90-pound Great Dane? If you cannot store the body, what other sources could you explore?

This case emphasizes the need for good communication with clients, preplanning for death, euthanasia, and body care before a crisis. How could this situation be handled differently, using the bond-centered veterinary practice ideas and verbal and nonverbal communication techniques discussed throughout this book?

Although justifiable solutions exist in this example, room is also available for the possibility of unethical choices. One such choice would be for you to cremate the body as a deliberate way of covering up any mistake you may or may not have made during Chester's care. Others might include modifying or altering Chester's case records, charging your clients for tests or procedures that were never done, telling your clients (on reaching them) that their cat was not doing well when, in fact, their cat was already dead.

To avoid this ethical dilemma, you might ask clients to sign a release when their animals are hospitalized. This release would give you the right to do what you think is best if you have to act quickly on behalf of an animal and your client cannot be reached within 24 hours, or some other reasonable time frame. This release might also ask about the owners' preferred method of body care.

Case 2: Treating Your Own Companion Animals

> Your own dog, Lady, is now 14 years old. She has been showing her age more visibly recently. It is becoming more difficult for her to get around, she's urinating in the house several times a week, and she's becoming finicky about eating. Her "bad" days are beginning to outnumber her good ones, and you know that the time to say goodbye is fast approaching. Lady has been with you through thick and thin and you know you want to be with her when she dies. However, you've been thinking of taking it one step further— you've been thinking it might be best if you euthanized Lady yourself.

The first step in this situation would be to examine your feelings about Lady's decline and inevitable death and to ask yourself *why* you feel that you should be the one to euthanize her. Are you trying to spare someone else the task? Are you attempting to prove to yourself that you can "handle it" or that you are "in control?" Are you afraid to let others see you grieve?

Thought should be given to the consequences for both you and Lady if you decide to do the euthanasia yourself. For example, it is doubtful that you can be emotionally present and comforting to Lady at her death if you are performing the euthanasia. What if difficulties arise during the procedure? Will your decisions about Lady affect how you feel about euthanizing animals in the future?

Before you make a decision about who will euthanize Lady, you might need to step back and contemplate how you will decide *when* Lady should be euthanized. For example, you may have a difficult time assessing day-to-day changes in Lady, just as your clients do with their pets. Therefore, it may be helpful to have someone who has not seen Lady for awhile take a look at her. That is, you may want to have Lady examined by another veterinarian. He or she may be able to tell you if you are making assumptions about her physiologic condition that cannot be confirmed. Without other input, you may feel later that you made too hasty a decision or that you prolonged her discomfort.

Most professionals in human medicine abide by a generally accepted principle which precludes physicians from treating their own family members, except in cases involving minor illnesses or injuries. Many reasons exist for this policy. It is impossible for anyone to be completely objective when treating family members, whether they be human or animal because it is not possible to completely separate your professional self from your "personal" self. Attempting to do so puts pressure on you to be both an objective, supportive professional and a family member who is appropriately concerned about a loved one. By choosing not to bear the responsibility of euthanizing your own animal alone, you may experience, in a very personal way, how it feels to trust others.

On the other hand, if you are proud of how you handle euthanasia and you have a less-involved support person who agrees to assist you, it may be right for you to go ahead with the procedure. In this case, you should also have a back-up plan if you change your mind. A plan for debriefing after your pet's death with someone who is understanding and trustworthy is also a good idea.

Case 3: Personal Involvement with Clients

One of your recent patients is a cat who was hit by a car. Shadow had multiple injuries, and it has been touch and go as to whether she would survive. Although Shadow now seems to be recovering, you have had lengthy discussions with her owner about whether or not to continue treating Shadow. You have also discussed euthanasia. During the course of these discussions, both you and Shadow's owner have self-disclosed some details of your personal lives to each other. You have come to respect and admire not only your client's commitment and attachment to Shadow, but also the personal side that has been revealed to you. Shadow's owner has told you that you are a wonderful person. You realize you've come to look forward to the owner's visits to Shadow.

During one of these visits, you are alone in the clinic near closing time. Shadow's owner asks you to go out to dinner. You are attracted to this person and may be interested in developing a more personal relationship. Should you say yes to the invitation?

In a helping relationship, it is not uncommon for one or both parties to feel some attraction to each other. When clients feel vulnerable, they may become more attached to those who offer support and understanding. Helpers may find this openness appealing and may feel needed, wanted, and appreciated by the people they are attempting to help. People who are new to helping roles may become unclear about the appropriate boundaries in a helping relationship.

This situation is one in which no dilemma exists. When clients are vulnerable, in the midst of crisis, any future personal relationships must be put on hold until their pets are no longer your patients and until the owners are no longer your clients. Within the context of a helping relationship, it would definitely be unethical and inappropriate for you to become romantically or sexually involved with a client while a pet is under your care. Doing so would be taking advantage of your client's vulnerability and the trust that has been placed in you. Based on reports of various human service professionals engaging in sexual relationships with their clients, it is clear that this ethical problem needs attention. Those who train veterinarians to be helpers should address this issue by creating an awareness of the problem and by providing strict codes of professional conduct.

What can you say to Shadow's owner? How can you decline the invitation in a way which will not offend or cause hurt feelings? In addition, how can you help the owner continue to feel comfortable having you as Shadow's veterinarian?

You might say, "I'm so flattered by your invitation. You and I have been through some emotional times with Shadow, and I have come to know you as a very caring person. It means a great deal to me that you think that much of me. However, it would be unfair to both you and Shadow for us to have a personal relationship right now. You need to be able to trust me and to know that I can remain objective about Shadow's care. I'm not sure I could do that if we were to become involved." Whether or not you continue your conversation by inviting your client to again pursue a personal relationship after Shadow's treatment ends will obviously depend on your own feelings and on the status of your other personal relationships.

On the other hand, what if the client who asks you out to dinner is not particularly vulnerable or in the midst of crisis? What if he or she has brought a pet to you for vaccinations or a simple yearly check-up? Looking at dating from a slightly different angle, what might be the consequences of dating a coworker, perhaps a member of your own staff? What ethical dilemmas might this situation pose? Many of these ethical questions are difficult to answer until you have actually experienced them.

Case 4: "Convenience" Euthanasia

> Linda Massey has made an appointment to vaccinate her dog Tiger. Tiger is a 4-year-old Springer Spaniel. When Linda arrives at the clinic she is angry and upset. It seems that while Linda was at work last week, Tiger destroyed the living room couch and tore up a large section of the living room carpet. This is not the first time such things have happened. Tiger has also chewed doors, torn down drapes, and dug holes in the yard. Linda tells you that she cannot deal with Tiger's destructive behavior any longer and doesn't think anybody else would be willing to either. Rather than taking him to an animal shelter and never knowing what would happen to him, she would prefer that you euthanize him now.

This example introduces the question of so-called "convenience euthanasias." The veterinary community is beginning to discuss this issue,[10,11] along with the overpopulation of companion animals.[12] The traditional position in veterinary medicine has been that the veterinarian's first obligation is to the client and that what the client wants done is what the veterinarian should do. Not all veterinarians agree with this position.

You clearly do have choices in this situation, but it is important to realize that each choice has potentially different consequences. Perhaps the worst situation is to be confused about the criteria you will use to make decisions about whether to perform a euthanasia. The first step in resolving your confusion might be to decide your own "bottom lines." For example, you could decide that, no matter what the circumstances, you will perform any client-requested euthanasia. On the other hand, you could decide that you will only agree to euthanize terminally ill or suffering animals. It is more likely, however, that your "bottom lines" may not be so clear-cut. In that case, you will need to consider what factors will be involved in your decision-making process and what information you will require from clients to make your decision. It is also important to consider all the potential consequences of your decision so that you can be prepared to handle and be comfortable with them. Decide also what alternatives you are prepared to offer clients. For example, are you prepared to offer to find homes for unwanted animals? Will you be willing to assist a client in finding a new home for a pet? If so, how can you accomplish this task? If not, to what other resources can you refer clients?

One factor that will probably be important in your decision is the owner's stated reason for wanting the euthanasia. What will you consider to be a justifiable reason for requesting euthanasia? Will euthanasia be justifiable if your client is moving and does not want to (or cannot) take the pet? What if the request is due to a behavior problem? What if the behavior problem is potentially resolvable, as is destructive behavior or housesoiling? What if the problem is aggression? Are you interested in obtaining the knowledge required to work with behavior problems? Are you prepared to refer behavior cases to a behavior specialist?

A second factor to consider will probably be your past history with the client. What if this is a new client whom you have never seen before? How will it affect your decision if this is a long-term client? What if it is a long-term client who has a history of getting rid of pets and getting new ones? What if the client has provided good care for their animals, but is a person you do not particularly like?

In addition, what will you need to know from your clients regarding the way in which they arrived at the decision to euthanize their animal? Because you are being asked to perform an irreversible act, you have a vested interest in knowing the way in which that decision was made. It is understandable that you would want more information from a client before you decide how to proceed. Based on who *you* are and what *your* needs are, will you ask just a few questions about the circumstances or will you want to gather a substantial amount of information? What if your client's decision was an impulsive one? What if your client has already pursued other unsuccessful alternatives? What if your client is not at all interested in other alternatives?

Will the age of the animal make a difference to you? A healthy 2-year-old dog has many years ahead, whereas a healthy 8-year-old dog has fewer. Is that a significant factor? You will probably want to consider each of these factors in light of the others. For example, would your decision be different if Linda's dog were 8 years old? What about a family who was moving and decided that their 12-year-old cat could not adjust to a new home? What if the reasoning behind their decision was that the 12-year-old cat was not using its litterbox for behavioral reasons?

A set of consequences will be associated with whatever decision you make. Examples of the possible consequences regarding both the animal's fate and your future relationship with your client (if you decide to refuse the owner's request) are listed in (Box 14-1). Both positive and negative consequences are possible. Obviously, if you decide to euthanize the animal, the animal's fate is no longer a question. Whether this choice is more likely to retain or to lose clients has never been studied. The most important consequence will be the way you feel about the decision and about

BOX 14-1

Possible Consequences of Not Euthanizing a Healthy Animal at the Owner's Request

Both positive and negative consequences are possible as a result of the decision not to euthanize a healthy animal. The client may:

- Have the euthanasia performed at another veterinary clinic.
- Take the animal to an animal shelter where it may either be adopted or euthanized by the shelter staff.
- Find another home for the animal.
- Decide to keep the animal and seek other alternatives.
- Become a long-term client due to the alternatives provided.
- Abandon the animal so it becomes a stray.
- Kill the animal themselves in an inhumane way.
- Never return to the veterinary clinic because it reminds them of their guilt.

yourself. If you euthanize, will you feel that you saved the animal from a worse fate? If you do not, will you feel that you have given the animal another chance or shifted the responsibility for euthanasia of unwanted animals to an animal shelter? Do you care whether you lose this client? With either decision, will you feel that you have betrayed your professional oath to "protect animal health and to practice (your) profession conscientiously?" How will your decision affect your feelings about euthanasia in general? How will your decision affect your staff or interactions with your own family?

If you do choose to euthanize the animal, give some thought to how the procedure can be made less stressful for you and for your staff. You can still ask the client if she wants to be present. In some situations, it may make it easier for you, your staff, the animal, and the owner (if present) to sedate the animal before euthanasia. Regardless of client presence, you and your staff can ensure that the animal dies with peace and dignity, surrounded by caring people. You can do so by applying the new paradigm of euthanasia discussed in Chapter 8, making the euthanasia a "ceremony" (in your own way) rather than a mechanical, clinical procedure.

A decision that would, without question, be unethical would be to tell the client that you will euthanize her pet and then not do it. If discovered, at the least, this action may provide a client with grounds to file a grievance or lawsuit against you. If you do so consistently, it may even be grounds for revoking your license to practice veterinary medicine.

To conclude this case example, we want to suggest that, just as a code of ethics exists for veterinary professionals, a code of ethics should also exist

BOX 14-2

One Veterinarian's Memory of "Convenience" Euthanasia

"We in veterinary medicine are not, on the whole, philosophers. We don't enjoy grappling with insolvable moral questions. And there is no end to them, in school or in practice. Reality dictates that most new vets work in someone else's practice; and as hired guns, they must do what they are paid to do, which is whatever the clients want done. Not only do they debark dogs and declaw cats but they are also asked to euthanize healthy animals that have developed bad habits or become inconvenient, as well as curable animals whose owners cannot afford, or choose not to afford, the treatment.

That was the real world, and I had been there already. I was a technician in a small-animal practice a few years before I worked for Jill Henderson. A small black-and-white terrier was brought in to be put to death. My boss "let" me do it, although it is not legal for a technician to euthanize animals (what would constitute malpractice in a euthanasia case, I do not know).

I remember Domino because he was my first and because he was sweet and obedient, because he wanted only to please.

It was a test of strength and will, a moment that I was only too aware could separate the sheep from the goats and determine my future. I talked to the little dog, patted him, carried him down the hall, and put him on the stainless steel table. I asked him to shake, and he raised his paw, pleased to do his trick, pleased to please me. I slipped a tourniquet around his leg, and when the vein stood out, I inserted the needle, released the tourniquet, and pushed the plunger. The dog slumped dead on the table.

For a moment I stood there in horror at my power—and in greater horror that I had been able to wield it. In the privacy of that small exam room, I cried. And then I picked up Domino's body and put him in the freezer for Animal Control's weekly pickup.

Domino's owners were moving away; they'd said they couldn't take him. They left him, alive, in my arms, and did not see him die so trustingly. I wish I could talk to them today, ten years later, and tell them that I still see that room, the reflection of the bright lamp off the shiny table, the black-and-white dog. I would tell them that it hurt. I hope they still think of him, and I hope that they hurt, too, for that is as it should be."

From Gage, L., and Gage, N.: *If Wishes Were Horses: The Education of a Veterinarian.* New York, St Martin's Press, 1992, p. 130. Used with permission of the publisher.

for pet owners. Some pet owners abandon, abuse, overburden, and stress their companion animals. Some breeders often alter the physical appearance of animals, causing them pain and discomfort to conform to arbitrary human standards. Some pet owners allow their pets to breed indiscriminately, thoughtlessly contributing to the pet overpopulation problem. Others do not license, vaccinate, or use leashes, doing little to prevent illnesses or injuries for their pets. Many treat veterinary professionals like persons without feelings, asking them to euthanize animals for less than justifiable reasons (Box 14-2).

We would like to see members of the professional veterinary community become more proactive and demonstrative about their own values and ethics when interacting with irresponsible pet owners, particularly in situations regarding convenience euthanasia. One of the most compelling arguments against human euthanasia is the belief that the privilege would be abused by those looking for an easy way to "get rid of" unwanted family members. As in human medicine, this area of veterinary medicine is worthy of considerable debate. Veterinary medicine must develop some effective guidelines governing this dilemma, especially if we are to act as role models for developing euthanasia protocols in human medicine.

Case 5: Intrusiveness

Mr. Brown is a law-enforcement official in your community. He and his black Labrador Retriever, Ebony, are a well known pair. Ebony is a scent-detection dog and is not only Mr. Brown's best friend, but also his working partner. Mr. Brown has relied on Ebony's company even more lately, since the unexpected death of his wife.

Late one afternoon, Mr. Brown brings a very sick Ebony into your clinic. From the history and Ebony's symptoms, it is pretty clear that she ingested ethylene glycol. Despite your treatment and assistance from specialists, Ebony dies a few days later. It is obvious that Mr. Brown takes Ebony's death very hard. Without Ebony, he feels that he has lost his professional identity and the special status that he enjoyed as Ebony's handler. He also feels somewhat responsible for her death and is still grieving the loss of his wife.

Although Ebony's cremains have been at your clinic for several weeks, Mr. Brown has not felt ready to pick them up. When Mr. Brown does finally come to your clinic several weeks later to get them, he doesn't look like his normal self. He has lost weight and appears disheveled. He can barely talk because he is trying very hard not to "lose control." You have talked with Mr. Brown before about grief and even referred him to a pet loss support group, but you know he has not attended the meetings. Now, your concern for him is growing. You would like to refer Mr. Brown to a grief therapist, but you are afraid he might find this insulting. After all, his profession expects that he be strong and in control. In addition, because Mr. Brown is somewhat of a local celebrity, you

reason that others, who are more qualified than you to talk
with him, will probably notice his deterioration and try to
help him. Should you rationalize away your concerns and let
him walk out the door without saying anything more?

This case illustrates many of the points that we have tried to make
throughout this book. The grief over the death of a pet cuts through all
kinds of stereotypes. When pets are integral parts of people's lives, their
deaths bring unavoidable grief. You and your staff may be the first to
recognize how deeply this loss affects some people. Both students and
practicing veterinarians seem to be continually fearful of invading the privacy of their clients. Historically, an unwritten standard of practice seems
to suggest that veterinarians need to guard against intruding into the private lives of their clients. One of the results of this unfortunate "rule" is
that veterinary medicine itself may have contributed to the trivialization of
pet loss by simply not acknowledging clients' feelings.

So how should you respond to Mr. Brown? If you ask him to come into
your office, have a cup of coffee, talk for a minute, and then make your
referral, what is the worst he could do? Tell you to mind your own business? Clients have probably said much worse things to you! The other side
of the coin is all the potential good that could come from your attempt to
help. Although his grief recovery is not your responsibility, it *is* your
responsibility to offer high-quality care (within the limits of your resources)
to Mr. Brown, as you did for Ebony. This care includes making referrals to
qualified human service professionals. Less potential for harm exists from
attending to client's feelings than from ignoring them.

Case 6: Honesty

Mike and Tanya Kopple choose cremation for their cat, Sasha,
after she dies of cancer. They want Sasha individually cremated with the cremains returned to them afterwards. You
agree to follow through with your clients' wishes and make
the appropriate arrangements with the local pet cemetery and
crematory.

After 10 days, you realize that Sasha's cremains have not
been returned to your office. After talking to the people at the
crematory and checking through their records and your own,
you realize that you neglected to write down any specific instructions regarding your clients' wishes for individual cremation. The agreement that you have with the pet crematory
states that, without written instructions designating a body
for individual cremation, all bodies receive mass cremation.
By default, Sasha had been cremated days ago, along with

many other animals, and her ashes had already been scattered on the grounds of the pet cemetery.

You know how upsetting this news will be for your clients. You think that perhaps, rather than telling the Kopples the truth, it would be kinder to obtain some cremains from the pet crematory, give them to the Kopples, and allow them to think the ashes belong to Sasha. You are also concerned about protecting yourself. Perhaps you should not admit your mistake. What if the Kopples switch veterinarians or, even worse, bring a lawsuit against you? What should you do?

In an attempt to spare the Kopples any further pain, you decide to give them some cremains and tell them that they are Sasha's. However, you neglect to update your staff regarding your decision. On the day the Kopples pick up Sasha's cremains, one of your technicians sees them as they are leaving. Casually, she offers her condolences on Sasha's death and also mentions how sorry she is about the mix-up with the cremation instructions. Confused, the Kopples return to you and ask for an honest explanation.

Honesty has been defined as the extent to which individuals and groups in organizations abide by consistent and rational ethical principles related to obligations to respect the truth.[13] In the world of medicine, honesty is a somewhat controversial ethical principle. Most everyone can agree that there is an inherent "rightness" to telling the truth; however, it seems that, because veterinarians are committed to working for the *benefit* of their patients (and clients), some are skeptical about the moral relevancy of the "truth for truth's sake" principle. For many, especially when a simple opportunity to "rectify" a mistake exists, telling the truth often seems to create more harm than good.

How honest you can be with clients depends on many variables. For instance, if you are a confident, skilled communicator with a sterling reputation and a thriving practice, you may not think twice about the risk that honesty creates. If, on the other hand, you are struggling to build a clientele and are not an experienced communicator, the risk created by telling the truth may seem greater. However, if you truly take time to consider all of the possible consequences entailed by lying to clients, a strong case for telling the truth can be built.

In general, the potential loss is greater than the potential gain when you engage in lying or dishonest behavior. In the case study related above, lying would surely cost you your clients and possibly do serious damage to your professional reputation, especially if, when the Kopples return to you after talking with your technician, you lie to them again. When you think through the consequences, your own short-term anxiety about telling the

Kopples the truth would be far preferrable to dealing with any possible long-term legal difficulties or the loss of your clients' trust. As Rodger Charlton states:

> The principle of informed consent requires respect for individuals and their autonomy, and so their right to be informed, and discourages a paternalistic attitude which deems that deceit may be beneficial for a patient's [or in this case, client's] welfare.[14] (p. 617)

Many kinds of deceit exist. For example, it is probably as dishonest to withhold information from clients as it is to lie to them. It is also dishonest to pepper your conversations with polysyllabic words and medical jargon or to instill false hope about any given situation. When ethical quandries arise, whatever choices you make about honesty, it is important to remember that blunt honesty is often as damaging as lying. As a helper, when you decide to be honest with clients, you must pair the information that you give them with sensitivity and the effective communication techniques described previously.

CONCLUSION

Ethical codes and rules of professional conduct grow from knowledge and experience. It is our feeling that the helping relationships that exist within the context of bond-centered veterinary practices are yet too new to be governed by an authoritative ethical code. To fully develop this code, numerous situations, beyond those discussed in this chapter, require thoughtful consideration. For example, if an owner cannot come to a timely decision, do you euthanize an animal who is in pain, but tell the owner that the animal died on its own? Do you agree to perform high-risk surgery, inflicting further pain on an animal, because the owner hopes that her pet will die in surgery, sparing her the decision about euthanasia? Do you deplete your blood supply by caring for an animal who has no hope of survival because the owner wants you to do "everything possible" to save his pet? Do you "blow the whistle" on colleagues or associates when you know that they have purposely misled or even lied to clients? Furthermore, what is your position on issues like pet overpopulation, leghold traps, tail docking, ear cropping, no-pet regulations in public housing, humane slaughter, the proliferation of puppy mills and pet shops, or the protection of endangered species? You must decide for yourself by what ethics to abide within your bond-centered practice. Ultimately, you must evaluate the personal risks and professional consequences associated with helping your clients—and with not helping them.

Quackenbush and Glickman[15] postulated that the very act of seeking medical care for pets indicates that a strong bond exists between the companion animal and the owner. Therefore, given what is known about the importance of pets in people's lives and about the grief that pet owners feel when their companion animals die, it may be time for you to stop asking, "Is it ethical for me to offer help when my clients' pets die?" and start asking, "Is it ethical for me to turn away without offering help when my clients' companion animals die?"

REFERENCES

1. Thompson, D., ed.: The Pocket Oxford Dictionary of Current English, 8th ed. New York, Oxford University Press, 1992.
2. Self, D.J., Schrader, D.W., Baldwin, D.C., et al.: Study of the influence of veterinary medical education on the moral development of veterinary students. J. Am. Vet. Med. Assoc., *198*:782–787, 1991.
3. Rollin, B.E.: Veterinary and animal ethics. In Wilson, J.F., ed.: Law and Ethics of the Veterinary Profession, Yardley, Pa., Priority Press Ltd., 1989, pp. 24–49.
4. Rest J.R.: Moral Development: Advances in Research and Theory. New York, Praeger, 1986.
5. Self, D.J., Jecker, N.S., Baldwin, D.C., et al.: Moral orientations of justice and care among veterinarians entering veterinary practice. J. Am. Vet. Med. Assoc., *199*:569–573, 1991.
6. Kohlberg, L.: Moral stages and moralization: The cognitive developmental approach. In Lickona, T., ed.: Moral Development and Moral Behavior. New York, Holt, Rinehart and Winston, 1976.
7. Gilligan, C., and Attanucci, J.: Two moral orientations: Gender differences and similarities. Merrill-Palmer Q., *34*:223–237, 1988.
8. Thornton, G.W.: Veterinarians as members of the humane community. J. Am. Vet. Med. Assoc., *198*:1352–1354, 1991.
9. Wilson, J.F.: Law and Ethics of the Veterinary Profession. Yardley, Pa., Priority Press Ltd., 1989.
10. Antelyes, J.: Convenience euthanasia revisited. J. Am. Vet. Med. Assoc., *193*:906–908, 1988.
11. Hart, L.A., Hart, B.L., and Mader, B.: Humane euthanasia and companion animal death: Caring for the animal, the client, and the veterinarian. J. Am. Vet. Med. Assoc., *197*:1292–1299, 1990.
12. Koweit, A.J.: Pet overpopulation. J. Am. Vet. Med. Assoc., *198*:1097–1296, 1991.
13. Murphy, K.: Honesty in the workplace. Forest Oaks, Calif., Brooks-Cole Publishers, 1992.
14. Charlton, R.C.: Breaking bad news. Med. J. Aust., *157*:615–620, 1992.
15. Quackenbush, J.E., and Glickman, L.T.: Helping people adjust to the death of a pet. Health Social Work, *9*:42–48, 1984.

Resource Appendix

We have three goals for this Resource Appendix:

1. To provide those who teach veterinary students with a suggested model for integrating information regarding the human-animal bond, pet loss, client grief, and communication techniques into the professional veterinary curriculum.

2. To provide readers with a brief list containing the names, addresses, and telephone numbers of some of the human-animal bond and pet loss-related services, supplies, and organizations with which we are familiar.

3. To provide brief bibliographies for several of the helping-related subjects introduced in this textbook in order to encourage readers to engage in further reading.

We sincerely hope that this information will help promote the growth of human-animal bond and pet loss-related classes, programs, and veterinary practices across the country.

APPENDIX A

Curriculum

Pet loss, patient death, grief, and euthanasia are threatening topics for most veterinary students.

We have found that teaching students how to deal effectively with emotionally threatening topics is similar to teaching people how to ski. Many ways exist, but some seem to work better than others. For example, if you are a skiing instructor, you can immediately take a class of beginners up the longest lift to the top of the highest mountain and let them discover for themselves how to get down. This method is usually known as trial and error. Although trial and error might actually work for some skiers, for others it can lead to exhaustion, broken bones, severe sunburn, and even an exaggerated fear of ever attempting to ski again.

Perhaps a better way to teach people to ski is to provide them with a step-by-step orientation to the sport. First, for example, you can make students knowledgeable about the goals and methods of skiing. Then, you can teach them the techniques that are most effective to use during the various phases of the skiing experience. Finally, you can provide students with opportunities to apply their newfound knowledge and skills by asking them to ski down the mountain while you carefully supervise and tactfully critique their efforts. This method, although more time-consuming for you, is usually more beneficial, in the long-run, for students. Not only does it provide students with the knowledge and skills necessary for skiing, it also provides them with a positive "emotional orientation" to the sport. It also empowers students by creating a foundation of excitement and confidence about skiing. With confidence as a stable base, most students find themselves feeling enthusiastic about practicing their skiing techniques repeatedly until the sport becomes almost second nature for them.

During our 10 years of teaching at Colorado State University (CSU), we have encountered some seasoned veterinarians *and* human service professionals who believe that today's veterinary students should learn how to face patient death and their own emotional responses through the process of trial and error—just as most of them did. Our clinical and classroom experience has proven, however, that most veterinary students appreciate being emotionally oriented to the issues surrounding companion animal death *before* they face their clients. Therefore, before students face clients during their senior year, we present a series of guest lectures and classes throughout the freshman, sophomore, and junior years within the required core curriculum. Every student receives this information.

During this orientation, there are usually a few students who are initially angry with us for forcing them to face the emotional side of their profession. We have found, however, that, when students are at the receiving end of well-planned educational experiences, even when the experiences are emotional, both reluctant and enthusiastic students learn to cope more effectively with their own emotions. Many also build a foundation of excitement and confidence about helping pet owners through times of pet loss and grief.

As educators, we feel that it is our ethical responsibility to approach threatening subjects such as pet loss, death, grief, and euthanasia in careful, thoughtful ways. To this end, we have implemented a fairly comprehensive curriculum that allows students to learn in a step-by-step fashion. For example, during the freshman year, we avoid overwhelming students by merely introducing the topic of pet loss. During the sophomore year, we build on the introductory material provided the year before and explore the issues of pet loss and client grief in more detail. Issues pertinent to patient death and euthanasia are examined in depth during the junior year and, during the senior year, students actually implement and apply what they have learned.

Some important points to bear in mind when teaching students about pet loss and grief are:

- The subject matter is bound to intimidate or upset some students. It may also trigger memories of their own losses and stir up old feelings of grief. Additionally, some students will not be able to reconcile their own value systems and the appropriateness of helping others during grief. Thus, students may display varying degrees of acceptance or resistance to the material.
- Instructors who teach this subject matter should be experienced counselors or veterinarians trained to provide grief education and intervention. They should have a clinical history of helping emotionally distressed clients, should be accessible to students, and should be willing to offer them ongoing support as they integrate the material.

A roster of the classes that we teach at CSU follows. Some of the teaching methods we use to teach veterinary students about the human-animal bond, pet loss, patient death, grief, and euthanasia are also described.

How the Subjects of Pet Loss, Patient Death, Grief, Euthanasia, Helping, and Communication Techniques are Integrated into Colorado State University's Professional Veterinary Medicine Curriculum

Freshman Year   *Two Hours Required*

Freshman Perspectives   *Two Hours, Entire Freshman Class*

This is a year-long class within the core curriculum that provides students with basic information regarding various topics pertinent to their careers in veterinary medicine. We present a 2-hour guest lecture. Our teaching goals during this lecture include introducing students to the field of human-animal bond studies and to Changes: The Support for People and Pets Program. Subjects covered related to the human-animal bond include attachment, consequences of the bond, current research, current status of the field, and future directions of the field. Information covered pertaining to the Changes Program includes the history of the program along with its clinical and educational goals.

Although the bulk of this class relies on an interactive lecture format, videotape and slide presentations illustrate how students can expect to be involved with human-animal bond studies and the Changes Program over the next 3 years. Several handouts are also provided to students.

Sophomore Year   *Three Hours Required*

Veterinary Ethics   *Three Hours, Entire Sophomore Class*

This is a semester-long class within the core curriculum that challenges students to consider several ethical dilemmas pertinent to veterinary medicine. We present a 3-hour guest lecture. The goal of our lecture is to educate students about how to help pet owners when the human-animal bond is broken. The main premise of the lecture is that, because veterinarians have the right and privilege to euthanize ill or injured animals, they also have a moral and ethical responsibility to conduct the procedure sensitively, keeping their clients' (as well as their patients') needs in mind. Subjects covered include a description of typical veterinary clientele, characteristics of highly attached pet owners, assessment of grieving (sometimes thought to be difficult) clients, normal manifestations of grief, ways in which grief can become complicated for pet owners, and the importance of offering clients the option of being present during their pets' euthanasias. The ways in which helping clients through the ordeal of pet loss can enhance the practice of veterinary medicine are also discussed.

The bulk of this class relies on an interactive lecture format, but videotapes, slides, overheads, and handouts are also used to illustrate the points made.

Junior Year	*Nine Hours Required, 20 Hours Elective*
Orientation to Junior Anesthesia Lab	*One Hour Required, Entire Junior Class, Approximately 20 Students Per Group*

Within the core curriculum, every junior student spends at least 1 week learning how to anesthetize animals. We provide an orientation session during the first day of the rotation. This interactive lecture centers on preparing students for the potentially emotional experiences of anesthetizing, performing cardiopulmonary resuscitation, and euthanizing animals. The focus of our orientation is on providing students with information about performance anxiety, anticipatory grief, and stress management.

Several handouts are provided to students. The ongoing support of the Changes Program is also offered.

Junior Seminar	*Four Hours Required, Entire Junior Class*

This is a 4-week course within the core curriculum that provides students with an overview of several areas pertaining to the practice of veterinary medicine. We provide a 4-hour guest lecture. The purpose of our lecture is to prepare students to effectively help grieving pet owners. To this end, we provide students with information regarding appropriate, sensitive protocols for conducting client-present small- and large-animal euthanasias, offering body care options, and following-up after companion animal death. Also included is information about writing and sending condolences, adopting new pets, and making referrals to human service professionals.

Teaching methods used in this class include slides, videotapes, demonstrations, props, handouts, and class discussion and participation.

Practice Management	*Four Hours Required, Entire Junior Class*

This is a 4-week course within the core curriculum that informs students about effective client relations and practice management techniques. We present a 4-hour lecture. The purpose of our lecture is to prepare students to communicate effectively with clients during various emotional situations. Included in the lecture is information about verbal and nonverbal communication techniques and communication theory, in general. Specifically, students are taught techniques for intervening in emergencies, delivering "bad news," and facilitating decision-making.

Teaching methods include the use of handouts, overheads, demonstration, and role-play. The highlight of this class for students is hearing from a panel of pet owners whose companion animals have either recently died or are near death. Among other topics, panel members are asked to relate specific information regarding what their veterinarians did that was (and that was not) helpful to them.

Junior Elective   *20 Hours Elective, Offered up to Four*
                                     Times Per Year, Approximately 15
                                     Students Per Class

This week-long class is not required or part of the core curriculum. We are the sole instructors and offer it on a limited basis each year. Usually, we have a waiting list because we purposely keep the class size small. The students who elect to take this course are usually very committed to establishing their own bond-centered practices.

Several concepts pertinent to a bond-centered veterinary practice are introduced and developed during this class. They include the TEAM model of helping, the principles of paraprofessional helping, the veterinarian's role in helping during client grief, and advanced communication techniques. Lecture time is dedicated to providing students with more in-depth information about loss and grief, suicide assessment, dealing with anger, dealing with guilt, home euthanasia, and helping specific populations like children, people who are disabled, and the elderly.

This class relies heavily on class participation. Teaching methods include small group discussions, role-plays, guest speakers, homework practice assignments, a "purposeful ending" exercise, and the completion of a comprehensive case study. The class is graded on a pass-fail basis.

Senior Year   *One Half Hour Required, 40+ Hours*
                                     Elective

Oncology Rounds   *One Half Hour Required,*
                                     Approximately Four Students Per Week

Senior students are required to complete a clinical rotation in oncology. We provide a weekly debriefing discussion with the clinicians, staff, and students assigned to the oncology service. The purpose of the discussion is to sort through the emotional experiences that inevitably arise when working with cancer cases. Many discussions focus on feelings about specific patients or on case management strategies that can be used when working with specific clients. Clinicians, staff, and students are encouraged to talk directly to one another, asking questions and giving each other both positive feedback and constructive criticism regarding the cases they have been involved with during the week. Changes counselors facilitate these interactions and also provide input from a counseling perspective.

Elective Clinical Rotation   *Forty Hours Elective, Offered Four*
                                     Times Per Year, up to Four Students
                                     Per Class

This week-long course is not required or part of the core curriculum. We are the sole instructors and offer it on a limited basis each year. We usually have a waiting list because we purposely keep the class size small. Students who want to be supervised while they try out the communication and helping techniques that they have learned previously elect to take this course.

Most students who are accepted into the senior clinical rotation have completed the elective during their junior year. Thus, they are well-prepared to interact with emotionally distressed clients. Throughout the course of the rotation, students team cases with clinicians, intervening as helpers or counselors. In this capacity, students educate clients about grief, support them during diagnoses and treatment procedures, facilitate their decision-making processes, and assist them during their companion animals' deaths or euthanasias. When possible, supervisors observe students' work through a one-way observation window located between the Changes Program's counseling office and an examination room. After being observed, students receive both positive feedback and constructive criticism from the supervisors and their classmates regarding their helping and communication techniques.

During the senior rotation, the concept of detached concern is emphasized. Many of the lectures focus on developing this technique. Topics such as unresolved grief, codependence, personal emotional "triggers," transference and counter-transference, the ethical dilemmas of helping, and establishing personal limits and boundaries are explored and discussed. Students are encouraged to make connections between their personal and professional lives with the hope that they will make commitments, not only to helping clients during emotional times, but also to helping themselves during stress. The overall goal of this class is to increase each student's level of confidence in regard to helping emotional clients.

In addition to live supervision through the one-way observation window, other teaching methods include role-plays, guest speakers, field trips, and the completion of a written bond-centered practice plan. The week ends with a debriefing exercise designed to draw closure to the cases students have experienced. Students receive a grade for their class based primarily on their participation, performance, and effectiveness. (Note: When students complete all required and elective courses in client relations, they graduate with 73.5 contact hours.)

Special Projects   *Hours Vary, Approximately Two*
                                      Students Per Year

This class is not part of the required core curriculum. We are the sole instructors. Senior students who have completed both the junior and the senior electives may choose to spend an extra week engaged in counseling duties with the Changes Program. Special projects may also include handling pet loss-related cases that occur during evening or weekend hours, intervening in emergencies, or completing special projects designed to enhance the services offered by the Changes Program.

Intern/Resident/New Faculty   *Four Hours Required for Interns and*
Training   *Residents, Suggested for New Faculty*

                                      Approximately 15 Participants Per Year

The purpose of this training is to ensure that veterinarians who are new to CSU understand and are aware of CSU's commitment to client relations and the bond-centered practice philosophy. This approach makes it easier for them to work with students, staff, and other clinicians who are similarly trained. During this training, new clinicians are informed about (and encouraged to use) CSU's established protocols for conducting small- and large-animal client-present euthanasias and for referring clients to the Changes Program. Participants are also provided with an overview of attachment, the manifestations of normal grief, and basic verbal and nonverbal communication techniques.

APPENDIX B

Resources

Human-Animal Bond-Related Organizations

The Delta Society
P.O. Box 1080
Renton, WA 98057–9906
Tel.: (206)–226–7357

Ask for their Pet Loss and Bereavement Packet, their Directory of Pet Loss Resources, or their Pet Loss Packet Supplements for Veterinary or Mental Health Professionals. The Delta Society can also provide information about community education programs, animal-assisted activity or therapy programs, and human-animal interactions in general. In addition, many of the books and videotapes mentioned in this Resource Appendix are available to either rent or buy from The Delta Society.

The American Veterinary Medical Association's (AVMA) Committee on The
   Human–Animal Bond
Contact the AVMA
1931 North Meacham Road, Suite 100
Schaumburg, IL 60173–4360
Tel.: (800)–248–AVMA

Animal Behavior Society (ABS) Board of Professional Certification
c/o Dr. Suzanne Hetts
Animal Behavior Associates
4994 So. Independence Way
Littleton, CO 80123
Tel.: (303)–932–9091
Fax: (303)–543–9645

American Veterinary Society of Animal Behavior (AVSAB)
c/o Current President (the current president is Dr. Gary Landsberg)
Doncaster Animal Clinic
99 Henderson Avenue
Thornhill, Ontario L3T 2K9 Canada
Tel.: (416)–881–2752

Human Service Referrals

The Delta Society Directory of Pet Loss Resources
(See address and telephone number listed previously)

Includes a state-by-state listing of local pet loss counselors and support groups as well as descriptions of services offered by various university-based pet loss programs across the country.

Pet Loss Support Hotline
University of California-Davis
Bonnie Mader, MS, Director
Weekdays, 6:30 to 9:30 p.m. Pacific time
Tel.: (916)–752–4200

Staffed by veterinary student volunteers.

Pet Loss Support Hotline
University of Florida
Thomas J. Lane, DVM, Director
Weekdays, 7:00 to 9:00 p.m. EST
Tel.: (904)–392–4700, Ext. 4080

Staffed by veterinary student volunteers.

International Association of Pet Cemeterians
5055 Route 11
Ellenburg Depot, NY 12935
Tel.: (518)–594–3000

Contact them for information regarding pet cemeteries.

American Association of Suicidology
2459 South Ash
Denver, CO 80222
Tel.: (303)–692–0985

Contact them for educational information.

American Association of Marriage and Family Therapists (AAMFT)
Contact AAMFT Referrals
1100 17th St. N.W., 10th Floor
Washington, DC 20036
Tel.: (800)–374–2638

Ask for a copy of their *Consumer's Guide to Marriage and Family Therapy* and a list of AAMFT members.

The American Association for Therapeutic Humor
1163 Shermer Road
Northbrook, IL 60062
Tel.: (708)–291–0211

Ask for their bibliography on humor as therapy and a copy of their newsletter called "Laugh It Up."

The Humor Project
110 Spring Street
Saratoga Springs, NY 12866
Tel.: (518)–587–8770

Ask for their information packet on the positive power of humor and their magazine called *Laughing Matter*. This organization also provides workshops, courses, and seminars.

Audio-Visual Educational Materials

American Animal Hospital Association (AAHA)
Contact AAHA's Member Service Center
P.O. Box 150899, Denver, CO 80215–0899
Tel.: (800)–252–2242 or (303)–986–2800
FAX: (303)–986–1700

Ask for their videotaped series on pet loss: $59.00 per set for members; $85.00 per set for nonmembers. Additional workbooks are $5.00 each for members; $7.50 each for nonmembers. Brochures are 30 for $15.00 for members; 30 for $20.00 for nonmembers. Books about pet loss can also be ordered from AAHA. (They have three books aimed at children and one book aimed at adults.)

"Art and Dusty"
Contact Changes: The Support for People and Pets Program
Colorado State University Veterinary Teaching Hospital
300 West Drake, Fort Collins, CO 80523
Tel.: (303)–491–1242

Videotape describing the grief felt when a pet dies and what veterinarians can do to help, 1991, 17 minutes.

"Broga and the Annison Family"
Contact Changes: The Support for People and Pets Program
Colorado State University Veterinary Teaching Hospital
300 West Drake, Fort Collins, CO 80523
Tel.: (303)–491–1242

Videotape describing an entire family's response to pet loss and to being present at their dog's euthanasia, 1993, 25 minutes.

"Charlie & Nita: The Elephant Man"
Contact The Delta Society Resource Library
P.O. Box 1080, Renton, WA 98057–9906
Tel.: (206)–226–7357

Videotape depicting the strength of the human-animal bond, 1990, 8 minutes.

"When Your Best Friend Dies"
Contact ABC Television Video Service
825 7th Avenue
New York, NY 10023
Tel.: (212)–456–1731

Videotaped segment about pet loss counseling that was part of ABC Television's "20/20" program. First broadcast 1985; rebroadcast 1988, 20 minutes.

For information about educational materials aimed at helping children and parents cope with pet loss, see Box 12-1.

Printed Educational Materials

Animals in Society Curriculum Guide
Contact the Center for Animals and Public Policy
Tufts University, School of Veterinary Medicine,
200 Westboro Road
North Grafton, MA 01536
Tel.: (508)–839–5302

Free to veterinary schools.

"Death of the Family Pet: Losing a Family Friend" pamphlet
Contact the ALPO Pet Center
P.O. Box 4000
Lehigh Valley, PA 18001–4000
Tel.: (215)–395–3301

Free to veterinarians.

"Pet Loss and Human Emotion: When the Question is Euthanasia" pamphlet
Contact the AVMA
1931 North Meacham Road, Suite 100
Schaumburg, IL 60173–4360
Tel.: (800)–248–AVMA

Receive one sample brochure free; order multiple copies at $0.20 per copy or $20.00 per 100 copies.

"The Loss of Your Pet" pamphlet
Contact American Animal Hospital Association's Member Service Center
P.O. Box 150899
Denver, CO 80215–0899

Tel.: (800)–252–2242 or (303)–986–2800
FAX: (303)–986–1700

Brochures are 30 for $15.00 for members; 30 for $20.00 for nonmembers.

For ordering information regarding educational materials designed to help children and parents deal with pet loss, see Box 12-1.

Condolence Card Companies

A New Breed
P.O. Box 266
Timnath, CO 80547
Tel.: (303)–482–0722

Eldorado Arts
P.O. Box 217
Eldorado Springs, CO 80025–9900
Tel.: (800)–248–2820

Paw Marx (formerly Woodgeard Graphics, Inc.)
R.R. 5, 12765 Rt. 34
Bryan, OH 43506
Tel.: (419)–636–7124

Casket and Urn Companies

Hoegh Industries, Inc.
P.O. Box 311
Gladstone, MI 49837
Tel.: (906)–428–2151

Peaceful Pets, Inc.
P.O. Box 1371
Cleveland, GA 30528
Tel.: (800)–422–3553

Pet Insurance Companies

DVM/VPI Insurance Group
4175 E. LaPalma Ave., Suite 100
Anaheim, CA 92807
Tel.: (800)–USA–PETS or (800)–872–7387

Medipet
Fireman's Fund
P.O. Box 94314
Seattle, WA 98124–6614
Tel.: (800)–528–4961

Memorials

Hundreds of animal-oriented programs and organizations accept donations in memory of companion animals. Most promote causes such as animal welfare, conservation, preservation, research, and public education. Some of these organizations, such as Ducks Unlimited and the National Wildlife Fund, are national in scope. Others, such as zoos, humane shelters, and service programs, are focused more locally in terms of the population they serve. If you live near a university veterinary school, check with the college to see which of their fundraising programs might interest you or your clients. You can also donate to your alma mater in memory of companion animals.

Develop a list of programs and organizations that you feel would be worthy of your memorial donations. Create a balance between national and local programs. Be sure to check with each organization on your list regarding the specifics of how to donate to them.

The following represents a sample list of programs and organizations that accept and appreciate donations:

Animal Assistance Foundation
Make checks payable to Animal Assistance Foundation
455 Sherman Street, Suite 462
Denver, CO 80203–4402
Tel.: (303)–744–8396

The primary goal of this organization is to fund efforts concerned with reducing pet overpopulation. A portion of the donations received is also used to assist indigent families with the cost of veterinary care for their companion animals.

American Humane Association, Inc. (AHA)
Attention: Animal Protection Division
63 Inverness Drive East
Englewood, CO 80112–5117
Tel.: (800)–227–4645; in Colorado: (303)–792–9900

Changes: The Support for People and Pets Program
Make checks payable to The CSU Foundation—Changes
Send to Changes: The Support for People and Pets Program
The Colorado State University Veterinary Teaching Hospital
300 West Drake, Fort Collins, CO 80523
Tel.: (303)–491–1242

Humane Society of the United States (HSUS)
2100 L Street, N.W.
Washington, DC 20037
Tel.: (202)–452–1100

The Morris Foundation
Send to Morris Animal Foundation
45 Inverness Drive East
Englewood, CO 80112–5480
Tel.: (303)–790–2345

A nonprofit organization that funds veterinary medical research to benefit animals. Make checks payable to Morris Animal Foundation. Include the name and address of the donor, the name and address of the person to whom a memorial note should be sent, and the name of the pet or person who is being memorialized through the donation.

APPENDIX C

Bibliography

The Human-Companion Animal Bond

Anderson, R.K., Hart, B., and Hart, L., eds.: The Pet Connection. Minnesota, CENSHARE, University of Minnesota Press, 1984.

Anderson, R.S., ed.: Pet Animals and Society. New York, Macmillan Publishing Company, 1975.

Davis, H., and Balfour, D., eds.: The Inevitable Bond: Examining Scientist-Animal Interactions. New York, Cambridge University Press, 1992.

Fogle, B., ed.: Interrelations Between People and Pets. Springfield, Ill., Charles C. Thomas, 1981.

Katcher, A.H., and Beck, A., eds.: New Perspectives on Our Lives with Companion Animals. Philadelphia, University of Pennsylvania Press, 1983.

Quackenbush, J., and Voith, V.L., eds.: The human-companion animal bond. Vet. Clin. North Am. [Small Anim. Pract.], 15. Philadelphia, W.B. Saunders, 1985.

Rowan, A.N., ed.: Animals and People Sharing the World. Hanover, N.H., University Press of New England, 1988.

Serpell, J.: In the Company of Animals. New York, Basil Blackwell, Ltd, 1986.

Sussman, M.B., ed.: Pets and the Family. New York, Haworth Press, 1985.

Pet Loss

Anderson, M.: Coping with Sorrow on the Loss of Your Pet. Los Angeles, Calif., Peregrine Press, 1987.

Church, J.A.: Joy in a Woolly Coat: Living with, Loving, and Letting Go of Treasured Animal Friends. Tiburon, Calif., H.J. Kramer Inc., 1987.

Kay, W.J., Nieburg, H.A., Kutscher, A.H., et al., eds.: Pet Loss and Human Bereavement. Ames, Iowa State University Press, 1988.

Kay, W.J., Cohen, S.P., Fudin, C.E., et al., eds.: Euthanasia of the Companion Animal: The Impact on Pet Owners, Veterinarians, and Society. Philadelphia, The Charles Press, 1988.

Lemieux, C.: Coping with the Loss of a Pet. Reading, Pa., Wallace R. Clark, 1988.

Mooney, S.: A Snowflake in My Hand. New York, Delta/Eleanor Friede, 1983.

Nieberg, H.A., and Fisher, A.: Pet Loss: A Thoughtful Guide for Adults and Children. New York, Harper & Row, 1982. (Currently out of print.)

Quackenbush, J., and Graveline, D.: When Your Pet Dies: How to Cope with Your Feelings. New York, Simon and Schuster, 1985. (Currently out of print.)

Quackenbush, J., and Voith, V.L., eds.: The human-companion animal bond. Vet. Clin. North Am. [Small Anim. Pract.], Philadelphia, W.B. Saunders, March 1985.

Sife, W. The Loss of a Pet. New York, Howell Book House, 1993.

Sussman, M., ed.: Pets and the Family. New York, The Haworth Press, Inc., 1985.

Loss and Grief—Self-Help

Colgrove, M., Bloomfield, H.H., and McWilliams, P.: How to Survive the Loss of a Love. Los Angeles, Calif., Prelude Press, 1991.

Davies, P.: Grief: Climb Toward Understanding. New York, Carol Publishing Group, 1989.

Deits, B.: Life After Loss: A Personal Guide Dealing with Death, Divorce, Job Change, and Relocation. Tuscon, Ariz., Fisher Books, 1988.

Harper-Neeld, E.: Seven Choices: Taking the Steps to New Life After Losing Someone You Love. New York, Clarkson N. Potter, 1990.

James, J., and Cherry, F.: The Grief Recovery Handbook. New York, Harper & Row, 1988.

Levine, S.: Healing into Life and Death. Garden City, N.Y., Anchor Books/Doubleday, 1987.

Lightner, C.: Giving Sorrow Words: How to Cope with Grief and Get on with Your Life. New York, Warner Books, 1990.

Manning, D.: Don't Take My Grief Away: What to Do When You Lose a Loved One. Harper–San Francisco, 1984.

Rando, T.A.: How to Go on Living When Someone You Love Dies. New York, Bantam, 1991.

Staudacher, C.: Beyond Grief: A Guide for Recovering from the Death of a Loved One. Oakland, Calif., New Harbinger Publishers, 1987.

Staudacher, C.: Men and Grief: A Guide for Men Surviving the Death of a Loved One. Oakland, Calif., New Harbinger Publishers, 1991.

Stearns, A.K.: Coming Back: Rebuilding Lives After Crisis and Loss. New York, Ballantine Books, 1989.

Tatelbaum, J.: The Courage to Grieve. New York, Harper & Row, 1980.

Tatelbaum, J.: You Don't Have to Suffer: A Handbook for Moving Beyond Life's Crises. New York, Harper & Row, 1989.

Loss and Grief—Children

See Box 12-4.

Grief Theory, Counseling, and Therapy

Bowlby, J.: Attachment and Loss, Vols, 1, 2, and 3. New York, Basic Books, 1969, 1973, 1980.

Cook, A.S., and Dworkin, D.: Helping the Bereaved: Therapeutic Interventions for Children, Adolescents, and Adults. New York, Basic Books, 1992.

Cook, A.S., and Oltjenbruns, K.A.: Dying and Grieving: Lifespan and Family Perspectives. New York, Holt, Rinehart, and Winston, 1989.

Feinstein, D., and Mayo, P.: Rituals for Living and Dying: How We Can Turn Loss and the Fear of Dying into an Affirmation of Life. Harper–San Francisco, 1990.

Knott, J.E., Ribar, M.C., Dudson, B.M., and King, M.R.: Thanatopics: Activities and Exercises for Confronting Death. Lexington, Mass., Lexington Books, 1989.

Kübler-Ross, E.: On Death and Dying. New York, Collier Books/Macmillan Publishing Company, 1969.

Kubler-Ross, E.: Death: The Final Stage of Growth. Englewood Cliffs, N.J., Prentice-Hall, 1975.

Linn, E.: I Know Just How You Feel . . . Avoiding the Cliches of Grief. Incline Village, Nev., The Publishers Mark, 1986.

Osterweis, M., Solomon, F., and Green, M., eds.: Bereavement: Reactionism, Consequences, and Care. Washington, D.C., National Academy Press, 1984.

Rando, T.A.: Grief, Dying, and Death: Clinical Interventions for Caregivers. Champaign, Ill., Research Press Company, 1984.

Roth, D., and LeVie, E.: Being Human in the Face of Death. Santa Monica, Calif., IBS Press, 1990.

Simos, B.: A Time to Grieve: Loss as a Universal Human Experience. New York, Family Service America, 1979.

Stroebe, W., and Stroebe, M.: Bereavement and Health: The Psychological and Physical Consequences of Partner Loss. New York, Cambridge University Press, 1987.

Worden, J.W.: Grief Counseling and Grief Therapy: A Handbook for the Mental Health Practitioner. New York, Springer Publishing Company, 1982.

Helping and Communication Techniques

Bolton, R.: People Skills: How to Assert Yourself, Listen to Others and Resolve Conflicts. New York, Simon & Schuster, 1979.

Bilodeau, L.: The Anger Workbook, Minneapolis, Minn., CompCare Publishers, 1992.

Bramson, R.M.: Coping with Difficult People . . . in Business and Life. New York, Ballantine, 1981.

Kennedy, E.: Crisis Counseling: The Essential Guide for Nonprofessional Counselors. New York, Continuum Publishing Company, 1986.

Small, J. Becoming Naturally Therapeutic: A Return to the True Essence of Helping. New York, Bantam, 1990.

Woititz, J.G., and Garner, A.: Life-skills for Adult Children. Deerfield Beach, Fla., Health Communications, 1990.

Zunin, L.M., and Zunin, H.S.: The Art of Condolence. New York, Harper Perennial, 1991.

Stress in the Helping Professions

Atkinson, H.: Women and Fatigue. New York, G.P. Putnam and Sons, 1985.

Beattie, M.: Co-dependent No More. New York, Harper–Hazeldon, 1987.

Elkins, D., and Brackenridge, S.: Methods of coping with stress and prevention of burnout in veterinary practice. The Compendium on Continuing Education [Small Animal], 14:157–161, 1992.

Elkins, A.D., and Elkins, J.R.: Professional burnout among U.S. veterinarians: How serious a problem? Vet. Med., 82:1245–1250, 1987.

Elkins, A.D., and Kearney, M.: Professional burnout among female veterinarians in the United States. J. Am. Vet. Med. Assoc., 200:604–608, 1992.

Freudenberger, H., and North, G.: Women's Burnout. New York, Penguin Books, 1986.

Hart, L.A., and Hart, B.: Grief and Stress from So Many Animal Deaths. Companion Animal Practice, March 1987, pp. 20–21.

Kelman, E.G.: Practice stress, burnout and rustout. In McCurnin, D., ed.: Veterinary Practice Management. Philadelphia, J.B. Lippincott, Co., 1988, pp. 320–339.

Lattanzi, M.E.: Coping with Work-Related Losses. Personnel Guidance J., 6:350–351, 1981.

Lattanzi, M.E.: Professional Stress: Adaptation, Coping, and Meaning. *In* T.F. Frantz, ed.: Death and Grief in the Family. Rockville, Md., Aspen Publishers, 1984.

Lazarus, R.S., and Folkman, S.: Coping and Adaptation. *In* Gentry, W.D., ed.: The Handbook of Behavioral Medicine, New York, Guilford, 1984, pp. 282–325.

Lief, H.O., and Fox, D.C.: Training for Detached Concern in Medical Students. *In*: Lief, H.I., Lief, V.I., and Lief, N.R., eds.: The Psychological Basis for Medical Practice, New York, Harper and Row, 1963, pp. 12–35.

Quill, T.E., and Williamson, P.R.: Healthy Approaches to Physician Stress. Arch. Int. Med. *150*, September 1990, pp. 1857–1861.

Schaef, A.W.: The Addictive Organization. New York, Harper and Row, 1984.

Whitfield, C.L.: Co-Dependence: Healing the Human Condition: The New Paradigm for Helping Professionals and People in Recovery. Deerfield Beach, Fla., Health Communications, Inc., 1991.

Zuziak, P.: Stress and Burnout in the Profession, Parts 1, 2, and 3. J. Am. Vet. Med. Assoc., *198*:4, pp. 521–524; 5, pp. 753–756; 6, pp. 941–942, 944; 1991.

Index

Page numbers in *italics* indicate illustrations; those followed by t refer to tables.